Rethinking Autism with Dolto: Syllable Soup

Rethinking Autism with Dolto takes up a principal legacy of Françoise Dolto's immense project—her conviction that autism is a regression to the archaic.

Dolto theorizes that the infant *in utero*, deep in dreams, is receptive to the audition of "phonemes" during the pre-conscious "archaic stage" of psychosexual maturation. That dream-work on words—an idiosyncratic prehistory at the onset of mental and emotional life—secures the unconscious circulation of affect and the ontogeny of thought long prior to speech, seeding associative thinking and facilitating self-regulation. Kathleen Saint-Onge uses the written work of four nonverbal autistic authors in seeking corroboration for Dolto's formulations, finding thoughtful self-reflections that relate the experience of living in silence with relentless anxiety while relying on regression as a defence. Dolto's unprecedented insights into the infant's earliest learning carry formidable implications for autism interventions, and for primary language and literacy. At issue is an enduring susceptibility to archaic echoes—the haphazard, securing return of pre-invested phonemes—in communicative exchanges, including reading and writing.

Rethinking Autism with Dolto considers unconscious processes as inherently reparative, heralding the responsibility education holds for human health, and supports a rethinking of autism that presumes competence. Readers are invited to new conversations in psychoanalysis, child development, education and linguistics through an exploration of the unconscious concomitants of first language acquisition.

Kathleen Saint-Onge is a researcher and educator originally from Québec, Canada. Interrogating the unconscious, affective roots of language, she earned her master's and PhD from York University, Toronto. Her previous publications include *Discovering Françoise Dolto: Psychoanalysis, Identity and Child Development* (Routledge).

Rethinking Autism with Dolto

Syllable Soup

Kathleen Saint-Onge

Routledge
Taylor & Francis Group
LONDON AND NEW YORK

Designed cover image: Getty | Kyryl Gorlov

First published 2024
by Routledge
4 Park Square, Milton Park, Abingdon, Oxon OX14 4RN

and by Routledge
605 Third Avenue, New York, NY 10158

Routledge is an imprint of the Taylor & Francis Group, an informa business

British Library Cataloguing-in-Publication Data
A catalogue record for this book is available from the British Library

ISBN: 978-1-032-65509-3 (hbk)
ISBN: 978-1-032-65514-7 (pbk)
ISBN: 978-1-032-65512-3 (ebk)

DOI: 10.4324/9781032655123

Typeset in Times New Roman
by KnowledgeWorks Global Ltd.

I dedicate this book to all those whose muted stories cannot be told for decades, or perhaps a lifetime.

* * * *

Anxietia: A hardy perennial with roots far too deep for pulling, and overgrowth soundly contained by durable borders made of comfortable rituals and familiar compulsions.

(KS 2011/2023)

Contents

Preface x

Introduction 1

PART ONE
Analysis **11**

Preamble for Part One 13

1 Conservation 21

Preliminary Words 21

A. Archaic 22
B. Affect 24
C. Anxiety 28
D. Environment 31

Notes 34

2 Circulation 37

Preliminary Words 37

A. Third 38
B. Passivity 41
C. Regression 44
D. Symbolization 47

Notes 50

3 Presentification 55

Preliminary Words 55

A. Phonemes 56
B. Traces 59
C. Witness 63
D. Exteriorization 66

Notes 70

Summary for Part One 75

PART TWO
Evidence 79

Preamble for Part Two 81

4 Primary Defence 91

Preliminary Words 91

A. Regression 96
B. Anxiety 102

Notes 108

5 Auditory Influence 113

Preliminary Words 113

A. Phonemes 120
B. Passivity 125

Notes 132

6 Resonant Experience 136

Preliminary Words 136

A. Exteriorization 142
B. Witness 148

Notes 154

Summary for Part Two 157

PART THREE
Practice 161

Preamble for Part Three 163

7 Name—Awaiting Echoes 172

Preliminary Words 172

A. Inscription 173
B. Reverberations 179

Notes 183

8 Library—(Re)Finding Echoes 185

Preliminary Words 185

A. Inscription 187
B. Reverberations 191

Notes 193

9 Transcription—Producing Echoes 195

Preliminary Words 195

A. Inscription 197
B. Reverberations 202

Notes 206

10 Forest—Following Echoes 208

Preliminary Words 208

A. Inscription 210
B. Reverberations 214

Notes 217

Summary for Part Three 219

Conclusion 222

Bibliography *228*
Index *239*

Preface

Every book owes its life to many people, only one of which is its author.

This book would not exist without the body of work of two world-renowned researchers: Sigmund Freud and Françoise Dolto. Freud's articulation of the unconscious is essential to understanding the earliest life of the human infant. Dolto, who was both a doctor and psychoanalytic therapist, leveraged Freud's discoveries during her long career working with children and infants—many with mutism and/or autism—to theorize the "archaic stage" of mental and emotional development that begins during gestation.

I am indebted to two formidable influences who share my love of language, and with whom I had the honour of working at York University in 2008–2016. The first is Heather Lotherington, Professor Emerita (Retired), an educator dedicated to research in multilingualism and early literacy. Heather is the best among the fine linguists I have admired and appreciated, beginning at McGill in the 1970s. Heather encouraged me to conceive the Major Research Paper for my Masters (2011) as a language memoir, reflecting on my emotional gains and losses between tongues; that text was revised and published as *Bilingual Being: My Life as a Hyphen* (McGill Queen's University Press, 2013). The second is Deborah Britzman, Distinguished Research Professor and FRSC, my wonderful doctoral supervisor. Deborah is a practising psychotherapist, an award-winning academic and writer, and a scholar of psychoanalysis recognized as an authority on Freud.[1] Deborah unsettles education by invoking the learner's emotional world, and she provided me with the best guidance possible, combining theoretical rigour with creative freedom. My dissertation (2016) was revised and published as *Discovering Francoise Dolto: Psychoanalysis, Identity and Child Development* (Routledge, 2019).

There are many other individuals at York, faculty and students, who helped shape my thinking. I am especially thankful to professors Mario DiPaolantonio, Alice Pitt and Daniel Yon, for their unwavering kindness and timely provocations; Lisa Farley and Aparna Mishra-Tarc, for their insightful reflections on Dolto; and Paula Salvio, one of my examiners, for concurring on the relevance of Dolto to autism.

I would also like to thank Judith Hamilton, of the Toronto Psychoanalytic Society, for sponsoring an instrumental workshop on Dolto in 2012. And I extend my profoundest gratitude to some unnamed reviewers of this project for their strong support; to Susannah Frearson, my editor, for her sustained advocacy; and to the fine team at Routledge, for being the standard-bearers for Dolto in English.

Hundreds of outstanding peers in the Peel District School Board—from which I have recently retired after 21 years of service—have inspired me with their dedication. In all, I have spent about 38 years teaching in one grade or another, full-time or part-time across four Canadian provinces, since obtaining my certification from McGill University in 1984. Being a part-time "grad student" while working full-time in classrooms, I benefitted from sharing invaluable daily experiences with my students and their families.

I also extend my sincere gratitude to four nonverbal autistic authors for their texts: Naoki Higashida, Ido Kedar, Tito Mukhopadhyay and Birger Sellin. I appreciate that "autistic authorship" is a contested notion, but surely a book about autism cannot, and should not, exclude autistic voices.[2] As to why I believe these authors *can* write—and that being unable to speak does *not* entail being unable to think—we are touching the very heart of the journey I am proposing.

I am incredibly thankful to my three adult children—Peter, Jacob and Sarah—and their life partners for their unconditional support. Special mention goes to my infant grandson, H., for reminding me daily of how much children can comprehend before they can speak. My gratitude also extends to my brother, Rick, and his wife for their warm friendship; and to my mother, Thérèse, now in her nineties, for her poignant chronicles from the slippery margins of time and space, before her words went away.

Some editorial notes are in order. I use "he" for the infant/child to distinguish "him" from the mother or Dolto ("she/her"). I generally prefer "autists" to the common expression, "person(s) with autism." All citations from Freud are from the Standard Edition (SE). Translations of Dolto and other French sources are my own.[3] I encourage readers seeking greater detail regarding how Dolto's work dovetails Freud's to consult my prior text on Dolto; I remain thankful to Anne-Marie Canu (a respected Dolto scholar) and Catherine Dolto (a physician and infant specialist) for their support during that project (2014–2018).[4]

The goal of the present work is to try to ease the suffering of autists through Dolto-inspired interventions, and to suggest new avenues for Freud in 21st-century pedagogies. As Dolto explains, humans are constructed in, through, and by language. The valuation of the "phoneme," as she posits it, follows naturally. Thus, this is the theoretical object I choose to use to demonstrate why, and how, Dolto theorizes regression as the first and foremost human defence—and autism as regression. Dolto points to something she considered ridiculously obvious: learning begins *in utero*, long before we are conscious. As a result, she incidentally formulates the affective origins of associative thinking in the sub-basement of cognition. Her (re)thinking about autism also reveals that literacy is potentially reparative. Could there be a stronger call to education?

The possibilities issuing from Dolto's work defy the imagination. Yet little of her work appears in English and it was only recently—35 years after her death—that Routledge released the first-ever English translation of her watershed text.[5] In fact, the task of translating Dolto is exceedingly complicated because she navigates uncharted theoretical waters, continually switches registers of formality, and invents words on an ad hoc basis. Dolto was original to her core, once quipping that, "If to live well we had to identify with our parents … we would still be Cro-Magnons."[6] In short, she was a fresh thinker who nurtured authenticity and independence in others. Thus the vibrant growth of Dolto scholarship worldwide will benefit from waves of interest among all sorts of different groups, and the dedicated efforts of all kinds of minds.

I write this book as a researcher, educator, mother, grandmother and concerned citizen. There is a fair bit here that will rub hard against the grain of standard approaches to autism, and I can already hear the multitudes of well-funded dissenters heading my way. But I write on anyhow, thankful to those willing to rethink autism a little to make a big difference. Above all, I write in solidarity with those who cannot speak and whose writing (even when it happens) is inherently suspect. Sound is such that it often needs to be amplified by many voices before it can be heard.

Notes

1 See Britzman 2011.
2 I also thank two nonverbal autists who shared their early history of reading with me, patiently typing their replies to my questions, one finger at a time: Jamie Burke (Syracuse, NY, 12 November 2016) and Jamil Shah (Oakville, ON, 4 December 2016).
3 I favour literalism in my translations of Dolto because I believe in the specificity, beauty and potency of her words.
4 There are over 1,200 citations in this book—that is a lot of page numbers and dates. I have done my best to ensure accuracy, and I hope that any small slips that will inevitably remain will not diminish the value of the work as a whole. Except where otherwise noted as "C. (Catherine) Dolto," all uses of the name "Dolto" herein will refer to Françoise Dolto.
5 Original in French: Dolto, F. 1984. *L'image inconsciente du corps.* Paris: Éditions du Seuil. New in English: Dolto, F. 1984/2023. *The Unconscious Body Image* (S. Bailly, Trans.). London: Routledge. Note that I refer to the French original (on which I have relied for over a decade) when citing this text herein.
6 1983.

Introduction

I wish to begin this book at "Mute Bridge." That is not the structure's actual name, but that is what is written conspicuously across the grey-brown arch carrying Bloor Street over the Humber River in Toronto. Nineteen times along the north face of the iron trestle scaffolding the concrete road above it, someone has graffitied "MUTE" in giant, white capital letters. It stands out among the colourful tags that any paddler can see as the lovely blueway slowly winds in a southeasterly direction, flowing beneath more major roads and rail lines before finally discharging into Lake Ontario.

The river is navigable in both directions, and the time it takes from mouth to bridge—or vice-versa—is about 45 minutes at the speed of someone searching for herons and deer. When the water is flat, as it is most mornings, a paddler can bob up and down almost indefinitely under that word, "mute," at least until the mosquitoes detect a human presence. The word serves up a stark counterpoint to the heavy traffic above and the subway line emerging from below the city on its own overpass, parallel to Mute Bridge.

Whatever possessed the artist to choose this word to scribe, again and again, on such a dangerous surface? It's easily four or five storeys at its centre, and some 12 boat lengths by my estimation. The work is even signed in the upper right corner, where a concrete pile anchors the bridge. For in the same font, size and colour, the author credited is—not without wit—"The Paint Cans."

It's been here for who knows how long—I can only vouch for four years. And who is the target reader? After all, few can see this graffiti other than by canoe, kayak or paddleboard. It isn't visible from the road above, and it's barely within range for passengers heading east on the subway, or condo dwellers above its banks, beyond the water-logged willows. No one swims here—it's too shallow and turbid. A small craft rental service operates here seasonally, but concrete slabs dropped during the bridge's construction make it a rather unappealing put-in for most vessels. As for the handful of fishers speckling the rocks, they are usually way downriver. Clearly, this message is aimed at a limited set of readers, yet considered significant enough for the writer to take appreciable chances recording it. Then again, perhaps every book is no different: intended for a small audience and published at some risk.

DOI: 10.4324/9781032655123-1

The word this artist chose, "mute"—repeated on high from one bank to the other—ironically seems to shout. But at whom? And by what twist of fate, after living in 30+ homes in four provinces, have I chosen this geographic location for my ventures? How, too, has it come to pass that a word that is so important for me on the "inside" has been given such prominence on the "outside"? It is an uncanny feeling, as if my presence had been anticipated by someone I don't know but, in this moment, need.

Mute Bridge has become my turn-around point most mornings from my launch at the mouth of the river. Daily, I seek its familiar message. A testament to the power of reading, it strengthens me as nothing else can, and it gives me the impetus to begin writing. It's as if I am completing something already started rather than initiating a project on my own. Rationally, I know that makes no sense. But emotionally, it makes perfect sense somehow. And here is Mute Bridge serving up another fine metaphor, in this arching gap between affect and logic that will, in fact, evoke the infant's mental and emotional situation, as we will learn with Françoise Dolto.

Dolto offers bold and brilliant theorization of how we might explain things because, as she often liked to say, «tout se passe comme si» [everything happens as if]. And in studying the infant with Dolto, we will experience something akin to the dark matter of space, whose existence can only be inferred based on how it affects nearby bodies. Admittedly, Dolto's insights are also subject to refusal because all that pertains to the unconscious seems scientifically suspect. Freud explains:

> Our right to assume the existence of something mental that is unconscious and to employ that assumption for the purposes of scientific work is disputed in many quarters. To this we can reply that our assumption of the unconscious is *necessary* and *legitimate* ... [because] psychical acts often occur which can be explained only by presupposing other acts, of which, nevertheless, consciousness affords no evidence.[1]

Freud resolves that, "conscious acts ... fall into a demonstrable connection if we interpolate between them the unconscious acts we have inferred";[2] in sum, "we should apply this process of inference to ourselves."[3]

In Part One: Analysis, comprised of three chapters, I describe Dolto's thinking about the infant's "coming to reality" (consciousness) from an unconscious state that commences sometime during gestation. I survey critical notions Dolto developed based on her reading of Freud, in chapters that will require the reader's patience because a vocabulary of Doltoisms needs to be introduced. From this grounding, we will examine the role of the instinct of conservation in early human life; the unconscious circulation that is central to survival; and the triangular progression by which an infant comes to reality. The reader will gain an appreciation of the lifelong need for affective self-regulation, and of the ontogeny of associative thinking that begins—surprisingly perhaps—*in utero*. In addition to appealing to a wide readership, this first part may be of particular interest to psychoanalysts[4] and specialists in infant development.

I believe it can be uncontroversially argued that both Freud and Dolto make one central point: all humans have a permanent component of their mental life—a reservoir—that is unconscious. As we mature (assuming good health), we develop our capacity for conscious control: for achieving tasks requiring a high level of motor skill; engaging difficult problems; solving organizational or technical challenges, and so on. Meanwhile, our unconscious capacities remain vibrant and largely unnoticed unless we sleep (i.e., dream)—or until life events threaten our survival and, so doing, undermine the stability of our conscious control. At such times, we will notice the continued influence of the unconscious and its curious feature of non-time, non-space—past and present blur, we are transposed to an elusive elsewhere, and we become susceptible to the sudden intrusion of fears, symptoms, and remembrances. Anyone who has been traumatized needs no explanation about how a past that seems long-gone can impinge on one's daily life, even decades on.

The simple truth is that the unconscious remains with us, even when we are operating consciously. As Freud explained, "unconscious ideation"[5] or "unconscious thinking … is also active in the day."[6] On the other hand, in our dreams—for which each of us has evidence, and which Freud's project investigated so eloquently—we revert to unconscious mental life. Yet even as we dream, we absorb bits of the world around us, especially sounds and sensations. For example, we may dream of a fire alarm to find our phone ringing; or dream of a broken leg to awaken with a cramped limb; or dream of a baby in distress to discover that a pet seeks our attention, etc. In other words, we all have examples of how, when we are unconscious, we are not entirely impervious to the environment—just mostly so. Another common experience is how material from the prior day may manifest in our dreams, albeit disguised. If I lose a key, I may dream that someone else has lost a key—or that I have lost something different. Such examples abound in our lives and may make dreams feel uncanny.

As for comas, these constitute an unconscious form of human existence by definition. And what of dementia? Millions of affected families (like mine) witness the nebulous grasp on reality that pervades in conversations: the confusion between past and present, the muddle of people and events, and the poor articulation that sounds like sleep-talking. And of course, everyone also acknowledges slips of the tongue, famously called "Freudian slips" for his study of everyday manifestations that give away the continued hold of the unconscious. In effect, we often betray precisely what we would prefer not to reveal. Every human is vulnerable to such unwitting disclosures—we literally cannot help it. And if we are honest, we also have instincts and feelings about things and people that logic cannot justify. I believe that only a small subset of humans is defensive at such a suggestion. Most of us admit to doing things on hunches, whether from a sense of pending fear or fortune. The unconscious is an ordinary fact of life.

There is a continuum from unconscious to conscious mental life, but the unconscious substrate always remains. And since the unconscious is first, and consciousness arises later and slowly, then the infant's primary opportunities for learning happen under the dominant influence of unconscious processes. With Dolto, then, we will focus on the unconscious impact of "phonemes"[7] in learning prior to consciousness—learning that is so precocious that we will need to include (astonishingly, perhaps) the prenatal period. Dolto's use of the term, "phoneme," is not identical to that of linguists but is instead much closer to the sense of a syllable. Functionally, it is a pronounceable, discernible chunk that includes a vowel and forms a word either alone or in combination with other syllables. In effect, it is what any ordinary speaker or hearer is most sensitive to in a language. And the observable fact that phonemes appear repetitively in different permutations in long strings of speech is a critical correlate.[8]

Temporal parameters will become clearer, but suffice it to say at this point that we will be studying the mental and emotional life of the infant from about the 24th week of gestation. And as will be apparent through Dolto's theorization, audition is key in this pre-conscious learning.[9]

I cling to the symbolism of Mute Bridge for dear life—this notion it seems to expound that what is mute can find a means to shout. Its message only gains in poignancy as I play with it further. For the Humber gets progressively shallower upriver, against the current, becoming impassable just north of Mute Bridge. The flow turns into a bubbling rush over jagged stones and no matter how much the paddler strives, the water exerts tremendous resistance. It seems we reach a limit we cannot recede beyond. Yet by turning around here, and heading back downriver with the natural course instead, the traveller easily arrives at the river's mouth.

Most days, invited by this author in the wilds, I find myself musing on the thin line between reality and dreams, the boundaries of self, and how we can be secured by nature. What is this comfort in anonymous life? For the scripted arch makes my life's project into my visible horizon, while echoing the work that beckons back home, at my desk. It's as if I could forget my goals if random reminders did not arrive. Perhaps I could, for this project is not easy at all, and the subject is as murky as the Humber. I cannot see its bottom either. But sometimes, I can feel it.

There are other paddlers here too, like one who anchors his rowboat for hours. There is the former world competitor who typically laps me three times, and future racers in outriggers practising their strokes. And there are others like me, slowly taking in who-knows-what. "See three deer back a bit?" "Yup." To be frank, the morning crowd is a silent one. No one tries to catch up to another to paddle together, let alone talk. There may be a nod, but most people pass as if the other were not there. It is a sign of respect to let people travel on their own. For everyone has come for grace in solitude, to witness surprises that only the undisciplined natural world can provide, amid what lives around but without us, in the relative mutism of a forest made quiet by the city surrounding it.

I frankly don't even bring my phone anymore after ruining one thanks to some poor planning. So there are treasures I witness alone, like the deer who surprised me around a bend so that we were barely one metre apart. Or the eagle with a two-metre wingspan who snatched a carp mere centimetres from my bow. Yet the importance of having witnesses to experience will be a central one as we consider the infant's learning in the months of silence preceding the capacity for speech—at the boundary between reality and dreams.

In Part Two: Evidence, comprised of three chapters, I present vital testimony—first-hand accounts—of the lived experience of autism by soliciting the reader's engagement with four authors who are each considered to be nonverbal and severely autistic.[10] Guided by some commonalities evoked in their works, I seek to inform and support the discussion to which Dolto invites us. The objective here is to explore autism through the insights of four individuals who can offer greater accuracy than any theorist or interventionist. As we will learn, at issue is an individual who is fully engaged in sophisticated thinking but who is marked by excessive anxiety and a passive disposition inhibiting conscious motor actions (including speech). Freud himself emphasizes how, "the conscious system normally controls affectivity as well as access to motility … the setting-off of muscular activity."[11] Thinking about unconscious primary processes and the infant's precocious, pre-conscious learning enables a clearer grasp of the nature of autism.[12] In addition to appealing to a wide readership, this second part may be of particular interest to autists and their communities.

The four writers selected are Naoki Higashida (born in Japan in 1992); Ido Kedar (born in the USA in 1996); Tito Mukhopadhyay (born in India in 1989); and Birger Sellin (born in Germany in 1973).[13] To be clear, each of these four writers can indisputably be witnessed typing independently thanks to an abundant public record where extracts from their lives, interviews and movies are freely available online. It is worth stressing that many highly regarded individuals and some of the most prestigious media organizations in the world have staked their reputations on the authenticity of these nonverbal authors.

Naoki Higashida has authored two autobiographies—one being a *New York Times* and *Sunday Times* bestseller translated into 30 languages. He is the subject of a Japanese documentary and an award-winning American movie (2020). Higashida usually produces texts using a keyboard by pressing letters with his right forefinger. He appears in the film, *Wretches and Jabberers* (2010).

Ido Kedar is the author of two books, including an original autobiographical novel relating his life as/through "Anthony." His memoir has been translated into Hebrew, Japanese, Polish, Russian and Spanish. Kedar is the subject of numerous interviews, including one for the *Los Angeles Times*. He produces texts using a keyboard by pressing letters with his right forefinger.

Tito Rajarshi Mukhopadhyay (who resides in the USA) has authored six books, including a volume of poetry. He lectures to live audiences and is the subject of documentaries by the BBC and PBS. Mukhopadhyay began writing at age six with a pencil and usually produces his texts using a keyboard by pressing letters with his right forefinger.

Birger Sellin's poetic memoir has been translated into numerous languages, including English. In 1994, a German movie was made about him which was translated into French (1998). He holds the distinction of having published the first-ever autism memoir, introducing a new genre of literature. Sellin produces texts using a keyboard by pressing letters with his right forefinger.

Through such invaluable testimony, we will confirm that while the lack of a capacity for initiating speech is the defining manifestation of nonverbal autism, the most debilitating symptom experienced is anxiety. Furthermore, it will be revealed that the inability to speak does not, in fact, entail an inability to think. The reason (as we will have cause to conclude) is that these processes are developmentally (obviously) reversed: thinking comes first, then speaking. So the latter process cannot preclude (or occlude) the prior one. To rethink autism, then, we need to turn some common interpretations inside out.

A note that, as these four autistic authors are all independent typers, I will refrain from a digression into the hotly debated topic of "Facilitated Communication" (FC) by which these four writers were scaffolded for years in the acquisition of that independence. As an educator in "regular classrooms" for most of my career, I have held notebooks, pencils, markers, crayons, tablets, white boards, chalk boards and iPads—and guided countless hands—to facilitate the learning of printing. I believe that cutting with scissors, for instance, can't even be learned except hand-over-hand. Numerous times, I sat right next to a neurotypical learner reading one word—even one letter—at a time, at a speed that made me struggle to stay awake. Glancing at my desk, I saw piles of marking waiting for me and parent forms to sort. But if I ever tried to mark, sort or walk away for even a second, the child would stop reading. Somehow, I had to be there, waiting for words, watching the same page, serving up bits of encouragement: "You're doing great!" "Keep going!" This happened routinely with so-called "unidentified" primary children in middle-class neighbourhoods. These learners, in other words, had no special barriers to learning, yet they needed my emotional participation to keep progressing. Learning always involves facilitation.

But before leaving the Humber to get to work in earnest, I suggest that a sunrise paddle teaches one more critical fact that is vital to retain as we explore the earliest infant learning: everything looks very different half an hour later. Pre-sunrise, a thin layer of fog on the water helps illusions abound. Herons look like driftwood (and vice-versa), logs on the bank resemble crouching deer, and the sky and water seem merged in a light violet-blue haze so that there is barely any horizon. The forest's fragrance, carried by the morning dew, is astonishingly textured before the sun comes up. Slimy edges betray the pungent presence of geese; the acrid smell of the deadest treetops announce cormorant nests; and the shallowest water reeks of fish and algae mere centimetres below. Before the sun rises, the paddler is also keenly aware of each sound crackling in the brush, resounding ever louder as echoes in the stillness, as daydreams make the tiniest racoon out to be a coyote…

But once the sun arrives, everything changes. As light reaches the surface of the river, each shape gains its definition. Tiny inlets appear between towering cattails where the bank once seemed unbroken. The herons and driftwood stop playing their games on the margins of reality and can be seen for what they are—and it's easy to distinguish the water and sky. Yet not only vision changes with light—sound and smell do too. Cicadas begin to consume the air waves until they drown out the tiny crackles in the branches. And the odours so easily carried by the morning dew dissipate. Before, geese, cormorant and fish could be smelled before being seen—now, they are first seen then smelled. Senses switch (as) priorities. Meanwhile, new delights appear. The egrets that seemed so boldly white as to serve as signposts along the river's edges, marking each turn, now shimmer with the same blue-violet hue that, only moments ago, was the sky's colour. Goldenrods, sunchokes and purple loosestrife, once invisible among the thicket of blurry green objects, now seem ubiquitous. And the entire watery expanse begins to reflect everything right beneath you, until it seems as if you are paddling among the tree-tops. When the water is perfectly still, it's as if there are two identical worlds, so that if you turn your head just right, you can almost forget which is which. And the paddler is much more likely to hear or issue a "G'morning!" to a passerby. The sun's arrival has changed the games completely.

In Part Three: Practice, comprised of four chapters, we will focus on the role of language in the infant's complicated mental and emotional journey between two worlds—the world of dreams and the world of reality, along a meandering trajectory from one to the other. In fact, the child will begin to gestate in an unconscious state. As birth approaches, he will begin to notice more of the world (perception)—and himself (proprioception). Yet upon being born, the child will not immediately become conscious. Further, anyone who has observed a premature infant can vouch for the fact that the infant is fully alive, a unique individual, even when born 12 (or more) weeks early. And every child—even full-term—requires the first months postnatally to recognize familiars, adjust to diurnal rhythms, develop reactions to pleasure and displeasure, and start to self-regulate. Dolto's notions emphasize the vitality of the continuous circulation of affect that is necessary for every child's indispensable unconscious security—his self-preservation—in this complex process. In addition to appealing to a wide readership, this third part may be of particular interest to educators and linguists.

Dolto's work centres on the crucial role of language—specifically, on phonemes. At issue is that phonemes become increasingly discernible for the infant in the womb, thereby becoming objects for the dream-work that informs nascent symbolization and roots thought. Henceforth, the phonemes of the mother tongue become carriers of unconscious affects, with huge repercussions for the child's ability to establish his unconscious security among his familiars in a timely manner—including the capacity for speech—once outside the womb. Freud explains that, "what is essential in dreams is the process of the dream-work."[14] And the work of dreams he elaborates—displacement and condensation—is crucial to grasping the unconscious role of phonemes. To refer to "dream-work," then, is to articulate how unconscious processes effect labour in the development and sustenance of our mental and emotional life. Thus, we will follow the rich returns of the dream-work scaffolding the infant's affective investments in the objects of his progressively broadening reality—the infant's learning.

The infant lives a rich, animated interior life at the onset of sensations—at the margins of day and night, reality and dreams. And though vision will become the dominant human sense if all goes well (enabling tremendous efficiencies), the growing prominence of vision will entail a lessened reliance on audition. The games will change. Yet the formative processes at work in our earliest days of human learning are stunningly potent and leave a permanent legacy in our mental and emotional life. So a better understanding of this primary mode of human learning should inform educational practices for all children. Surprisingly, however, unconscious processes are never mentioned in schools. During nearly 40 years as a teacher, I never heard them invoked—not once. And only a handful of universities worldwide include any consideration in their teacher training. Why is education so unconcerned about unconscious influences in early learning? This final part aims to help fill this gap.

For it is a reality of our species that we are born incompletely formed, with a neurological system that will take some 24 months beyond birth to develop properly. Thus, our earliest education will be experienced while we are barely (if at all) conscious. It will be nurtured and impacted by repetitive experiences provided by our immediate environment that are inscribed while we are still in mid-formation: our loved ones (i.e., sources and means of affect); our geography (i.e., habituation to climate, food, etc.); our mother tongues, and so on. It is precisely this capacity for postnatal growth that enables human beings to survive in such a remarkable diversity of habitats. We would not be human without this prolonged infancy that turns our vulnerabilities into possibilities—as we continue to grow adaptively in the first months outside the womb, contingent on the presence of others, until we can assume independence. In sum, we are human because of our pre-conscious learning.

Through these final chapters, then, we will explore how some educational practices pertaining to language and literacy might enlist the child's unconscious capacities to secure a greater engagement, as we study the lifelong sequelae of the archaic stage of psychosexual maturation on child development—principally, on affective self-regulation and associative thinking. We will privilege a universal design for learning that informs non-invasive, non-mechanistic interventions that are mindful of what all humans share, whether or not we are autistic—namely, the continuous circulation of unconscious affect that underwrites, lifelong, our mental and emotional capacities. And we will articulate the inextricable, unconscious role of language by stressing the importance of the phoneme in our passive education and the enduring reliance on regression—that oldest and strongest human defence. Central considerations here will include the distinct function of the mother tongue; the reparation of free reading in liberating affect; how critical writing practices can support individuation; and why the natural world is unconsciously securing. We will thus end where we began—in the woods.

In sum, what follows is an attempt to study what is learnable about the role of unconscious processes in infant development that can help us better understand nonverbal autism—as well as what is learnable about nonverbal autism that can guide instructional design for language and literacy in early education. The style of each part is substantially different due to engaging such distinct corpora: Part One, Dolto (with Freud); Part Two, four nonverbal autists (with Dolto and others); and Part Three, educators (theorists and researchers). There is some intentional overlap at the joints between parts to emphasize crucial concepts as they build, and to enable each part to be at least somewhat comprehensible independently.

In exploring the infant's learning style, we will focus on the staggering role language plays in learning prior to consciousness, while the infant is immersed in an auditory milieu. We will thus meet the infant on the long, winding developmental bridge between being unconscious and becoming conscious—i.e., during pre-conscious learning—wherein the precocious audition of language from the environment inscribes unconscious security. Dolto refers to this language landscape as a "sonar heritage,"[15] and her thinking about phonemes inspires the present subtitle, *Syllable Soup*.

In truth, if I did not start at Mute Bridge, perhaps I would not start this book at all. The problem is that thinking about human life before thought begins is disorienting. It is incredibly compelling to revert to silence and not even attempt that first word. But if I bring any special capacity to this work, other than my research inclinations, it is that my own challenging childhood history (about which I have written elsewhere)[16] has often made me subject to regression. So the discomfort of losing conscious landmarks and surrendering to archaic moorings is familiar. I believe that this is the basis of my "right to write" on this topic—my membership, such as it is, among the narrators of silence.

As it turns out, language acquisition is dominated by unconscious processes, driven by the instinct of conservation, that commence *in utero*—and it is this unconscious aspect of language learning to which the present work is attempting to contribute. I think the material herein will be of interest to a wide audience that includes autists, parents, aides, advocates, therapists, academics and researchers in education and linguistics. And I sincerely hope that it helps to generate a productive (re)consideration of early learning prior to the onset of the capacity for speech. In our first days, after all, every human being is an *infans*—one who cannot speak. We all begin as mutes.

Notes

1 1915a, 166–167 (emphasis his).
2 Ibid, 167.
3 Ibid, 169.
4 Readers of Jacques Lacan may find the discussion herein to be of particular interest given that Dolto and Lacan were contemporaries who often interacted. In my previous text on Dolto, where I take up their intersects in some detail, I stress that she valued Lacan for drawing attention "to words and their meaning for the child's unconscious prior to reading and writing" (in Djéribi-Valentin & Kouki 1998, 276); I also discuss there how Lacan found Dolto's flower-doll compelling (see Chapter 10).
5 Freud 1896d, 151.
6 Freud 1900b, 613.
7 For an engagement with phonemes in the traditional linguistic sense, see Chapter 5.
8 The significant and extensive implications for the Deaf are regretfully beyond the scope of the present project, though I take the opportunity to advance a few insights tangentially throughout the text.

9 "Preconscious" (no hyphen) is a Freudian term that "qualifies the operations and contents … that are not present in the actual field of consciousness … but that are differentiated from the contents of the unconscious system by remaining accessible to consciousness" (see Laplanche & Pontalis 1967/2004, 321); for "the preconscious system is situated between the unconscious system and consciousness" (ibid). However, "if we take 'unconscious' in the sense [of] … that which escapes consciousness[,] the distinction between preconscious and unconscious is erased" (ibid). In fact, in the perinatal infant's mental and emotional life, what is unconscious versus preconscious is impossible to distinguish. So I use "pre-conscious" (hyphenated) to designate what is prior to the reliable establishment of consciousness.

10 "Nonverbal autism" is a high-frequency phrase that turns up 15–20 million search hits on any given day. It refers to someone who is unable to speak, though other forms of communication may be possible, such as gestural and/or behavioural signs. My use of the term, nonverbal autism, adheres to common usage in general parlance and in educational systems. Of course, the four autistic authors are technically "non-speaking" rather than "nonverbal" since they can write; yet they self-identify (and are clinically identified) as "nonverbal autistic." The discordance between expressions anticipates our discussion.

11 1915a, 179.

12 In his therapeutic interventions with the first patient of psychoanalysis, "Anna O" (i.e., Bertha Pappenheim), Freud identified the sequelae of impeded affective circulation in her difficulty with conscious (intentional) movement—including speech—acute anxiety, echolalia and mutism (in Breuer & Freud 1893a, 42). I believe the parallels with the symptoms of nonverbal autism should draw our attention.

13 Kedar and Mukhopadhyay write in English. I extend my sincere gratitude to Anthea Bell (Sellin's translator); and to David Mitchell and KA Yoshida (Higashida's translation team).

14 1933a, 8.

15 Dolto 1981, 286.

16 2013.

Part One

Analysis

Preamble for Part One

As I write this preamble, my hearing is being tested. I face the joint liabilities of ageing and decades of employment in loud spaces. Online, countless articles warn that hearing loss can lead to social isolation. At least in terms of audition, then, it seems as if the older adult is living the infant's life in reverse. Prenatally, the infant's hearing was constrained by bodily tissues and water. But postnatally, he gains the capacity to attend to sounds—including language—that ease his social inclusion and draw out his voice from his silence.

Let us journey with the infant for a moment. Birth has not yet arrived, but his body is preparing. His brain and organs are developing, and rhythms of sleep and semi-wakefulness become observable. In fact, many characteristics of the young human antedate birth. In neonatal wards worldwide, even the most fragile infants find their own unique ways to show they love being cared for and spoken to. For every newborn tries to begin responding to the world and needs the world to start responding to him. There is an engagement of dependency from the first moment of human life, hence a need for communication. Human survival—the continuation of the species—depends on it.

Freud theorized the five stages of psychosexual development that the human infant will traverse from birth to maturity (oral, anal, phallic, latent, genital). Whether one is aware of (or agrees with) Freud's entire project, this contribution is widely considered indispensable. Even Piaget endorsed Freud's basic framework: "The time has come to forget both official prejudice and parochial attitudes, and to incorporate the living part of Freudian psychology, i.e., the method and the facts, in psychology as a whole. The facts are indisputable."[1] In elaborating the psychosexual stages, Freud theorized a flow of unconscious energy—experienced as unconscious affect[2]—originating in early life that continually circulates as a kind of fuel for psychosexual maturation. It is as if a rich reservoir of unconscious affect drives the processes whereby we, as biological organisms, gradually gain the capacity to instrumentalize our bodies (ourselves) for success in reality.

Psychosexual maturation, as Freud demonstrates, entails withdrawing the unconscious affect attached to a prior stage and transferring it to suitable "objects" of the next stage through a kind of diffusion—displacement—by means of unconscious associations. This process serves a vital function in human health by venting

DOI: 10.4324/9781032655123-3

(liberating) affect. Freud is narrating how each member of our species—born vulnerable and incomplete (with brain development needed outside the womb)—begins to "feel" human through a continuous circulation of unconscious affect that inscribes (substantially idiosyncratically) certain objects as crucial pathways for our survival.

To be clear, objects are not necessarily material things.[3] For example, milk is an object for the infant, securing survival. But the name of the mother is also an object because it unconsciously evokes the one sustaining survival. Even an association to that word is an object since, despite associative distance, it recalls unconscious security. Therefore, each stage in psychosexual maturation compels a shift in unconscious objects of love as affect is displaced towards new objects (if all goes well). By logical reduction, every invested object of a later stage inherits unconscious affect from its association to a prior loved object. Even when living in present reality, then, our beloved objects carry unconscious traces of our unique past.

Dolto worked with countless patients whose traumas during World Wars I and II led her to infer an even earlier time in psychosexual development, as she reflected on unconscious transferences that seemed rooted sometime prior to what she called the "umbilical castration"[4] (i.e., birth). She then used her observations to sketch the child's psychosexual development during a passage she called "the archaic." And though she was reluctant to make explicit claims about theory, I believe it is evident from her body of work that she effectively theorized what precedes the oral stage: the archaic stage.

In the archaic stage, all objects are dream objects—liquid objects—because the gestational infant is unconscious and only gradually gains the capacities that will eventually enable consciousness. Further, during psychosexual maturation in the womb, even the objects of reality have a liquid quality: his nutrition, his watery comfort, and sound as it begins to permeate—i.e., words. Dolto's therapeutic work with young patients was remarkably successful precisely because she believed that every human being is receptive to language during the archaic, wherein the parents' language is "more subtle than liquid."[5]

Dolto's critical assumption, then, is that unconscious affect attaches to phonemes as "liquid objects" for the infant's dream-work. Dolto also insisted that for the infant, everything is language: the mother's heartbeat, his heartbeat, his mother's voice and words, the words around him (crucially, his father's or mother's other), and other ambient sounds. On this view, even anxiety, love and fear are language. And since there is a trace of the unconscious affective investments of the previous stage in each succeeding one, each of us lives out "archaic object relations"[6] all the time without realizing it consciously. For example, our love for an author, language or occupation invariably carries our silent history of archaically invested objects. The past, in a real way, is still (always) present.

Crucially, investing unconscious affect in new objects can be impeded by challenging life events at any stage. For example, the breastfed infant whose mother is unexpectedly hospitalized suffers a sudden "oral castration" (i.e., weaning). This is experienced as trauma in that the object on which survival depends—his mother (his milk)—has been removed without giving him a chance to transfer the affect on which survival depends to a new object. While we might expect infants to accept another form of food in the interest of survival—and some do—it is not unusual to find an infant refusing nourishment altogether instead. At work is an unconscious process of "regression" to an earlier time, prior to the oral stage, when eating by mouth was not needed because food was provided by the placenta and absorbed passively. Unconscious affect is withdrawn, then, to preserve the unconscious affect that is already secured, in what is effectively the opposite of displacement: condensation. And we arrive at a significant reflection: unconscious regression is our first defence as human beings—and the infant's only defence.[7]

Following Freud, Dolto elaborates regression to the archaic—i.e., to archaic stages of the organization of libido.[8] She describes it as a "regression of the feeling of the subject to an archaic image of his body that could not be surpassed … or renounced without the subject losing his notion of continuity, his existential security."[9] At issue is that nothing in a subject's present affective life can bring him pleasure at least as intense as the lost pleasure associated with this archaic image.[10] And as the infant has not yet surpassed the archaic stage, regression is simply to a deeper unconscious state wherein he engages even less of his nascent reality. Dolto believes regression is necessary to the conservation of health,[11] and that recovery from autism is therefore possible, since "all that is living is still living in language."[12] Thus arises the vital role of the phoneme.

To restart psychosexual maturation following regression—i.e., to get unconscious affect to recirculate in the direction of maturation—it will be necessary to locate objects that unconsciously recall the mother: for example, her smell, voice or words. This is a way of drawing the infant's unconscious investments towards new objects through association, thereby sustaining the affective circulation that secures survival. As Dolto puts it, "The unconscious process of survival is to consume a partial object coming from another that represents the mother."[13] Let us keep in mind that the infant at this stage is incapable of conscious action. He cannot actively search for objects of any kind. He can only wait for objects to arrive, for a form of reconnaissance of their unconscious association with the mother, thus inviting his unconscious affective investment. It is not a question of the infant seeking suitable objects, then, but rather of being lured by the objects around him (i.e., presented to him). For the infant in the archaic stage encounters objects while he is dominantly unconscious and passive.

At birth, beloved objects representing archaic unconscious security might be easily lost amid the rush of newness. This is particularly true for a child who reaches birth regressed due to an unnarratable history that was nonetheless survivable—thus survived. Perhaps the gestational infant or mother were unwell during gestation. Dolto notes that even anxiogenic events affecting the mother can provoke regression in the infant—such as the death of the mother's parent or the infant's father, war, forced migration, and so on.[14] Yet if the child survives, his unconscious history through the archaic stage of psychosexual maturation is likely to be physically unnoticeable at birth—he will "look" unaffected.

The famous researcher on infants, Margaret Mahler, concurs on this point: "Disturbances of the symbiotic phase may go unrecognized."[15] Nonetheless, the child who has regressed often—or for an extended time—during the archaic stage will have a diminished capacity to locate objects in reality that are continuous with his invested objects of dream-work. Further, his predominantly passive disposition will prevent his active search for suitable objects. As a consequence, his unconscious affect will be less easily transferrable to objects of reality during the oral stage. The result will be an infant who is harder to secure, experiences devastating anxiety, and adheres to patterns of his past (including passivity and repetition) to keep investing objects of dream-work rather than the lures of reality.

Crucially, the infant's self-preservation—his lifelong potential for healthy psychosexual maturation and the happiness that comes with it—depends on having as much affect as possible circulating forward freely. And as the archaic marks the source of unconscious affect—its fountainhead—archaic objects harbour the strongest affect. We can infer, then, that unconscious associations to archaic objects will retain the greatest force for (re)fueling psychosexual maturation.

In either case—whether a new object for affective investment cannot be found, or a prior one has been lost before its affect could be transferred—the instinct of conservation compels the continued circulation of unconscious affect by whatever means possible. In brief, in the drive for survival, affect that cannot be invested to secure conservation is, simply put, conserved.[16] I offer that we can thus consider unconscious affect to be naturally resorptive.

Unconscious affect that cannot be transferred onto new objects that secure survival is withdrawn—i.e., reinvesting prior objects—until a suitable new object can be secured. For in the archaic, previously invested objects are objects of dream-work, so they remain deep within us as perpetual sources of unconscious security, impervious to any actual destruction or loss in reality. To restate, the infant who reaches the oral stage then regresses to the archaic will become reinvested in objects of dream-work. The result is that every regression will make progressive psychosexual maturation more difficult. On the other hand, prior objects of affective investment (if they can be "located") can be instrumentalized (i.e., presented, offered) to lure forward investments and help exit regression.

Here, then, is the archaic triangulation comprising the roots (origin) of the famous Oedipal triangle. The infant is alive in an unconscious relation (dream-work) with another who provides the means for his survival. As Dolto explained it repeatedly, mother and infant are one and the same in the infant's unconscious. For the infant, it is not a case of *being with* the mother but rather of *being* the mother since all he experiences is *as-if, with, and through* her. The infant (i.e., "first") is unconsciously blurred with his indissociable "second" as a «moi-mamère» [me-mymother],[17] to use Dolto's coinage. That said, this "second" is nonetheless distinguishable from any "third" object (e.g., food, father, word, voice, etc.), especially nearer to the horizon of reality. This "third" is associated with the mother yet ever-changing, as objects arrive from beyond the womb for the infant's dream-work.

In short, the mother is an environment for the arrival of everything—and any "third" is unconsciously invested by virtue of its association with the "second." In this context, Dolto invokes an archaic mother and archaic father—archaic parents that precede any sense of the actual parents. For in the archaic, the mother and father are experienced in dream-work, without clear boundaries (but with abundant associations) between them. As such, they are easily combined (condensed) in dream-work. So the "third" blends with the "second" unconsciously. And when the infant later starts to distinguish his mother ("second") from himself ("first"), he will then be, just like his father ("third"), associated with his mother but not her—as "first" and "third" blur.

Such are the highly fluid positions of archaic triangulation that take place in dream-work at the onset of human psychosexual maturation. And since unconscious affect is always in circulation so long as we live, archaic triangulation always finds a way to continue. Like a rushing river dammed in one place seeking another outlet, it compels a path however it can, using unconscious associations as means of displacement. As Dolto stresses, this «situation triangulaire»[18] is the source of the child's unconscious security, as affect is conserved by continuous circulation between objects that guarantee his survival. We also note how Dolto's project closely dovetails Freud's work on dreams because we find evidence of displacement and condensation in the archaic.

Here, in the context of the archaic triangular situation, a profound paradox emerges affecting language. The mother tongue is primarily associated with the mother's voice. But words are also other than the mother, in that they enter dream-work from various sources; words are thus also associated with the other-of-the-mother (i.e., father). This is why (as we will see) Dolto believes that refinding the symbolic (archaic) father is the therapeutic key to recovering lost (trapped) affect and helping a child exit regression. It's because the dreamed other-of-the-mother is unconsciously the archaic witness to the indissociable infant-mother. Thus, the infant's most invested words—first phonemes, like first dreams—serve as landmarks for recovering archaic investments.

From this archaic register, the infant struggles to achieve the unconscious affective transfers to reality needed for psychosexual maturation. If all goes well, he invests unconscious affect in objects of reality that are continuous with his archaic investments via the mechanism of association by which affects are displaced unconsciously. Thus, his affective investments gradually gain associative distance from his archaic objects (becoming associations of associations, and so on), while nonetheless remaining in continuity with them. For affect has an economy and it is invested for the sole purpose of survival—while what enables survival generates (by definition) "pleasure." This notion of an affective economy confirms how and why the lures of reality need to be good enough to draw out the infant from his dreams of unspeakable archaic bliss. For as Dolto notes right from the start of her project, "pleasure can never be renounced without an exchange for another pleasure."[19] On the other hand, if all does not go well, the infant will return to a prior mode of being—undiscernible physically—by regressing to an anterior stage wherein his unconscious security is assured because it once was.

The flourishing of proprioception and perception as the infant nears term presents countless new possibilities for affective investments. Whatever is most closely associated with the mother more easily inherits affect, and repetition gives some objects greater prominence. However, the umbilical castration (birth) marks a complete upheaval of his circumstances along with a sensory awakening. Through rapid changes, it will be more difficult for the infant to find unconscious echoes of objects that are continuous by association with his prior unconscious investments. Further, with the progression towards consciousness, space/time and gravity will complicate matters (e.g., delays in feeding, the mother's voice at a distance, the body grounded differently, etc.). And soon, passivity will no longer be enough to secure objects. For in the oral stage, the infant will need to commence the active "call and response" essential to his new conditions for survival.

I believe we can now begin to appreciate the staggering value of the mother tongue in offering innumerable liquid objects that are unconsciously invested because of their archaic relation to the mother and the frequency with which they are encountered. Phonemes thus acquire special value in securing the unconscious circulation of affect, as Dolto stressed lifelong. We should also note that, of the five senses, hearing is the most continuous in function from the womb to beyond it, in that the other senses are relatively unexercised in the womb. This gives audition a special role in securing archaic continuity through a wild abundance of objects that are, in turn, naturally associated with each other through sound as a fact of every language (e.g., in English: kind – kindness; ear – fear – dear, etc.). We thereby advance a critical summation: the fetus dreams in a long-established auditory world.

Ultimately, then, psychosexual maturation progresses two steps forward and one step back—much better if the exchange of pleasure is palpable so that anxiety is minimized. As Dolto explains it, in the oral stage, the phonemes the child begins to babble serve two functions precisely because they are unconsciously already invested: first, they are experienced as a kind of "food," as self-feeding (self-securing) through taking in some invested objects of dream-work; second, as the child hears himself speak, his self-uttered phonemes recall the mother's continued presence so that he will once again be (like) her, returning his archaic dreams of security. The infant in the oral stage will receive unconscious affects from the archaic and, reciprocally, regression during the oral stage will reinvest archaic objects. The infant will float back and forth imperceptibly for weeks.

Dream objects will be slowly reified through the developmental process of transferring unconscious affect to real objects that carry unconscious traces of the archaic. So doing, things (actual objects) will become associated with their names (liquid objects). In everyday terms, we will say that the infant is developing language comprehension. At the same time, reality will offer familiar objects that are already invested with unconscious affect—like the mother's most repeated words—that will keep entering dream-work, as they have for months. Freud explains that the capacity for becoming conscious develops precisely through "thing-presentations" receiving unconscious affect through their associations with "word-presentations";[20] meanwhile, dreams use residues of "verbal presentations."[21] For when the child reaches that bridge between the unconscious and consciousness, travel is open in both directions.

In fact, we don't even need a theory to know that this is true because of the common human experience of the transference of dream material to thought—and vice-versa. We wake up with solutions to long-standing problems; we remember where a lost object was placed; we recall an important idea we had forgotten; and a dream about others (good or bad) illogically changes what we think about them. Conversely, snippets of our conversations with loved ones, weighty news, and even random words we read or heard the day before find their way into our dreams. In addition, we can be jolted from near-sleep by the dread of a single thought, something not to forget to do or bring tomorrow—just as a single word uttered in a meeting or on a bus can throw us into daydreams that disconnect us temporarily from reality.

Freud explored the continuity between unconscious dream-work and conscious thought in his highly popular texts on dreams, jokes and slips—as well as in his work on word-things and DaVinci.[22] As Freud explains it, "conscious systems of thought … are merely projections … translations … from the unknown, unconscious."[23] As for the infant, then, words seed his fetal dreams—and his fetal dream-work seeds his thoughts. So the infant's thoughts are derivatives of his archaic dream-work. Such is the mental and emotional situation of every infant traversing the archaic stage—and of one who reaches the oral stage but regresses (whether briefly or routinely) to the archaic. Yet it is only by progressing steadily through the oral stage that the child will be able to articulate his first word. The powerful and decisive conclusion is that thought antedates speech. The infant is mute but thinking.

The following pages offer 12 overlapping essays through which we will analyse in greater detail the theory surveyed above to get a better grasp on the infant's development in the archaic, and on the role of familiar phonemes in psychosexual maturation. Chapter 1 focuses on the dominant influence of the instinct of conservation in human development. Chapter 2 is centred on the unconscious circulation of affect by which the fetus becomes capable of nascent emotional and mental activity, investing in liquid objects subject to dream-work. Chapter 3 follows the gestational infant's growing capacity for symbolization, as objects that are unconsciously invested prenatally facilitate investments in objects postnatally. Throughout, we will also reflect on the nature of unconscious triangulation while the infant is passive, and on the vital process of association.

By way of an apology, I admit that these essays are not linear in the least. In each, we never begin with a question and end with an answer. For Dolto's work charts the rich, vibrant and fluid space between dreams and reality. Thus, our movement through her theory will necessarily be more like a fruitful wandering on a vast water-soaked land, sometimes covering our steps again, to try to find what we can. Most enigmatically, while travelling with Dolto, we will end up journeying uncomfortably close to the sacred terrain of philosophers as we contemplate the infant's existential anxiety, and where thought and "self" begin. But Dolto was an unassuming genius who chose to spend her time in clinics rather than polemics. Inspired by her, I suggest we roll up our sleeves and get down on the ground with the infant instead, to play with a single notion: Dolto's belief that autism is a regression to the archaic.

Notes

1 1962, 184.
2 Freud explains that "we call the original affective impulse an 'unconscious' one" (1915a, 178); and he uses both expressions, "unconscious affect" and "unconscious emotion" (ibid). Freud elaborates the three vicissitudes of unconscious affect: "either the affect remains, wholly or in part, as it is; or it is transformed into a qualitatively different quota of affect, above all into anxiety; or it is suppressed, i.e., it is prevented from developing at all" (ibid). He stresses that "if the instinct did not attach itself to an idea or manifest itself as an affective state, we could know nothing about it" (ibid, 177).
3 Note that liquid objects defy any simple delineation of part versus whole.
4 In Djéribi-Valentin 2005, 516.
5 In Caldaguès 1982, 61.
6 In Dolto & Roudinesco 1986/1988, 12.
7 Freud uses the term "regression" to designate an involution or withdrawal of libido (1909b, 45; 1912, 102; 1914a, 74–75 & 82). Such withdrawal is possible because of the indestructibility of unconscious paths (1900b, 553f). Thereby, "primitive stages can always be reestablished" (1915b, 286). For Freud, regression is "a return to anterior forms of development of thought [and] object relations" (in Laplanche & Pontalis 1967/2004, 400); and to "an anterior mode of organization" (ibid, 401). For as Freud explains, "unconscious material … brings its own modes of working along with it" (1940[1939], 167). He elaborates: "The flight from unsatisfactory reality … takes place along the path of involution, of regression, of a return to earlier phases … from which at one time satisfaction was not withheld … to stages of development that are earlier in time [wherein] the original and primitive methods of psychical expression are employed" (1909b, 49). Furthermore, Freud emphasizes how "it is only dreams that can tell us about the regression of our emotional life to one of the earliest stages of development" (1915b, 286).
8 In Guillerault 1997, 116.
9 Ibid, 265.
10 Ibid, 142.
11 Ibid, 265.
12 1987, 77.
13 In Dolto & Winter 1986, 125.
14 For example, in Dolto 1971, 214 and Halmos 1994, 33.
15 1965, 561.
16 The preeminent French dictionary of psychoanalysis renders Freud's term, "self-preservation," as «pulsions d'auto-conservation» (Laplanche & Pontalis 1967/2004, 148). On that basis, I believe we are free to use "conservation" or "auto-conservation" right along with "self-preservation." Relatedly, that dictionary notes that using "instinct" (in French or English) for Freud's *trieb* (in German) is "an inaccuracy of translation" (ibid, 203); yet "instinct" has been in circulation for over a century. At issue is that translation yields losses, since perfect correspondence is rare—but also gains, as multilingualism produces new associations in thought. In fact, psychoanalysis has long endured controversies around terminology; Élisabeth Roudinesco astutely calls translation, "the sea serpent of the history of the movement" (1982, 348). Dolto was unrestricted by the boundaries of French, liberally coining new terms, and the terminological disruptions she provokes open fertile grounds for thinking.
17 In De Sauverzac 1985, 127.
18 In Caldaguès 1982, 215–217.
19 In Marette 1940, 153; Marette was Dolto's maiden name.
20 1915a, 209–215; also 1896e, 232.
21 1900a, 49.
22 1910; I elaborate this connection in my previous text on Dolto.
23 1907/1962, 150 [Meeting of 20 March 1907].

Chapter 1

Conservation

Preliminary Words

The instinct of conservation is real and not some theoretical fiction. Whether one prefers Freud's lucid analyses or those of literally thousands of other writers invoking an instinct for self-preservation in their works on diverse subjects, the fact remains that all biological organisms seek to survive. Survival is the most basic instinct of everything that lives—and the human species is no exception. Freud's elaboration of instincts is an unprecedented weaving of the biological with the psychological, as he describes how humans first develop under the primary and dominant influence of the instinct of conservation, and how this growth trajectory nonetheless enables us to refine neurological structures that will enable consciousness and the complex achievements of a healthy adult brain. Freud's project follows the sequelae of instincts in psychosexual maturation as a slow shift from unconscious to conscious life, whereby the unconscious remains beneath consciousness as a reservoir of immeasurable strength—and as a powerful thread to our prior, pre-conscious personal histories.

Therefore, the unconscious is real and not some theoretical fiction either. Dolto puts it bluntly: "The unconscious is not an obscure, *mute* receptacle of *useless psychical representations*."[1] As the instinct of conservation is a fact of life, and as the unconscious is a personal resource within each of us driving psychosexual maturation from its onset, then we can expect that the infant—who is, by definition, pre-conscious (i.e., prior to consciousness)—will demonstrate the clearest evidence of unconscious processes. Furthermore, since the instinct of conservation originates at the onset of life, our infant is functionally older than his birthday suggests, as Dolto notes: "Seven months, that is nonetheless 9 and 7: sixteen months of life."[2]

The economist and Nobel laureate, Daniel Kahneman, theorizes a decision-making model to explain why we often ignore rationality (our "System 2") in favour of what he calls, "System 1": "System 1 has been shaped by evolution to provide a continuous assessment of the main problems that an organism must solve to survive … we have inherited the neural mechanisms that evolved to provide ongoing assessments of threat level."[3] He adds, "Emotional arousal is associative, automatic, and uncontrolled, and it produces an impulse for protective

DOI: 10.4324/9781032655123-4

action … System 1 cannot be turned off."[4] Kahneman does not cite Freud here, but he certainly invites our interest because his research clearly seems to validate the sustained residence of unconscious processes deep within us, and the reality that humans are subject to the instinct of conservation.

Provocatively, Dolto once stated in an interview, "As for precocity, I really have no idea anymore where it is … It really seems to be right from the first day of life."[5] With this caveat in mind, we will travel with Dolto through the archaic stage—as a kind of experiment in thought, so to speak—to the onset of unconscious capacities in the infant, at some unspecified earlyish time during gestation which we permanently leave open. Our infant is still months away from consciousness and thus fully driven by the instinct of conservation within the archaic triangular situation—his condition of highly fluid dream-work—in what Dolto usefully referred to as a "larval" Oedipus Complex.[6]

Dolto's words disclose a deeply uncomfortable aspect of her work that needs to be aired before referencing her any further because it holds such astounding moral and ethical implications. I am not Dolto's apologist, but I strongly believe that we should not employ her work for any larger conversations about "when life begins"—and furthermore, that doing so would grievously misrepresent her lifelong dedication to therapeutic objectives. It's only that in theorizing the early development of the mental and emotional life of the infant—and inferring some gestational antecedents—Dolto could not help but incidentally land on some socio-political terrain both distant and different from her own self-declared destination: "I have come for this, to witness for you the unconscious."[7]

A. Archaic

Survival is a simple-enough story at its core: the instinct of conservation drives the wish to live, and all that is associated with survival is good. In an unconscious state of non-time, non-space, the infant begins life by absorbing everything that enables his self-preservation within the "me-mymother"—i.e., the unique mode of inter-relational health[8] that is gestation. Sometime early during physiological development *in utero*—at a time we hold as an unanswerable question—we "locate" the imperceptible shore of unconscious existence. And from the moment that unconscious capacities begin to function, says Dolto, we can speak of the unconscious mooring of the subject to life[9]—of an unconscious existence[10] in the archaic stage of desire.[11]

This "archaic epoch"[12] is marked by repeated experiences, among the most prevalent being heartbeats (the infant's and mother's), which Dolto describes as "a rhythmic two times, the basic sign of vegetative life."[13] As nutrition reaches the child and waste matter is removed—all through liquid media—the child grows thanks to innumerable archaic rhythmic exchanges.[14] We cannot know when or what of these exchanges infuses his dreams. For our idiosyncratic archaic history,[15] as Dolto puts it—our "archaic heritage,"[16] as Freud called it—remains absolutely unnarratable and intimately bound in silence. All we know is that, under the influence of the instinct of conservation, every infant develops unconscious capacities (we cannot know exactly how) and he begins to dream (we cannot know exactly when), using some input (we cannot know exactly what) that reaches him through his nascent perception and his increasing proprioception.

Freud makes a clear case about dreams that has withstood over 100 years of scrutiny: dreams secure our wishes. Freud explores the two main mechanisms of dream-work—displacement and condensation—and concludes that, "dream language ... forms part of a highly archaic system of expression."[17] In turn, what Dolto finds is that in the archaic stage, dreams are indeed the infant's system of expression. Dream-work that accompanies the unconscious archaic experience of surviving is unconsciously securing the wish to live, offering the gestational infant what Dolto calls "archaic symbolic satisfaction";[18] this satisfaction is experienced unconsciously in the "archaic subbasement"[19] of human life—far beneath consciousness—within a "unitary structure in the interior."[20] And, like any basement, the home to be built upon it will depend on it.

As with every stage of psychosexual maturation, there will be variations between individuals in how the archaic stage is lived. For while all humans are subject to "an unconscious logic of the precocious stages,"[21] Dolto stresses, there will be differentiation at the individual level because, "archaic, unconscious libidinal organization is idiosyncratic."[22] Nonetheless, in whatever way the archaic stage unfolds, if we are born—i.e., if we live—then our archaic passage symbolizes our survival such that the umbilical separation will be experienced as a wound,[23] Dolto explains. Further, since we cannot have survived without that archaic passage, it's as if we need to keep it with us. So our idiosyncratic archaic history is inscribed deep within us, and we will carry that unconscious record without any conscious realization.[24] As Dolto elucidates, based on hundreds of therapeutic interventions over five decades, "the archaic always continues to exist within us ... constantly there is a level that is archaic."[25]

At birth, immeasurable reservoirs of unconscious affect—the "libidinal wealth"[26] at the "source of life"[27]—gradually begins to be unconsciously transferred to objects of the oral stage that sustain our wish to survive (if all goes well). Affect is transferred successively as we move through further psychosexual stages as a result of which, Dolto notes, "every other is an object of the transference of relations much more archaic."[28] Conversely, for psychosexual maturation to proceed, it will be vital for "archaic pleasure to be surpassed."[29] Dolto sums up the infant's archaic transference situation in her trademark, highly condensed style: "The archaic affect of the fetal epoch leaves its living traces in narcissistic organo-emotional representative associations."[30]

Of course, the archaic is a theoretical construct that isn't, strictly speaking, provable. Given this, it might be easy to dismiss it as a hypothetical fabrication except for one thing: if we assume the archaic stage, then countless facts about infancy and psychosexual maturation become clearer. To stress, then, the archaic has the same experimental status as black holes. It must be assumed—inferred—to be true in order to explain what is known to be true. And while there is wide public recognition for great physicists who correctly theorized aspects of the cosmos hundreds of years in the past—sometimes, at the cost of their lives—theories of psychosexual maturation are often regarded with grave suspicion.

Yet the fact of psychosexual maturation is that long before birth, the infant is a living being capable of dreaming; his dreams use some of the sensory material around him (and in him) as liquid objects; these dream (liquid) objects predispose his later affective investments in actual objects of his environment; and the gradual transfer of affect from dream objects to real objects is the primary means for coming to consciousness. In effect, then, knowledge about unconscious processes should provoke a radical paradigm shift in our relations with infants. For parents emerge first and foremost as teachers—as every infant's first teacher. Everything the parent says or presents to the infant constitutes the most important learning of all—formative learning that will facilitate (or not) affective investments that will make the real world feel unconsciously secure. And the conjunction of the infant being closer to reality while being able to take in more of reality is not a coincidence either. Everything that is already loved (i.e., unconsciously affectively invested) continues to be—but what is new must somehow become associated with what is already loved.

Can we pinpoint exactly when unconscious capacities begin? No, we cannot. Can we predict which objects from the environment will enter dream-work as liquid objects to become invested with unconscious affect? No, we cannot. Can we locate unconscious processes? No, we cannot. Most likely, unconscious activity originates in some (or several, or all) of the lower brain structures that form early during gestation and are well on board by the second trimester. Perhaps there is additional involvement of the enteric nervous system, which also develops early *in utero* as "the only organ that contains an intrinsic nervous system that is able to mediate reflexes in the complete absence of input from the brain or spinal cord."[31] Some day, unconscious functions may be localized. But if the field of astronomy sets an example, that discovery could take hundreds of years. In the meantime, there is much to do that cannot wait for neurological specificity—and does not require it. The infant needs us to stop missing the forest for the trees.

For without the archaic, we will miss how the oral stage inherits an idiosyncratic history of dream-work on liquified objects that acquire materiality. Without the archaic, we will miss how the infant is an instinctive being for whom the assurance of unconscious pleasure enables consciousness. Without the archaic, we will miss how complex affective processes in the womb have momentous consequences for psychosexual maturation. And without the archaic, we will miss the chance to consider the sequelae of being regressed during transitions from the archaic stage to the oral stage. We will need to be willing to accept uncertainty to experience discovery. For the archaic calls us—just as it calls the infant—to awaken our capacity for adventure.

B. Affect

In 1888,[32] Freud defined transference as the displacement of an infantile scene onto the present[33] and a means of displacement in the service of primary processes.[34] He explains that transference is an exchange of unconscious affect that is present in all relationships.[35] Freud also describes how the transference is "a universal phenomenon of the human mind"—one that "dominates the whole of each person's relations to his human environment."[36] In brief, it is the means by which unconscious phantasies are externalized.[37] And externalizing his dreams—his unconscious phantasies—is precisely the preoccupation of the infant in the archaic stage. Dolto herself refers to the operational fact of the transference[38] as an unconscious dialectic[39] and an emotional resonance[40] between human beings. She adds that it is an infraverbal expression[41]—a primitive human exchange[42] before and beneath speech—that serves as an "archaic witness to a system of affective relays."[43] Critically, the affects of this earliest stage leave traces in the child—and in the adult he becomes.

In 1895, Freud theorized affect as both the result of, and evidence for, primary processes: "The affective process approximates to the uninhibited primary process";[44] and "where there is affect there is a primary process."[45] Recalling that affect has an economy (i.e., it can be invested, or not), Freud also speaks of "quanta of affect."[46] And by analysing the transference of affect in his clinical work, Freud observes the "incomparable strength of the first affective ties of human creatures,"[47] and of the "perennial first inclinations of dream-life"[48]—i.e., the lifelong impacts of our earliest unconscious affects. Freud also stresses that not only affect[49] but somatic stimuli influence dreams.[50]

So we can reasonably infer that the gestational infant in the archaic stage dreams of whatever he begins to feel in his own body, for example, and also of whatever he begins to hear with increasing clarity. April Nowell, a paleolithic archaeologist, astutely remarks that, "one significant advantage of extra-uterine brain growth is that the developing brain is shaped by experiences in infancy and early childhood."[51] To this we can now add that intra-uterine brain growth is also being shaped by early experiences. For the environment provides objects for dream-work during the archaic stage that will influence the infant's capacity to shift affect to real objects during the subsequent oral stage.

Let us sum up the situation so far. From early in the infant's gestational development—likely sometime in the first trimester, but certainly by the second—he becomes capable of unconscious activity that is characterized by dreaming. As he matures in the womb, his capacities for perception and proprioception are enhanced, thereby enabling some of the actual objects of his world—his food, heartbeats, repetitive sounds and words, his mother's voice, even his mother's anxiety—to become objects of dream-work in the way that dreams always take in some random, unpredictable objects of our world. Unconscious affect that is attached to the objects of dream-work then makes these objects more likely to receive investments of affect in reality. A word his mother often speaks—for example, her significant other's name—may serve the infant as a dream object countless times, inscribing it with quanta of affect.

As the infant nears reality, he develops an improved awareness of his environment and better audition. And when he finally exits the womb and hears that word more clearly, affect will be more readily transferred onto that real object and its associated objects—for example, onto the father and his name, his mother's voice, the phonemes of the mother tongue, and so on. We can now understand that the transference of affect from dream material to the proximal objects of reality constitutes the most significant scaffold in the infant's transition from the archaic stage to the oral stage. And we should keep in mind that the developmental goal is for the infant to emerge from the archaic stage with the capacity to invest as much affect as possible into the objects of the next stage, the oral stage.

I believe that we can also begin to fathom the origins of the infant's emotional world. The affect originating in unconscious processes in infancy is the precursor of emotions. But whereas in reality there will be love and hate, for instance—i.e., all kinds of positive and negative emotions—there is no negative in the unconscious. For the archaic transference situation compels a critical turn: there is only affect or its absence. In other words, affect circulates or it is impeded (in a given direction). And since unconscious affect needs to be continuously displaced as long as we live, the affect that cannot be transferred onto new objects will necessarily be reinvested in prior objects. On the one hand, then, a forward movement of affect onto new objects by associative displacements (diffusion) leads to a spread of affect that enables learning—i.e., our investment in new objects. On the other hand, affect that is reinvested in prior objects—regression—condenses (re-concentrates) affect onto limited objects, resulting in less associative branching so fewer pathways for displacement—that is, a lessened capacity for learning from our environments.

Dolto observes in even the youngest child some «réactions affectives.»[52] We are dealing with an "affective economy,"[53] she states. Normatively, then, the infant will transfer affect from his archaic dreamscape to his actual landscape. But if he cannot, Dolto stresses, then we will need to seek the "economic reason for non-insertion."[54] What Dolto is highlighting here is that the infant is unconsciously securitized during the archaic stage in a continual "intimate affective mute colloquium."[55] For he is held within a fused, indissociable "me-mymother" where affect keeps circulating with another who is as-if himself, and the pleasurable give-and-take fuels his dreams as a guarantor of his survival.

This dream-work is perfectly sufficient during the archaic stage—a herald of human success. And yet, it will soon no longer be enough. At issue is that the infant's physical trajectory is unrelenting, and his psychosexual maturation needs to proceed in tandem. Parturition will trigger a rapid increase in growth and all kinds of sensory capacities will come on board in quick succession. To be successful with everything from swallowing milk, to developing wakefulness, to responding to his name, the infant will need to feel sufficiently securitized through transferring unconscious affect to objects in reality. But a deeply regressed, fully passive position—however it eludes appearances—will limit his potential for such successful transferences and may even foreclose critical developmental windows.

It seems that we have reached a conclusion of some substance: the infant's welcome—in the largest sense—is crucial in facilitating the free flow of affect from dream objects to the objects of reality. We are speaking here of a process that is functionally a drawing out of the infant from his entirely unconscious state towards a reliable capacity for consciousness via familiar, repetitive objects that lure his forward investments. For success, we will need to meet the infant on his grounds at least as much as he has come to ours, in the manner of creating open channels for water to naturally flow. For in one more paradox, the infant will be most successfully awakened by reminders of when he was asleep—as if continuing the dream of perfect bliss.

Here, we pause to note Freud's insistence on the principal purpose of dreams being the satisfaction of the oldest wish, to sleep—i.e., his "discovery of the omnipresence in dreams of the wish to sleep."[56] By this, Freud draws our attention to the principle of inertia[57]—about which he wrote in some of his earliest publications—as being critical to our understanding of the circulation of unconscious affect, and indispensable to any consideration of nascent development (i.e., primary narcissism): "Discharge represents the primary function of the nervous system … For among the paths of discharge those are preferred and retained which involve a cessation of the stimulus: *flight from the stimulus*."[58]

In fact, these first days and weeks will be instrumental in scaffolding the infant's displacements of affect—sight unseen—in the oral-stage situation we will have prepared for him at birth. We should thus endeavour to populate his real world with echoes of his dreams—familiar moorings—that recall the situation wherein, up to now (and thanks to which) he has survived. As Dolto states categorically, even shockingly, "It is altogether the first days and the first weeks of the life of a human being that will have influence."[59]

By studying the archaic stage, we come to appreciate that there is a quality of life imported into reality from our earliest dreams—a quality we literally can't live without. The archaic filters the affect that future psychosexual stages inherit—while our passage in the archaic leaves permanent traces that unconsciously affect the love and work that evolves from our first beloved objects, and thus it profoundly impacts who we become. As for the infant in the archaic stage, he may be mute but he is listening—to his own body, to his mother's body, and to the world around him. Further, by the time he exits the archaic stage, even though he is just born, he already has a history of invested objects—a beautiful, elaborate dream world that secures his wish of survival. The task, then, is for his familiars to earn his investment in the reality in which he finds himself.

Yet once again, perhaps there is no real need for a theory to understand how and why our archaic dreams influence so much. Common examples abound from the oral stage that follows, for which the mouth is the site-means of pleasure. We all have affect invested in a special spice, soup, fruit, recipe, etc.—something our parents or grandparents prepared, or a food particular to our home area, or our favourite season, and so on. How far would we go to taste it again, exactly as it is supposed to taste? How much would we pay to re-experience it precisely as we once knew and loved it? In effect, we all have our versions of Proust's madeleine—a food, single ingredient, or style of baking/cooking (perhaps a family secret)—whose taste instantly transposes us, bringing back people and places long forgotten so saliently as to make our mouths and eyes water. A single sampling confirms the authenticity of the food. If anything is askew, then someone else is in the kitchen, or we have landed in the wrong restaurant or city. In fact, human experience is full of compelling evidence that the oral stage leaves its mark lifelong. The archaic stage is just that much earlier—and its affects are that much more powerful due to their proximity to their unconscious source. Beginning in the archaic stage, our infancy, we will fuel our dreams on little crumbs of unspeakable somethings that stunningly set us on a course of life and love.

C. Anxiety

"Precocious libidinal stages" are a proven fact,[60] Dolto believes, as "the libidinal sub-basement of relations of dependence ... that stays in later libidinal organizations."[61] Dolto is speaking about how psychosexual maturation begins very precociously, before the infant is born into social relations of dependence. She describes the infant's unconscious state during this archaic stage as a perfect continuum or "habitus" of security and unity.[62] In fact, the infant is dreaming. This dream state is so pleasurable that Dolto views anxiety as a "resistance"[63] to further psychosexual maturation. The notion is stunning: the satisfaction obtained through dream-work in the archaic can make it more challenging for the infant to successfully surpass the umbilical castration to engage the oral stage. So the infant may "stall" psychosexually—become "fixated"—not intentionally, of course, because he is incapable of conscious intention. It's just that his wishes are already being met.

In fact, infant fixations at the oral stage are common—for example, when the infant resists being weaned from the breast. Of course, the infant is older at this point and capable of some conscious intention (conscious resistance). It will certainly not be easy to coax his abandonment of the customary objects of pleasure for his mouth—the site (means) of pleasure in the oral stage—to the new objects we offer (e.g., new foods, a cup, etc.). So as we observe during the oral stage, this renunciation of prior-stage objects is a mental and emotional challenge. Dolto coins the term "symboligenic castrations"[64] to stress the sense of generation (production)—in that successful renunciations of invested objects of the prior stage result in net gains that enable healthy progression. Further, Dolto believes human survival depends upon this endogenous castration anxiety.[65] Saying so, she draws our attention to a complicated truth about infancy: symboligenic castrations are necessary to facilitate the new object relations that each successive stage depends on; but abandoning prior objects of investment generates anxiety that increases our need for security. So Dolto views existential anxiety as a developmental trial that every infant must surmount.

Freud explains that even at a very early age, we can witness a "kind of partial fixation."[66] Evidence of oral-stage fixations abound in our world—and not just among infants. There is strong case to be made, for example, that cigarettes and coffee are oral fixations. "Fixation" simply means the perseverative affective investment of the objects of a given stage despite progression to a subsequent stage. In the case of the infant in the archaic stage, the problem is that we obviously cannot see what the infant is fixated on in his dreams. And when he is born, we cannot observe fixation either—it is invisible. In fact, the trials and outcomes of the archaic stage remain imperceptible and unnarratable until—as Dolto discovered in clinic—remnants of that passage surface in therapy years later. The newborn may linger in the archaic, perfectly content, relatively impervious to the lures of reality. We also need to recall that in the liquid dreamscape of the archaic, the infant has no notion of a world differentiated from himself.[67] So he remains encapsulated in his mental-emotional world, even though he may have already left his physical capsule—the womb.

The infant may appear intact but, in truth, he may not quite be ready in terms of his psychosexual maturation for the world he is supposed to begin awakening to. He has, in brief, experienced the umbilical castration while fixated in the archaic stage. Freud described the "wish to sleep"[68] as a primitive form of pleasure wherein "satisfaction is obtained from the subject's own body and extraneous objects are disregarded."[69] This is actually a perfect description of the infant's archaic situation, as Dolto is elaborating it. Of course, it is a generally accepted fact that "the foundations of self-regulation lie in the infant's capacity to develop homeostasis in the first few months of life."[70] And we know that the first weeks of life outside the womb are crucial to establishing the developmental and relational processes on which the infant's new conditions for survival depend. Yet nascent self-regulation (e.g., cries, movements, head turns, wakefulness, etc.) requires the infant to manifest a capacity for consciousness. We recall Freud's stress on how "sexual instincts are unwilling to renounce their substitutive satisfaction so long as it is uncertain whether reality will offer them anything better."[71] So what in the world would lure the infant to abandon his archaic libidinal position?

The longer the child remains fixated, the more challenging his psychosexual progression will be. Returning to the oral stage once more—where we can observe what is happening—I believe we all know how hard oral habits are to quit: the earlier we started, and the longer the habit has been installed, the more difficult it is to abandon. Our entire physiological, mental and emotional systems seem habituated to the oral fixation. In the archaic, we cannot view the infant's beloved objects. But we can extrapolate the nature of fixation at the archaic stage, where affect remains in circulation inside a porous mental and emotional world that is entirely undifferentiated from the actual world. Dolto explains that affect that cannot circulate gets trapped, and affect that remains trapped is lost to life—perhaps indefinitely, or for years. For in the absence of the capacity to "liberate affects"[72] through the "intermediary of the transference"[73]—i.e., to achieve a «libération libidinale»[74]—the result will be what she calls «escargotage» [literally, "snail-ing"].[75] Her visual expression deliberately denotes a kind of winding around and around of affect without the possibility of outward displacement. Freud used the term "strangulated affect"[76] to denote this same problem of unusable, trapped affect.

Since affect is supposed to flow through subsequent stages as unconscious reservoirs are tapped and energy is deployed in the service of healthy psychosexual maturation, strangulated affect reduces the potential for the individual in the short- and/or long-term. This notion of a reduced capacity, and of inaccessible affect that cannot be put into circulation, does not serve conservation well. In fact, we can readily infer that the anxiety generated by trapped affect represents a flagrant threat to survival by restricting future affective investments on which much depends—such as our self-regulation, social relations and happiness. Thus, as Dolto's clinical work demonstrates, infants can be engulfed in truly "mortifying anxiety."[77] During a famous interview in 1987, Dolto is asked if one can speak of the existential anxiety of the baby. "Surely,"[78] she replies.

Throughout psychosexual maturation at the archaic stage, powerful reserves of unconscious affect are surging—like pressure behind a dam—in preparation for the massive affective displacements needed during the pending oral stage (facilitated by language, as we will see). So while the infant may be fixated in the archaic stage, affect is flooding and seeks an outlet. Yet without the capacity to transfer affect to new objects, affect will be reinvested in old objects and the inward spiralling will continue. The longer this fixation goes on, the more difficult an exit will become. As Dolto explains it, "when pulses [of affect in circulation], upon their appearance, find an interdiction exterior to the subject, the idea is repressed but the affective charge remains and provokes anxiety … which we call 'primary' anxiety."[79] So affect that is impeded because the infant is regressed (foreclosing possible associative pathways to new objects) provokes primary anxiety. In turn, this anxiety makes it even harder for the infant to exit the archaic stage because he needs archaic security to counter the anxiety. In coming to terms with anxiety and fixation, then, I believe we also come to realize how repetition (at any stage) can be inscribed as a means of safety.

Yet we have arrived at another paradox, as Freud explains it: "Withdrawal from reality is the main purpose of the illness but also the main damage caused by it."[80] In sum, anxiety is both the cause and result of fixation. In effect, anxiety is an incredibly strong trap. That is why, when discussing psychosexual stages, Dolto speaks of «évolution libidinale.»[81] Like always, her word choice is deliberate because rather than thinking strictly of development, the term "evolution" compels us to factor the influence of the environment scaffolding the infant's growth through the objects it presents that are then available for dream-work. Dolto describes the goal of successful psychosexual maturation like this: "The unconscious economic objective … is the neutralization of castration anxiety … The castration complex is a … success for the libidinal dynamic of the subject."[82] So affect needs to keep flowing somehow—it must be vented, liberated through circulation. In Freudian terms, what is required is a "translation of a quantity of pulsional energy"[83] from the objects of one stage to those of the next.

The renowned psychiatrist and pediatrician, Stanley Greenspan, once commented, "More than anyone else, Freud focused the attention of Western thought on emotions as motivators of behaviour. Any attempt to understand the origins of our most important mental abilities must therefore begin with his revolutionary concepts."[84] And revolutionary they are. For with Freud, and with Dolto in his wake, we discover that existential anxiety is endemic in our species. Anxiety tests our potential for putting as much unconscious affect as possible into free circulation in our lives, insofar as such transfers through subsequent psychosexual stages are the guarantor of our emotional health and future happiness. With Freud and Dolto, we discover that an affective economy drives psychosexual maturation. Thus, in order to minimize anxiety and maximize adaptability, the human infant needs to invest his conscious acts with his archaic unconscious inheritance.

D. Environment

The indissociable "me-mymother" is the infant's affective "environment" during the archaic stage of psychosexual maturation. Insofar as the unconscious infant cannot be separated from his mother during early gestation, the infant has no so-called "boundaries of self." And prior to parturition, since the infant cannot fathom a world beyond the mother, he has no boundaries between himself and the world either. Closer to term, as proprioception and perception improve, we can observe his pre-conscious capacities using diverse technologies: his body becomes palpable to his own hands, for example; and his audition discerns voices and music. But in the liminal zone between being entirely unconscious (i.e., when dreaming begins in the first weeks of life) and his preconscious activity (i.e., when cycles of wakefulness emerge in the last weeks of gestation), the fetus slips in and out of sleep. Thus, he lacks boundaries between his unconscious and preconscious states. And as objects arrive while he is in these ever-shifting states, objects lack hard boundaries as well. His indissociable, fluid environment is the source of all his objects—his mother is his environment. There are objects within her, or repeatedly associated with her—while other objects are only loosely associated with her, or come and go. We can reasonably conclude, then, that objects will have different "associative distances" to the mother—and to each other.

Keeping to audition for the sake of simplicity—and because it is relatively continuous as a pre- and post-natal experience—the mother's heartbeat and the name of his father (or significant other) will be a more familiar liquid object than the voice of an elder seen monthly, or a fire truck siren heard on occasion. Yet the environment provides objects for the infant's dream-work that change how he will encounter reality—his future. That is why we can earnestly state that the infant is engaged in precocious learning in the womb during the archaic stage. And insofar as he is indissociable from his mother, and she is indissociable from the world, his mother—and the/her environment—is his teacher.[85] It is critical to notice here that this is passive learning since the infant cannot seek objects in his environment. Instead, he waits, sometimes sleepily and sometimes quasi-wakefully, unable to choose objects or control which will enter his dream-work. In brief, the first learning of every human being is necessarily a passive education dependent on the environment.

There is valuable corroboration for the gestational infant's passive education from new research on olfaction. Scent is considered an "odor object"[86]—i.e., a "liquid," porous object without hard boundaries. Further, there is consensus that, "olfaction is probably the first sense … chemosensory systems are expressed in every living animal known, and chemosensitivity emerges very early in ontogeny."[87] Of particular interest to the archaic stage is this elucidating point: "Although humans appear less directly driven by olfactory input than many other animals, odors play an important modulatory role in human attraction, mood, dietary preferences, and detection of danger."[88] So it is inferable that the gestational infant can detect danger by scent. The mother's anxiety, her worry or suffering—and/or threats against her—are all palpable for the infant. Dolto explains that "there are also smells of anxiety because anxiety has a smell … the smell of anxiety is, in the unconscious, linked to the security of existing."[89] So we begin to see contemporary confirmations of what Dolto theorized decades ago about the infant's unconscious life in the archaic.

The renowned psychologist and neuroscientist, Rachel Herz, states that, "Humans understand the scent of fear, as well as happiness, in one another."[90] Herz adds:

> Our olfactory system is the first sense to develop. In fact, we have a fully functioning sense of smell by the time we are twelve weeks in the womb … we can begin to learn about odors well before we are born, and we do. The way we come to know various aromatic chemicals during this prebirth period is through what our mothers consume … Several studies have shown that what a mother consumes while she is pregnant will influence her baby's flavor preferences after he or she is born.[91]

And from this relatively new field of scientific study on olfaction, we find another critical concordance to the archaic: "Odors most likely are never sensed in the absence of background odors."[92] So there is a necessary triangulation whereby an object is detectable only by reference to another object—i.e., objects (only) become perceptible within an environment. Contemporary researchers also effectively confirm human precocious learning in the archaic when they speak of "traditional associative olfactory memory,"[93] attesting to the role of association; and when they describe how "olfaction is a highly emotive sense,"[94] attesting to the role of affect.

Such early capacities for smell, associated affects and associative pathways for memories should stun. In fact, we are witnessing the dawn of associative thinking during the archaic stage of psychosexual maturation. We are also discovering how/why we remember by association—it is an archaic skill of ours, hard-wired from our fetal life. All this is possible because of the development very early in gestation of structures such as those of the so-called "lower brain": "The key limbic structure to interact with our olfactory center is the amygdala. The amygdala is the brain's locus of emotion";[95] and "like all limbic structures, the hypothalamus [also] interacts with the olfactory system."[96] Here then, a century later, is at least the beginning of a confirmation of Freud's work on unconscious processes, and an affirmation of Dolto's elaboration of the archaic stage of human infancy.

Our passive education during the archaic stage—the original condition in which we survive, unconscious, in an indissociable environment—marks the first moment of learning. Crucially, this passive education is affectively driven and associative in nature. Dolto defines the archaic transference situation as a triangular formation in dream-work—a «co-moi papa-maman» [co-me father-mother].[97] As discussed, this blurry archaic triangular situation is, in a nutshell, a "me-mymother" (i.e., a pre-self indelibly associated with a "like-me"), encountering another object (i.e., a liquid "third" arriving in the environment). Further, it is a fact of gestation that the infant experiences the world in/with his mother, his mother-food,[98] such that even in the womb, "the mother is already associated to the food she makes appear."[99] We already know that in the archaic, the mother is also associated with her smell and with diverse objects of audition in her environment. In fact, the mother is associated with everything. For the infant has no input whatsoever that is not coming through his mother.[100] Everything, including his affect, circulates through her.

Dolto reminds us of Freud's key discovery that "libido is linked to the pleasure principle."[101] The infant's precocious learning in the archaic, then, is intrinsically bound with affect, to the blissful dreams in which he survives thanks to his all-providing environment. Freud himself stressed this: "Libido is an expression taken from the theory of emotions … [while] the chief characteristic of libido is mobility, the facility with which it passes from one object to another."[102] To restate, taking in our first objects in the archaic stage is only possible in/with an affective environment—i.e., in the dreamed presence of a "like-me" through which everything arrives, our "co-living with the mother."[103] Of vital importance, this pattern then becomes the mode for lifelong passive learning that continues, unconsciously, via rogue transferences in all human relationships—with a privileging of language.

That's why Dolto issues this caution: "Healing takes more than displacement, it takes a relation for the transference to put libido back into circulation."[104] For as we understand it now, displacements of unconscious affect—the transference—will require triangulation because that is the means for displacing unconscious affect that is established in the archaic stage. It won't be sufficient to simply lure to reality using associations to dream-work. Rather, the transference will always require triangulation with a "like-me" who unconsciously recalls the indissociable relation of "co-living" that inscribes the archaic transference situation. The other object—the "third," the word—can only help recover affect and restore affective circulation if there is, foremost, this indispensable "second."

Dolto is effectively theorizing the operational mechanics of psychoanalytic therapy (the "talking cure"), if you will, as well as anyone's recovery from regression. The "second" may be any trusted individual whatsoever; but if the transference happens, it is because (in ways immune to conscious control) that individual somehow unconsciously and affectively reconstitutes the archaic "like-me." Dolto explains it concisely: "The human being has his roots in his relation to the other, his first other, in the communication of unconciousnesses."[105] As a result of the archaic stage, then, Dolto believes that even in adults, "it is also possible that the affects of pregenital stages … need, in order to be expressed in the transference, a reciprocity of behavior."[106] Dolto adds that this unconscious desire for the "like-me" also drives social relations: "Elective affinities between human beings derive from these perceptions, holders of subtle accords between them, that make them recognize each other as similars."[107]

With Dolto, we discover that precocious learning begins in, and because of, the archaic transference situation—a triangulation with a "like-me" that enables engaging a "third." The infant's learning is thus the joint result of affect and association: transfers of unconscious affect are facilitated, and the engagement with new objects is scaffolded by associations to prior objects tracing their origins to dream-work. We also discover that our passive education is the archaic forerunner of our (later, conscious) active education. This notion of the mother as an affective environment facilitating precocious learning drives Dolto to coin the verb «mamaïser» [to motherify], as "whatever is *mamaïsé* will deliver securitizing continuity."[108] So the gestational infant's history of education begins in the archaic stage as an unconscious encounter with random objects provided by an indissociable environment, where affective continuity is the guarantor of his survival as a passive, highly precocious student of life. Driven by this originary, inscribed desire for unconscious security on which his conservation depends, the infant is far from a classroom indeed—and yet, he is already far down the road of learning.

Notes

1 In Marette 1940, 15 (emphasis hers).
2 Dolto 1987, 178.
3 2011b, 90.
4 2011b, 323.
5 In Coronel & De Mezamat 1997a.
6 In Marette 1940, 93; also Dolto 1981, 126 and De Sauvernac 1988, 156.
7 In Halmos 1994, 328.
8 In Guillerault 1997, 13.
9 Ibid, 138.
10 In Marette 1940, 15, 30 & 30f; Faure-Poirée & Djéribi-Valentin 1999, 41.
11 In Marette 1940, 30; Dolto 1981, 296–297; Djéribi-Valentin & Kouki 1998, 255.
12 In Guillerault 1997, 157.
13 In Lévy 2002, 105; also Dolto 1984, 90; De Sauverzac 1987, 70; Halmos 1994, 94–95, 257 & 350.
14 Dolto 1981, 251; De Sauverzac 1988, 144; Halmos 1994, 257.
15 In Djéribi-Valentin & Kouki 1996, 31.
16 1896/1954, 180; 1921, 127; 1937, 240 & 241; 1940[1939], 167.
17 1913, 176.
18 In Guillerault 1997, 42.
19 In Djéribi-Valentin & Kouki 1998, 92 & 103.
20 In Halmos 1994, 29.
21 In Dolto & Winter 1986, 97.
22 Dolto 1979, 170.
23 In Caldaguès 1982, 213; Djéribi-Valentin & Kouki 1996, 362; Kouki 2005, 27.
24 Regarding the use of the term "libidinal" here (and in a few other citations)—and the evident interchangeability of expressions pertaining to unconscious affect—Laplanche

and Pontalis explain that for Freud, "affect is the qualitative expression of the quantity of pulsional energy" (1967/2004, 12); and they stress that "the notion of affect … postulates a quantitative theory of investments" (ibid). They add that, for Freud, what is at issue is "an energy of investment" (ibid, 199) and an "unconscious energy" (ibid). While Laplanche and Pontalis admit that "it is difficult to give a satisfying definition of libido" (ibid, 224), it is nonetheless primarily a "quantitative concept" (ibid, 225) that Freud describes, in his own words, as "an expression borrowed from the theory of affectivity" (ibid) and as "the energy … of pulsions" (ibid).

25 In Manier & Kouki 2003, 52.
26 In Marette 1940, 58.
27 In Dolto & Winter 1986, 126.
28 In Djéribi-Valentin & Kouki 1996, 208.
29 In Ledoux 2006, 326–327.
30 In Djéribi-Valentin & Kouki 1998, 90.
31 Gershon 1998, viii.
32 1888, 48.
33 1900b, 546 & 567.
34 1900a, 184.
35 Ibid, 177.
36 1925[1924], 42.
37 1914b, 150–151.
38 In Guillerault 1997, 79; also Dolto 1971, 201.
39 In Guillerault 1997, 42, 244 & 269; Djéribi-Valentin & Kouki 1998, 107.
40 In Guillerault 1997, 79.
41 Dolto 1971, 195.
42 In Djéribi-Valentin & Kouki 1998, 103.
43 Ibid, 90.
44 1895, 357.
45 Ibid, 358.
46 Freud in Laplanche & Pontalis 1967/2004, 12; see also ibid, 325 & 448–450.
47 1930, 209.
48 Ibid.
49 1900a, 8 & 487; 1900b, 467.
50 1900a, 235; 1913, 169.
51 2021, 28.
52 In Marette 1940, 148.
53 Ibid, 12.
54 Ibid, 161.
55 In Guillerault 1997, 41.
56 In Strachey 1900, xix (the introduction to Freud's watershed work on dreams).
57 1895, 296.
58 Ibid (emphasis his).
59 In Dolto & Winter 1986, 74.
60 In Djéribi-Valentin & Kouki 1996, 69.
61 In Djéribi-Valentin & Kouki 1998, 103.
62 Dolto 1956, 32; Dolto 1981, 256, 290 & 299; Caldaguès 1982, 20; Dolto 1988, 17; Halmos 1994, 29; Djéribi-Valentin & Kouki 1996, 209 & 362; Guillerault 1997, 41 & 184; Kouki 2005, 22 & 86.
63 In Djéribi-Valentin & Kouki 1996, 27.
64 Dolto 1984, 78–90.
65 Dolto 1981, 227.
66 1909b, 46.

67 In Marette 1940, 27.
68 1900b, 570 & 590; 1901a, 680.
69 1909b, 44.
70 DeGangi 2000, 2.
71 1909b, 49.
72 In Faure-Poirée & Djéribi-Valentin 1999, 47–48.
73 In Marette 1940, 148.
74 Ibid, 202.
75 Dolto 1985d; Guillerault 1997, 220.
76 1893d, 39; 1909b, 18; 1914b, 156.
77 In Djéribi-Valentin 2005, 796–797; Potin 2008, 218.
78 In Ribowski 1987/2004.
79 In Marette 1940, 16.
80 1909b, 49.
81 In Marette 1940, 153.
82 Dolto 1940/1965, 7.
83 See Laplanche and Pontalis 1967/2004, 12.
84 In Greenspan & Benderly 1997, 40.
85 The notion of the environment as a teacher is central to the Reggio Emilia approach to education. Dolto antedates that approach and is speaking of an unconscious environment. Nonetheless, Part Three considers this concordance.
86 Wilson & Stevenson 2006, 19 & 22.
87 Ibid, 4.
88 Ibid.
89 In Djéribi-Valentin & Kouki 1998, 112.
90 2007, 18.
91 Ibid, 33–34.
92 Wilson & Stevenson 2006, 8.
93 Ibid, 9.
94 Ibid, 139.
95 Herz 2007, 3–4.
96 Ibid, 10.
97 In Halmos & C. Dolto 1994, 39; also ibid, 27; Dolto & Winter 1986, 166; Dolto 1988, 14.
98 In Guillerault 1997, 200.
99 Ibid, 49.
100 Any implications for In Vitro Fertilization (IVF) are beyond the scope of this book.
101 Dolto 1981, 122; also Dolto-Marette 1947, 795.
102 1940[1939], 151.
103 In Djéribi-Valentin & Kouki 1998, 64.
104 Dolto 1956, 34; see also Dolto 1940/1971, 239; Dolto 1977b, 43; Dolto 1981, 269; Dolto 1986a, 188–198.
105 In Djéribi-Valentin & Kouki 1998, 63.
106 Dolto 1981, 191; in Dolto's thinking, the notion of a «semblable» [similar] is best understood as a "like-me."
107 In Guillerault 1997, 243–245.
108 In Halmos & C. Dolto 1994, 191; also Dolto 1981, 281; De Sauverzac 1985, 158; Guillerault 1997, 157; Djéribi-Valentin & Kouki 1998, 126.

Chapter 2

Circulation

Preliminary Words

Sometime between the onset of life and the start of the second trimester, the fetus becomes capable of unconscious activity that is both emotional and mental. It is "emotional" because it is driven by affect. It is "mental" because it is characterized by dream-work that randomly incorporates some objects of his world. It is an "activity" because it comprises movement—one that signifies life as it continues throughout his survival, as a current beneath consciousness. This movement is a circulation of unconscious affects. Therefore, from the early onset of unconscious processes in gestation, the infant is dreaming while his affect circulates in an indissociable relation with another—who is as-if himself, so to speak, and whose affect is also circulating. It is a joint system where everything moves fluidly, from incoming nutrients to outgoing waste. As a fact of gestation, the "me-mymother" is a veritable hub of continuous circulation. So the infant's archaic dream-work, his perfect wish of survival, is inscribed by circulation from the beginning. This circulation of affect is—and leaves its traces in—the unconscious security of being alive.

From hereon, during further psychosexual maturation, Dolto states, every child "imagines himself in an activity that valorises him and sustains his «allant-devenant» [going-becoming]."[1] And when affect cannot easily be invested in new objects, so that circulation in the direction of the next stage is impeded, Dolto notes that "anxiety is a result not a cause of the failure of going-becoming."[2] For this circulation is essential to the unconscious securitization that life continues, as the "transference of objects of archaic fixation onto new objects all along the *déroulement*[3] of affective life."[4] This continuous circulation of affect in/with an indissociable other while deep in dream-work inscribes in each human being an "altogether unconscious imaginary dialectic."[5] In sum, the archaic stage is our first experience of being human, and it leaves a powerful legacy. As a result, our unspeakable, archaic desire for security—our wish to live—will be susceptible to unconscious transferences, as Dolto describes beautifully, "as a movement sufficient to symbolize the promise of the other to follow, a semblance of wind."[6]

DOI: 10.4324/9781032655123-5

A. Third

The Oedipus Complex is an unconscious triangular situation that helps to explicate the trials of each of the stages of psychosexual maturation, and its roots are in the archaic stage of infant life. Dolto puts it this way: "We are born in a triangular situation…[so] the child needs this triangular situation to continue [in order] to develop."[7] In the archaic stage that is experienced during gestation, the infant is completely unconscious at first, only gradually gaining (nearer to term) the capacity for enhanced proprioception, and for perception of the objects of his world, that will eventually make reliable consciousness possible. So the very deepest roots of the Oedipal triangle are somewhere in dream-work.

The archaic triangular situation is constructed completely unconsciously,[8] Dolto explains. As the child advances developmentally towards term—still inextricably bound to his indissociable (m)other, that "two" that feels like a "one"—he becomes increasingly able to slowly distinguish the other of the mother (the one who is usually but not necessarily his father) as a "third." Thus, "any other perceptible by his mass or by effecting emotional variations on the mother … is, like him, felt to be in dyad with the mother … qualifying and quantifying her dyad."[9] Dolto further describes this archaic triangulation of the indissociable "me-mymother" with a "third": "A common interest unites them emotionally. It is the beginning of a situation of three … [that is] two united relative to a third (the thing)."[10] In a useful shorthand, she adds, "one and one makes three."[11]

Here is a remarkable turn in the mental and emotional life of the human infant, as an experience enters (arrives, registers, etc.) from the outside, as other, within the indissociable "me-mymother"—the beginnings of the capacity for triangulation. The "me-mymother" is united through this unconscious common interest, as triangulation becomes the means for extending affective circulation through displacement (by association) to all kinds of other objects that can serve as "thirds." In effect, the infant in the womb begins to learn because of the archaic triangular situation. And as the infant's abilities develop, this vital capacity for triangulation supports his growing awareness of what is other to the "me-mymother," and this will facilitate his eventual separation (individuation) from it.

All the infant's first encounters with the world will be within this "triangulated climate,"[12] Dolto says. The "me-mymother" experiences objects of common affective interest together, as "objects are sometimes carriers of love."[13] Here, it is important to notice that continuous circulation through any triangular formation ensures a return—i.e., no net loss of affect. Dolto describes existential anxiety as the inability to find in the environment suitable objects of transference.[14] That is why restoring triangulation offers relief: "Communication with another permits the one who suffers to reunify himself, to re-find his cohesion."[15] Put another way, "the subject of desire represents a third of the Oedipal triangle,"[16] Dolto says, so "without other encounters in which to recognize themselves, all humans suffer."[17]

Archaic triangulation is also how the infant "achieves the consciousness of himself as master of his acts by the 'me-not you' … The 'me' arrives at the moment of the completion of the nervous system, which cannot happen before 23 months and generally not after 28 months."[18] Dolto is affirming the predominant influence of the unconscious in the child's mental and emotional life throughout the entire archaic stage right through the oral stage. And it is the role of the "third" that makes individuation possible: "For the fetus, there is no mother without another, that is to say, without the father … The father, for the child, is first a varying state of the mother and of himself, a discontinuity felt as qualitative on the continuous foundation felt to be quantitative."[19]

As Dolto explains it, these are "triangular perceptions that permit a subject to feel himself."[20] In a leap forward of a few weeks to parturition (i.e., the umbilical castration), when the infant will enter the oral stage, the unconscious archaic triangular situation—the sharing of a common interest with an indissociable other—will be the precursor of the instrumental conscious capacity for joint attention. While in a leap backwards some weeks (or years, in adults), this archaic triangular situation will forever hold the capacity to restore unconscious securitization, a deep healing. And from contemporary research on joint attention, we find powerful agreement:

> The emotional and cognitive impact of being the object of others' attention in early child development … begins to serve a critical organizational function in the dynamic process of human development by no later than two months of age. Accordingly, perception of attention to self stimulates infants in a way that triggers a cascade of developmental cognitive and affective processes involved in differentiating self and other.[21]

While still in the womb, as triangulation becomes an established pattern in (for) the infant's mental and emotional life, he experiences a particular repetitive "third" with a strong affective influence over the mother—i.e., the father (or significant other). This "third" is like himself by virtue of being in/with the mother but also being other to her. As Dolto clarifies, in the blurry dream-work of the archaic stage, both maternal and paternal security are included in the mother,[22] every mother is also a father,[23] and the father is the one who occupies the thoughts of the mother.[24] Dolto stresses how crucial the role of the father is as a pathway to differentiation, calling it the "symbolic role of the third, that is to say the father in the dyadic mother … of the mother and her child."[25] Without separation, circulation continues by reinvesting old objects, in what Dolto calls "transference that is more and more sticky"[26]—and psychosexual maturation stalls.

It is a cornerstone of Dolto's thinking that during gestation, differentiation through the "third" in triangulation is primarily achieved by audition. For the father (or highly significant other) is mainly experienceable through his voice and phonemes, through his repetitive arrival in the mother's environment, and her affect in his presence and/or during their conversations. This notion supports two further considerations. First, insofar as the symbolic father is the "third" largely through his words, words can serve as "thirds" for the transference, with huge repercussions for literacy. Second, insofar as the symbolic father enables the infant's separation from the dyad, any "social third" or "lateral person" can prevent the loss of individuation.[27] Dolto explains: "It is the «parole» ['speech'; 'words'] of a third that presentifies[28] for a subject, an absent person."[29] For the "third" acquires its value from its association with the "second"—the indissociable "like-me" of survival. As a result, finding a "third" restores the circulation of affect, and this triangulation returns the "second" and its assurance of security. As Dolto elaborates it, "there is a presence restituted only in language, but always by a third."[30]

This is why rather than working alone with young patients, Dolto famously conducted her aptly called "choral clinics" with witnesses:[31] "The analyst enters as a third, freeing the child."[32] Dolto reasoned successfully that choral clinics greatly enhance the speed and efficacity of therapy with children because it "returns the original triangular relation."[33] Dolto actually first introduced her notion of the "third" as a «présence affective» in 1940,[34] almost a century ago. What Dolto is saying is that including a "third" in therapeutic work makes a significant difference because archaic triangulation is a lifelong means of unconscious securitization as well as the first mode(l) of learning via a "common interest." And she finds evidence for archaic triangulation in every aspect of a child's interactions: "The child is always an interlocutor with another, who is an interlocutor with another. It is always a triangle."[35]

Freud detected "thirds" in triangulation in dream-work, noting how "mediating ideas" are needed.[36] Freud analysed how words serve as "nodal points,"[37] enabling affect and ideas to "call up the other"[38]—even if, as he pointed out, we cannot always figure out what the "third" is (or was). As he stated flatly, "the *tertium comparationis* often eludes us."[39] And thinking about how the "third" restitutes affective circulation—the transference—brings Dolto to her unprecedented theorization of phonemes. In her signature style—condensed yet elliptical—she muses on the role of language as the "third," while the infant is dreaming in the womb:

> Verbal pre-language transitional phonemes have something paranormal … at once perennial thing and confused language of the relation child-mother or child-father: materialized language, phantom of unspeakable words, unconsciously conjugated with a sensory havingness that seems to answer from a beingness in a passive state that would passively conduct to the subject being.[40]

The role of the phoneme in the archaic stage inscribes the power of words to effect healing—and it is the basis for the effectiveness of the "talking cure." As Dolto elucidates, "the word is a transitional object that the child acquires to never be separated from it. "[41] Thus, "the word is the best transitional object for the transference"[42]—and words are «objets transitionnels subtiles.»[43] The conclusion is that individuation, our sense of self, depends on some phonemes heard that once served as "thirds" in our idiosyncratic histories, following the path of the (symbolic) father, all while we were dreaming, unconsciously secure within a vibrant archaic triangulation. Thanks to precocious audition, then, affectively invested phonemes forever hold the potential to restore the emotional climate of the archaic transference situation, returning our unconscious security. The implications for the mother tongue—and mother tongue attrition—are astounding.[44]

B. Passivity

The gestational infant, who is in the earliest stage of psychosexual maturation, is entirely passive. He cannot control his nascent proprioceptive or perceptual abilities; he cannot control which objects arrive in his environment (i.e., in his mother or in her environment); and he cannot control the nature of his dream-work on any of those objects. In fact, we all live passively part-time when we sleep, for much-needed restoration—and our unconscious processes continuously keep working passively beneath consciousness. The difference for the gestational infant is that, with his unconscious capacities unbridled by consciousness and his physical state of utter dependency, he lives passively full-time. He remains passive throughout the archaic stage and well into the oral stage.[45]

In privileging the role of audition during gestation, Dolto describes passivity as a state of sustained expectation lived in a "fetal purée of significance … a purée of words."[46] She is evoking both the liquid quality of words and the sheer quantity of objects that language provides for dream-work. Dolto refers to the "genius of passive pulses,"[47] "oral passivity,"[48] and "oral passive survival."[49] Freud himself spoke of "quiescent cathexis" as "energy inherent in the unconscious wish,"[50] and of "instincts with a passive aim."[51] Dolto elaborates how prior to reality, the infant "hallucinates while sleeping,"[52] in a "dream-like, quasi-hallucinatory mode."[53] By this, he secures pleasure via the continuous circulation of unconscious affect in the archaic triangular situation.

Dolto explains that the infant in the archaic stage is passively susceptible to offers of objects for his dream-work through audition. He "ardently waits,"[54] she states, for he is "born waiting for human communication from the outside,"[55] and looking for "the road of a listening."[56] Her word, "road," reminds us that the "third" (starting with the symbolic father) charts the pathway to individuation. In other words, the infant first begins to experience "thirds" while passive. And it is while he is passive, too, that he will unconsciously secure a "second" ("like-me"), Dolto insists, for the infant "unconsciously attracts those who protect him."[57] Enigmatically, Dolto is compelling us to consider a powerful capacity by which humans somehow secure for themselves—unconsciously—the transference as a means for (re)finding the archaic triangular situation.

"Passivity exists,"[58] Dolto states bluntly. She further believes that "we should value what is passive in a child,"[59] because "passive pulses foster intense intellectual activity and receptivity."[60] And passivity is highly conducive to the development of thinking. As she puts it, "in passivity, the child is extremely receptive, even if he is not very expressive."[61] He "registers everything arriving,"[62] she observes. With Dolto, then, we discover that passivity is paradoxically richly productive. For "the third is always what will enable the transference,"[63] she confirms.

Interpreting Dolto's thought using her own shorthand, the reason is that the "third" returns the "second"; and the "second" returns unconscious security—proof of life, if you will. For affect transits unconsciously along well-worn pathways from a "third," by association, to that archaic blur of maternal and paternal security experienced in/with the indissociable (m)other of the original triangular situation in dream-work, long before any nascent sense of the real parents. And Dolto's unwavering conviction regarding the infant's passive receptivity, his innate unconscious strength, is at the forefront of her practice: "There is somewhere a subject with his own desire, veiled, who watches in his passive pulses for the moment when he will be found by someone."[64]

But what if new objects cannot easily be experienced somehow? What if a disturbance during gestation briefly interrupts or slows psychosexual progression? Perhaps it is the infant's own condition (unseen, undiagnosed); or his mother's illness (perhaps unnoticed); or an environmental or nutritional contaminant (detected or not); or even his mother's anxiety (e.g., family death, threat, war, famine, migration, trauma, fear, etc.); and so on. Due to the unmitigated dominance of the instinct of conservation during the archaic stage, the gestational infant will experience regression as a result, withdrawing unconscious affect defensively in a natural resorption that serves as a means of conservation. Dolto elaborates how, for the infant in the archaic stage, passivity is not merely the only way to engage new objects, it is also the only way to *not* engage objects. It is a "passive defence,"[65] she expounds, one that leads to regression as a "dynamic involution,"[66] and a "fall back to restart."[67]

During any of the later stages of psychosexual maturation, there can also be a "fall into passivity."[68] Dolto therefore defines a passive defence as a means whereby (wherein) "we continue with another to exist,"[69] in a "dream of existence"[70]—a "subtle link beyond space and time."[71] Poignantly, she notes that a fall to passivity returns the archaic triangular situation as "a refuge in our mute sayings in the silences that scan them."[72] Yet in this notion of falling back to restart, I believe we can sense a fresh hope for progression. That hope is exactly what Dolto resounded throughout her life: the unconscious is a *re*-source—a powerful means of recuperation.

Some contemporary studies on habituation can help elucidate our understanding of passivity:

> The habituation response of the fetus is most usually elicited by the presentation of a sound stimulus and observed by a change in heart rate or movement. The repeated presentation of the sound stimulus leads to a decrease in the magnitude of the fetus's response and eventually no response is observed. The fetus first habituates to a sound stimulus at 22 – 24 weeks gestation. The number of stimuli (sound presentations) required for habituation decreases as gestation advances … The habituation response of the fetus is adversely affected by conditions which may affect its brain, for example: the health of the mother … [the health of] the fetus … and environmental agents.[73]

Such research affirms the vital role of precocious audition in the arrival of objects during gestation, in that the fetus hears by at least the second trimester—perhaps even earlier, since by then he is already capable of habituation. It also corroborates what Dolto postulated about regression: the infant's capacity to experience objects will be negatively impacted by adverse conditions in the womb. In addition, we confirm Dolto's prediction that what is familiar and repetitive becomes a "habitus," as the infant reacts differently to what is new. Of course, we cannot know if it is unconscious or preconscious audition that achieves habituation—especially as the infant slips in and out of sleep. But it is evident, just as Dolto theorized, that the infant is ardently waiting for new objects, somehow able to tell new ones from old ones—and, furthermore, that learning (i.e., experiencing new objects) prior to birth, when he is not yet conscious, will change the infant's response to (and engagement with) the (later) objects of reality.

Dolto's emphasis on a retreat to "silences that scan" is indispensable. Regressed and passive, the child waits for a "third," a pathway, a road out. While waiting and dreaming, he is lured by objects that echo his archaic unconscious affective investments (through some associations to them). Dolto explains the problem of regression as one wherein language did not "arrive on time."[74] At stake is an infant who is in distress in some unnarratable way. For regression—quite literally being a disruption to progression—is provoked by something, however fleeting or undetected. Suffering, the infant withdraws affect to defend himself passively, to conserve resources in the unconscious drive for self-preservation. And to emerge from regression—i.e., to resume progression—he will need to achieve unconscious security through new objects (by association) for continued triangulation. Without this, regression cannot be prevented: affect is resorbed, reinvested in prior objects along existing pathways. As the infant falls deeper into self-securing dream-work, he has greater difficulty investing in new objects. Regression becomes much more challenging to exit and affect gets trapped.

The result, notes Dolto, is a child who is "left with unsymbolized desires and unspoken suffering."[75] This is a state Dolto movingly calls "affective starvation,"[76] as "children enter autism passively, no longer asking for anything."[77] So doing, by "slow renunciation,"[78] they "regress to anonymity and phantasy relations with sensations, in a private battle against solitude."[79] And even when psychosexual maturation is advanced, regression still manifests in (as) silence, as mutism entails a "metamorphosis to passivity."[80] We pause to absorb the sweeping breadth of Dolto's critical thinking as it emerges here, following a decades-long trail of clinical evidence: autism is a regression to passivity.

Long before any primitive capacity for "flight or fight," then, the infant has only one defence—hide. This leaves him vulnerable to his environment, his "securitizing sensorium,"[81] because he can do nothing to change it. In a truly original insight, Dolto believes this vulnerability remains until "the age of confirmed deliberate walking"[82]—that is, "the confirmed conquest of mobility."[83] For autonomous displacement reduces the infant's dependency on his environment by giving him the means to change it, if only one step at a time. But like the infant learning to walk, we need to take care not to get ahead of ourselves.

C. Regression

Like rogue slips of the tongue, everyday words reveal truths we (in)tend to forget. In English, for example, we *fall* asleep, we *slip* into a coma, or we *lose* consciousness. French has parallel expressions (to lose, to fall, etc.), conveying the same sense of subterranean capacities—of something beneath the surface of the self. Survivors of trauma know especially well how it is possible to walk around in broad daylight without feeling quite "here" but somewhere farther back—receded and submerged. Triggered, we may manage to put one foot in front of the other and mechanically perform in our lives, but we withdraw emotionally and have trouble thinking—and we suddenly feel terribly tired. The world near us seems distant, while the distant world of our trauma seems so near. The highly respected infant researcher, Margaret Mahler, writes that "states of panic seem to be the immediate trigger"[84] for regression. And Daniel Kahneman, writing on non-rational influences in decision-making, speaks of the "paralyzing effects of loss aversion."[85] While Freud himself referred to "the instinct to sleep,"[86] of "sleep as a defence against the external world"[87]—even, of "attacks of sleep."[88] In sum, withdrawing (from) consciousness is a common human defence.

If psychosexual maturation is advanced beyond the first stage, regression will be to some prior stage. But for the infant in the first stage, the archaic, regression can only be to an earlier time in that stage—i.e., towards being even more deeply unconscious. For as gestation advances towards term, the infant becomes capable of forward investments because objects become more palpable as perception and proprioception develop; objects present or happen repeatedly in his environment (mother); and/or the mother has strong affective investments in them herself. Regressing, the child withdraws some of the affect invested in these objects and sinks deeper into dream-work for the purpose of self-preservation. The net result is a loss of acquisitions and a reanimation of an idiosyncratic prior history with objects.

Unconscious affect continues to circulate unceasingly, however, as long as we live. It transfers along some sort of elusive pathways that are usefully construed as waterways, according to Freud's drive theory. Freud invokes tributaries and channels,[89] "an instinctual stream,"[90] and displacements along roundabout, connecting or indirect paths.[91] Dolto adopts Freud's watery metaphors as she describes how libido flows like a sea;[92] but if impeded, libido resumes a path previously employed,[93] or it meanders, depending on the terrain and quantity of flow.[94] Dolto adds that any excess flows through spontaneous breaches at the point of least resistance.[95] In short, affect is naturally displaced unless it is blocked or detoured somehow.

Freud's unprecedented elaboration of dream-work[96] is incredibly pertinent to our comprehension of the infant's mental and emotional life during the archaic stage. Unconscious affect circulates to new objects by progressively branching out at nodes, creating fluid networks of associations—i.e., displacement. On the other hand, if circulation is impeded, affect (re)surges onto prior objects (higher nodes), as "such of those elements as allow any point of contact are *condensed* into new unities"[97]—i.e., condensation. And the most condensed unity is that blur of three, the first unconscious transferential configuration—i.e., the archaic triangular situation.[98]

Sleep is a daily regression,[99] Dolto explains, while regression at other times is a "defence against the loss of relational protection,"[100] since humans react by withdrawing.[101] At various times in the clinic, she observes "libidinal regression,"[102] "archaic regression,"[103] "regressing tension,"[104] and even "momentary regression."[105] For Dolto, regression is reparative because it reinvests liquid objects of dream-work that are self-securing, thus providing "archaic symbolic satisfaction."[106] She elaborates on how there was "a trial of his history to which the subject could not renounce without at once losing the notion of his continuity, his security of existing."[107] At issue is the indispensable continuity of affective circulation:

> Regression is driven … by the loss of a specific object of libidinal fixation that happened to be necessary … the one who has suffered this trauma, invisible for others … can only attempt to refind himself … in another time or in an imaginary space different than his actual corporeal schema from which the anxious subject desolidarizes himself.[108]

Dolto's language is always original: regression makes the subject feel less solid, less real. Elsewhere she states that the subject "regresses to refind the possibilities that are buried in the precocious stages."[109] And insofar as the most precocious stage is the first, wherein the infant is dreaming and the archaic triangular situation begins, Dolto is once more upholding the unconscious as a resource for recovery.

Critically, regression can be caused by the loss of an object—but regression does not cause the loss of an object. Rather, regression causes the loss of affect from an object—paths dry up, so to speak. The withdrawn affect is reinvested in objects that have already assured survival, enabling unconscious securitization. As Dolto sees it, "a positive opportunity for recovery makes regression a necessity."[110] So she believes that "regression is or can be a positive process … [since] every event that provokes a subjective disorganization returns the subject to the search for libidinal investments that were previously acquired and … imaginarily conserved as a place-time of existential security."[111] Reinvesting in objects of a prior stage in «évolution libidinale,»[112] as Dolto describes it, provokes "a resurgence of unconscious affect that reactualizes the archaic object of fixation."[113] As such, withdrawal is a regression effected by the negation of the affective suffering.[114] And as affect is pulled (drained) from paths for dispersal back towards fewer nodes, regression causes "chain reactions of de-structuration."[115]

The psychiatrist and author on neuroplasticity, Norman Doidge, writes that "'going dormant' is a common strategy when a cell, or a more complex organ or organism, finds itself in a situation in which its normal ways of adapting to the environment fail."[116] He adds the following:

> While the sympathetic system is often called the fight-or-flight system, the parasympathetic is sometimes called the rest-digest-repair system … The

> parasympathetic system also turns on a "social engagement system" which allows us to connect to other human beings, and use them to sooth and support us, and help us to regulate our own nervous system.[117]

I offer, then, that the transference is precisely this: an unconscious social engagement system for self-regulating affect. Further, this 'rest and reparation' defence is just as we predict with Dolto: long before humans are capable of "flight or fight," the only defence is "hide"—regression.

The difficulty, Dolto explains, is that the passive, regressed child can become trapped for a considerable length of time in this "stagnant dynamic situation."[118] She stresses that regression is "a process of refolding … necessary to the conservation of his health … [but] this subject has remained trapped there."[119] Dolto stresses that "regression becomes a trap that is seldom spontaneously reversible,"[120] as the individual gets "stuck in profound regressive symptoms."[121] The problem is that being withdrawn, one is less susceptible to objects. So Dolto is clear: recovery requires regression and "a call beyond."[122] Of note, pathways for progression following regression will be different than they were prior to it. For pathways are foreclosed since it would be un-economical for self-preservation to keep reinvesting in an object that has already triggered regression. Thus, some new object in the environment must lure investments forward again by offering a fresh archaic echo of a very old object.

Recent findings reveal that "temporary regression can occur in a normal subject due to impoverished input."[123] I believe this suggests that regression has a momentum of sorts—once it starts, there is a diminished engagement with objects (impoverished input), leading to further regression. I believe we can also feel what Dolto means by a spiral of trapped affect: "The spiral inflects its movement, enrolls upon itself … and inverts, without ever ceasing, if nothing comes from the exterior to this individual to break the vicious cycle."[124] Bernard Rimland, the renowned psychiatrist specialized in developmental disorders, asserts that new research "raises the possibility of prenatal injury,"[125] and/or of "adverse prenatal conditions."[126] Potentially, then, a gestational infant may suffer an undetected trial that provokes regression. We cannot know its duration or severity, or whether it occurred repeatedly. But even when/if the infant resumes progression after regressing, a lag remains—time lost to progression. And recalling that anxiety is a result, not a cause, of failed psychosexual maturation, we discover the special vulnerability of the child who experienced regression during gestation.

At parturition, despite looking fine, the regressed infant is unprepared from a mental and emotional standpoint, manifesting a form of unnoticeable prematurity. For he is unconsciously withdrawn, passive and anxious. To remain secure following the prenatal trauma he suffered (but survived)—and that remains invisible, outwardly undetectable—he retains a securitizing dependence on dream-work. He also has well-worn paths for withdrawing—i.e., a dependence on regression as a defence. An effective lure will need to be associated with the oldest unconsciously invested objects—but we can't know which—because only these have a sufficient condensation of affect to reach back to the archaic triangular situation. For a paradox is installed at the onset of human learning: we only come to reality on the promise that we can hold on to our dreams.

D. Symbolization

It was Dolto's firmest belief that "nothing is only organic, with the human being, everything is also symbolic."[127] For gestation is not merely a physiological fact, but one that inaugurates new life for a "symbolic being."[128] As such, she described a «fonction symbolique»[129] as "foundational of the human being,"[130] attesting to the instrumental role of the unconscious in our mental and emotional capacities. As dream-work on objects delivers unconscious security in the archaic stage, the infant experiences pleasure—delivery of the wish to survive—via the continuous circulation of affect from his invested objects to newer ones, and through all their associative pathways. So the symbolic function, she explains, secures "granted desires … necessary for the pre-subject's cohesive structuration."[131] And insofar as archaically invested objects will help to secure the infant when reality arrives, months later, Dolto speaks of "pleasure in its symbolic function of securing affect and remembrance."[132]

Jean Piaget, among the most influential psychologists on child development, writes that "symbolic thought is … mainly found in dreams and daydreams … it is a form of thought whose roots are essentially 'unconscious.'"[133] Piaget states that "all thought, even the most rational, is both conscious and unconscious."[134] He adds that "every symbol is at the same time conscious and unconscious."[135] Piaget is clearly acknowledging the unconscious scaffolding of conscious thought. He also speaks of how "there is complete continuity between unconscious associations and intelligent activity."[136] Furthermore, he stresses that "all symbolism implies interest and affective significance, as does all thought."[137] Piaget even attributes to Alfred Binet, the psychologist who invented the first IQ test, a similar assertion: "Binet came to the profound conclusion that 'thought is an unconscious process of the mind.'"[138] Piaget believes that "in their content, children's dreams seem to be closely related to symbolic play." [139] He also notes that "the sleeper, having lost consciousness of his ego, is … in the same situation as the baby."[140] In infancy, then, symbolization begins as an affectively driven, unconscious mental activity. Yet in the context of his own insights on developmental delays in children, Stanley Greenspan—writing four decades after Piaget—astutely remarks, "the idea that feelings underlie cognitive learning is still a radical one."[141]

Masao Ito, a leading researcher on the cerebellum (which develops in the first trimester) writes that "current research on the cerebellum is rapidly advancing our understanding of how this remarkable structure can govern unconsciously the implicit component of our mental activity."[142] And Colwyn Trevarthen, the eminent psychobiologist, reports on fetal proprioception and perception:

> Fetuses filmed by ultrasound exhibit well-directed touching movements to their surroundings, and to their own body from 20 weeks, halfway through gestation,

> and they touch regions of the body that are receiving new sensory innervation, engaging with sensory feedback and "feeling" newly developed proprioceptive and somesthetic monitoring input ... Clearly, the foundation for whole-self co-ordination of intentional movements is laid down in the prenatal development of the brain and body.[143]

Trevarthen notes that "the neonate shows the beginnings of this special human cooperation in mental creativity or 'story-making' ... [and] the baby expects companionship";[144] and he observes "infant intersubjectivity."[145] Of course, we cannot circumscribe unconscious processes to the cerebellum, as we can reasonably expect that multiple organs will contribute to the prenatal development of something so crucially human as our mental and emotional capacities. But prenatal development is evidently preparing the infant for what the neonate is capable of: mental creativity and co-operation. I believe we also detect evidence here of the "me-mymother"—the indissociable formation at the origin of the infant's mental and emotional life, the unconscious start of intersubjectivity. For as Dolto predicted, the infant is not just *with* his mother but *as-if* her. And in the infant's first experiences outside the womb, he is observed "taking her intentions as his own."[146]

The symbolic function, as Dolto elaborates it, assures affective continuity between objects of dream-work and objects of reality. Thus, our archaic dream-work influences our progress towards consciousness because, in the incessant drive for self-preservation, the infant needs the world beyond the womb to feel sufficiently secure for his affective investments. Dolto stresses how symbolization is what unconsciously secures reality: "The symbolic function is in play, constantly keeping watch over the child."[147] She reflects on the enigma that space and time (i.e., reality) are vouchsafed by unconscious processes that not only precede but elude reality: "The importance of the symbolic function resides without any doubt in the fact that it escapes all delimitation in time and space."[148] Dolto also believes that since unconscious affect flows continuously, as the herald of survival, the infant cannot help but symbolize: "From every repeated signal, a human can make a symbol."[149] In actuality, the infant is unconsciously, unstoppably, driven to develop thought.

The process of symbolization effectively confirms that thought circulates affect. As Dolto describes it, "the symbolic function therefore implies the notion of recognized similitude";[150] for it entails a "putting into resonance of his affectivity, by a similitude of being, of the affect or thought evoked in him."[151] Dolto is emphasizing here how affect and thinking are indissociable in unconscious activity—and also, how the symbolic function necessitates a resonance with another human. This is, in truth, the basis for the success of psychoanalytic therapy—that through words shared with a trusted other (who echoes the archaic transference situation), it is possible to travel back in someone's affective history to release trapped affect and put it back into circulation, enabling healing "by associative thought-activity,"[152] as Freud described it. In turn, this also means that the regressed infant, whose affect is withdrawn along some pathways, can still symbolize by circulating affect through remaining pathways via rich associations on prior objects: he still develops thought. However, since symbolization is vital to securitization in reality, regression (i.e., the difficulty of engaging and transiting affect to new objects) leaves the infant feeling insecure in reality.

We should also keep in mind that every archaic experience is different. No two pregnancies are alike; the mother's internal and external environments change over time; even identical twins differ in cycles of sleep and wakefulness; and dream-work on objects is unpredictable and unrepeatable. So Dolto is not speaking of universal symbols in dreams or infancy, and she cautions: "Let us beware of symbolic dictionaries."[153] Rather, the symbolization of affectively invested objects is an unspoken narrative unique to each one of us because, as she stresses, "unconscious organization is idiosyncratic."[154] It stands to reason, then, as some words hold more affective charge than others, that our associative pathways offer a kind of archaic geography of our history.

In her own inimitable style, Dolto sums up the staggering importance of discovering affectively driven unconscious processes in the infant in the archaic stage: "This precocious symbolic function which, at the parasitic fetal stage, results from the symbolic function of the human being is one of the current discoveries that is the most significant."[155] In this context, we need to remember that the principle mechanisms of dream-work, displacement and condensation, both utilize associative pathways: displacement disperses affect via associative pathways, while condensation draws back affect via associative pathways. So we can rightly expect that symbolism, which begins in dream-work, will make use of associations too.

At this point, I believe we can infer the dominant influence of associative thinking in cognition in the infant, with a strong influence remaining throughout childhood. In adulthood, associative thinking retains its potential beneath rationality—and as a pathway to unconscious affective investments that are evidenced in dreams, slips of the tongue, and psychoanalytic therapy. A further inference is possible: as first objects are experienced unconsciously when the infant is with his indissociable "like-me," symbolization begins when an object is a source of pleasure due to being experienced with another who shares an affective similitude. To stress, it is the sharing of affect—i.e., that affect is being shared—that establishes similitude. From this, we can further infer that the precursor for the vital conscious skill of joint attention, on which future learning depends, develops as a natural outcome of the infant's archaic engagement with fluid objects during dream-work in the womb.

Freud describes how words become objects for dream-work in the first place: "Words are often treated in dreams as things";[156] they are therefore subject to condensation and displacement.[157] The words which are "deepest" in archaic pathways (the oldest liquid objects of dream-work) necessarily carry the most affect. Freud elucidates: "The greatest intensity is shown by those elements of the dream for whose formation the most extensive condensation-work was required."[158] Affect is displaced by dispersing through associative pathways from the most archaic objects to the objects of reality, and consciousness adds layer upon layer—associative distancing. The result is that adult dreams (and word association with adults) is laborious—whereas in children, as Freud noted, "the dream produces a direct, undisguised fulfilment of that wish."[159]

Since symbolization is unceasing, Freud concludes that even rationality is merely "ordinary thought, unconscious, with occasional intrusions into consciousness."[160] Freud details how "unconscious ideation,"[161] or "unconscious thinking[,] … is also active in the day."[162] And there is no hard barrier either: "Wish fulfilment is in the chain of intelligible waking mental acts";[163] while our adult thoughts are "elaborations" of our unconscious wishes, as "the "secondary elaboration of dream-content is identified with the work of waking thought."[164] Freud observes that even "quietly thinking" can affect dreams.[165] He also stresses how, in "unconscious mental activity, processes operate that are of quite another kind from those perceived in consciousness,"[166] being "more comprehensive and more important than the familiar activity that is linked with consciousness"[167]—for unconscious processes are of a "more primary nature"[168] and "make use of symbolism."[169]

Symbolization begins unconsciously as the mental and emotional activity that will generate conscious thought. As a result, thought begins in pathways with their roots deep in the archaic triangular situation, and affect transits from here along continuous paths for circulation, through progressive branching via associations, to invested objects that keep conferring archaic security, thereby assuring self-preservation. Dolto's explanation is clear and concise: "Symbolic filiation confers existential security."[170] A regressive position entails lessened security in reality but symbolization endures because it is a continuous unconscious process, so thought still develops abundantly. So long before coming to reality—and many months before speech is possible—the infant is mute but thinking. Dolto's evidence and conviction in regards to precocious symbolization leads her to a powerful conclusion, that autism is "proof of the symbolic function in humans."[171]

Notes

1 Dolto 1987, 31.
2 Dolto 1981, 199. Readers of the ever-popular Donald Winnicott will notice a similarity to his famous phrase, "going on becoming" (aka "going on being") (1956/1992, 188 & 303). In 1956, Dolto first refers to «continuité» (1956, 28). In 1957, she reiterates it (Dolto in Guillerault 1997, 277, 285 & 288) and also mentions «allant-devenant continue» [continuous going-becoming] (ibid, 267, 286 & 291); «continuation de l'intégrité biologique» (ibid, 260); and "continuity" as «sécurité d'exister» (ibid, 265). «Allant-devenant» appears in a paper in 1947 (Dolto 1981, 124, 125, 130 & 199), but it may have been inserted for a later edition in 1981 (ibid, 96f); it also appears unequivocally (as «allant, devenant») in a widely distributed publication in 1956 (1956, 28). To avoid belaboring a point of little interest for most readers, I will simply affirm my belief that Dolto's expression is her own. I also sense a significant divergence in approaches between these two contemporaries because Winnicott stressed the trajectory *towards* consciousness, whereas Dolto stressed the trajectory *from* an unconscious state. I consider some additional intersects with Winnicott in my previous work on Dolto.
3 I cannot bring myself to translate here because Dolto's vocabulary is so textured. Technically, the word means "unfolding." But in English, we lose "roule"—roll. Her word is literally "unrolling," evoking the "un-snailing" of affect.
4 In Guillerault 1997, 34.

5 Ibid, 42.
6 In De Sauverzac 1988, 13.
7 In Halmos 1994, 333; also Caldaguès 1982, 215–217.
8 In Caldaguès 1982, 216.
9 In Djéribi-Valentin & Kouki 1998, 87.
10 In Djéribi-Valentin & Kouki 1996, 84; also ibid, 373.
11 F. Dolto 1989, 39.
12 In Djéribi-Valentin & Kouki 1998, 64.
13 Dolto 1987, 134–135.
14 In Guillerault 1997, 72.
15 In Lévy 2002, 13.
16 In Djéribi-Valentin & Kouki 1998, 186–187.
17 In Kouki 2005, 65.
18 In Djéribi-Valentin & Kouki 1998, 64.
19 Ibid, 86.
20 In Lévy 2002, 92.
21 Mundy 2016, 155.
22 In Halmos 1994, 172; Djéribi-Valentin & Kouki 1998, 87.
23 Dolto 1971, 178; Caldaguès 1982, 126; Dolto & Winter 1986, 166; Dolto 1988, 14 & 77; Halmos 1994, 27.
24 In De Sauverzac 1985, 125; Dolto 1987, 43.
25 Dolto 1987, 43.
26 In Manier & Kouki 2003, 170; also De Sauverzac 1985, 193; Halmos 1994, 263.
27 In Halmos 1994, 263; Hamelin & Rabaté 2011.
28 Makes real; reconstitutes.
29 In De Sauverzac 1987, 203.
30 Ibid.
31 For example, Juan-David Nasio in Authier-Roux 2000, 21–22; the witnesses were fellow psychoanalysts or analysts in training.
32 In De Sauverzac 1988, 36.
33 In Charial, Eliacheff & Valentin 1999, 50–53; also Dolto 1977b, 28; Coronel & De Mezamat 1997b.
34 In Marette 1940, 166.
35 In Ribowski 1987/2004.
36 1900a, 235.
37 1896a, 198f.
38 1900a, 236.
39 1913, 177.
40 Dolto 1984, 64.
41 In Dolto & Nasio 1987, 24.
42 In Caldaguès 1982, 136; Dolto 1987, 109; De Sauverzac 1987, 195–196; De Sauverzac 1988, 133.
43 In De Sauverzac 1988, 128.
44 Donald Winnicott is credited with having coined the expression, "transitional object," in 1945 as being, "in the intermediate area of experience, between the thumb and the teddy bear, between oral erotism and the true object-relationship … [including] the infant's babbling … along with the use of objects that are not part of the infant's body" (1971, 2). I believe the overlap of terminology is an artefact of their primary subject group, infants. Dolto intends an archaic object of dream-work experienced in the infant's body prior to oral eroticism (and babbling)—the phoneme as a subtle, liquid, transitional object.
45 I reflect extensively on oral passivity in my previous text on Dolto.

46 In Lévy 2002, 106.
47 F. Dolto 1989, 14.
48 In Marette 1940, 30.
49 Dolto 1981, 27.
50 1900b, 594.
51 1913, 181; also 1912, 107.
52 Dolto 1981, 274.
53 Dolto 1940/2013, 17; also Dolto 1940/1971, 1; Caldaguès 1982, 157 & 161; De Sauverzac 1988, 146; Manier & Kouki 2003, 185; Kouki 2005, 75.
54 In Marette 1940, 114.
55 Dolto 1981, 272.
56 In Halmos 1994, 17; Manier & Kouki 2003, 154.
57 In Marette 1940, 112.
58 In Djéribi-Valentin 2005, 296; also Djéribi-Valentin & Kouki 1996, 305.
59 F. Dolto 1989, 26.
60 In Caldaguès 1982, 114; F. Dolto 1989, 14.
61 In Caldaguès 1982, 114.
62 In Marette 1940, 109.
63 Dolto in Faure-Poirée & Djéribi-Valentin 1999, 39.
64 Dolto 1984, 275.
65 Dolto 1965, 16; Dolto 1977a, 90; Dolto 1978, 50; De Sauverzac 1985, 154–155; Halmos 1994, 21; Halmos & C. Dolto 1994, 140; Manier & Kouki 2003, 233.
66 In Djéribi-Valentin & Kouki 1998, 97.
67 In Manier & Kouki 2003, 233.
68 In De Sauverzac 1987, 261.
69 In De Sauverzac 1985, 149; Guillerault 1997, 24–25.
70 Dolto 1984, 222.
71 In Kouki 2005, 53.
72 Ibid, 92–93.
73 Hepper 2013, 591.
74 There are obviously some serious implications for profoundly deaf infants. Dolto urged hearing parents to learn Sign and use home signs in the interim. She stressed that "every child, even the profoundly deaf, must hear (feel) his name symbolized as early as possible" (in Lévy 2002, 108)—for "the most phobic and most persecuted is a deaf child" (ibid, 85 & 111; Djéribi-Valentin 2005, 703; also Dolto & Winter 1986, 94).
75 Dolto 1981, 269; Caldaguès 1982, 139–140; Dolto 1985a, 527; Dolto 1986a, 117; Dolto & Winter 1986, 87 & 111; Dolto 1987, 96; De Sauverzac 1987, 36; Dolto 1987/1998, 54; F. Dolto 1989, 183–185.
76 Dolto 1981, 23.
77 Dolto 1971, 184; Dolto 1977/1984, 191.
78 Dolto 1971, 70; Guillerault 1997, 37.
79 Dolto 1981, 23; Caldaguès 1982, 148 & 151–152; De Sauverzac 1985, 70; Kouki 2005, 21 & 64.
80 Dolto 1981, 144.
81 Ibid, 299.
82 Ibid.
83 In Djéribi-Valentin 2005, 640.
84 1965, 557.
85 2011b, 340.
86 1940[1939], 166.
87 1907/1962, 223 [Meeting of 23 October 1907].
88 1896/1954, 180.

89 1900b, 479–480 & 483; 1905, 232 & 237.
90 1905, 232.
91 1900a, 311; 1900b, 532; 1913, 167–168; 1917[1916–1917], 350.
92 In Marette 1940, 14.
93 Ibid, 19.
94 Ibid, 18.
95 Ibid, 19.
96 To stress, displacement and condensation are the principal mechanisms of dream-work; see Freud 1900a, 177 & 1909b, 36 (see also Laplanche & Pontalis 1967/2004, 197).
97 1933a, 20 (emphasis his).
98 Those familiar with Melanie Klein's "combined figure" may see a parallel, but I believe the gap with Dolto is substantial. Klein speaks of a mother containing the penis and a father containing the breast (e.g., Bott Spillius et al. 2011, 271). In contrast, Dolto narrates a symbolic object of dream-work conveying maternal and paternal security. Also, Klein's combined figure is a parental dyad whereas Dolto includes the child in an archaic triangular situation. My prior text on Dolto expands on this.
99 In Halmos & C. Dolto 1994, 139.
100 In De Sauverzac 1985, 19; Manier & Kouki 2003, 190–191.
101 In Guillerault 1997, 20.
102 In Marette 1940, 223.
103 In Guillerault 1997, 89.
104 Ibid, 17.
105 Dolto 1981, 226; also ibid, 163; Guillerault 1997, 24 & 144.
106 In Guillerault 1997, 42.
107 Ibid, 17 & 24.
108 In ibid, 112.
109 In Manier & Kouki 2003, 225.
110 In Marette 1940, 224–225; Dolto & Winter 1986, 110; De Sauverzac 1988, 90; Halmos & C. Dolto 1994, 140–144; Guillerault 1997, 16, 42, 165 & 265; Manier & Kouki 2003, 225.
111 In Guillerault 1997, 25.
112 In Marette 1940, 153.
113 In Djéribi-Valentin & Kouki 1998, 99; also Guillerault 1997, 42.
114 Dolto 1987, 20.
115 In Guillerault 1997, 70.
116 2015, 103.
117 Ibid, 111–112.
118 In Guillerault 1997, 18 & 72.
119 Ibid, 25.
120 In ibid, 11, 26, 75, 114, 118 & 128; Faure-Poirée & Djéribi-Valentin 1999, 38 & 41.
121 In Faure-Poirée & Djéribi-Valentin 1999, 11.
122 In Manier & Kouki 2003, 225.
123 Hyltenstam & Viberg 1993, 27.
124 In Kouki 2005, 88–89.
125 Rimland 1964, 185.
126 Ibid.
127 Dolto 1984, 178.
128 In Caldaguès 1982, 41.
129 In Djéribi-Valentin & Kouki 1996, 48.
130 Dolto 1981, 270 & 296.
131 Ibid, 279.

132 Dolto 1986a, 158–160; Dolto 1981, 286.
133 1962, 170.
134 Ibid, 171.
135 Ibid, 172.
136 Ibid, 190.
137 Ibid, 171.
138 Ibid, 172.
139 Ibid, 182.
140 Ibid, 201.
141 In Greenspan & Wieder 1998, 110.
142 2011, 212.
143 Trevarthen 2011, 80.
144 Ibid, 85.
145 Ibid.
146 Ibid, 96.
147 Dolto 1981, 292.
148 Dolto 1986a, 158; also Kouki 2005, 21–22.
149 Dolto 1986a, 158; Kouki 2005, 21–22.
150 Ibid.
151 In Potin 2008, 192.
152 1893c, 15.
153 In Caldaguès 1982, 208.
154 Dolto 1979, 170.
155 In Djéribi-Valentin & Kouki 1998, 95.
156 1900a, 183
157 As described in Laplanche & Pontalis 1967/2004, 418.
158 1900a, 213
159 1916b, 159
160 1895, 373.
161 1896d, 151.
162 1900b, 613.
163 1900a, 122.
164 1900b, 499.
165 1905, 288; also 1900a, 235; 1913, 169.
166 1913, 171.
167 Ibid.
168 1900a, 177.
169 1900b, 352.
170 In Halmos 1994, 243; also ibid, 44; Caldaguès 1982, 37.
171 Dolto 1985a, 534; also Dolto 1981, 286; Dolto 1984, 83; Kouki 2005, 29–30.

Chapter 3

Presentification

Preliminary Words

The archaic stage legates an unconscious inheritance to the oral stage. The infant has already begun to symbolize on objects prenatally, and these unconsciously invested objects facilitate his investments in objects postnatally. Thus, through continuous affective circulation reaching back along associative pathways to the archaic triangular situation, he unconsciously experiences his wish for survival being fulfilled in reality. Such is the work of the neonate for which Dolto aptly coins the verb, "to presentify."[1]

The sense that matters most in the first hours, days, weeks and months will be audition[2] because its functioning is the most continuous from the womb to the world, and many liquid objects of dream-work have been supplied by sound. Throughout her project, Dolto reiterates how "audition is prior to vision";[3] and that throughout the archaic, the infant inhabits a "sonar climate."[4] Thus, once the infant reaches the oral stage, audition best "lures"[5] his affective investments in reality. As Dolto narrates it, the fetus lives an "extraordinary social life"[6] in a "listening relation"[7] with his mother, so the infant has a natural "unconscious desire" for communication.[8]

From being fully dependent on the indissociable "me-mymother" for his objects, the infant begins his slow progression towards choosing and using his own objects. "Birth is a liberation," says Dolto, as "we are born into liberty."[9] And whereas birthing typically centres on the physiology of the mother and infant, Dolto focuses on the newborn's mental and emotional transition:

> Sounds … interweave with the perception of his body in tension with needs, or in phantasms of desire … These sonar signifiers … retain the child in reality through an ephemeral articulation of a perception that has come from the exterior world to which he remains attached, that is, fragments of phantasms.[10]

I believe Dolto's thinking dovetails Freud's on how dream-work offers "consolations."[11] For in entering reality, still unceasingly driven by the instinct of conservation—self-preservation—the infant maintains unconscious security

DOI: 10.4324/9781032655123-6

through tethers of dream-work that reach new objects (enabling new pathways for affective circulation), since this is what guarantees his wishes being "fulfilled in a hallucinatory fashion,"[12] as Freud explains. Freud stresses that in this affective economy, we necessarily "only exchange one thing for another,"[13] since "unconscious wishes are always active and cannot be influenced."[14]

Dolto explains that "audition tempers anxiety"[15] in the womb—and therefore, it continues to do so in the progression towards consciousness. She elaborates: "Audition exists *in utero*, not sight … [and] conditions of presence and absence … depend on audition only."[16] Dolto is emphasizing how the availability of pre-invested liquid objects confers that securing presence on which the infant's archaic survival depends—and how, in turn, this endows language with a highly significant, indispensable role in unconscious securitization in reality:

> Language … [and] the *reconnaissance* of the self and the other elected as co-being of pleasure … are supports for the presentification of the other in space and time, the other momentarily absent whose objects are a co-existential having(ness) of security in the solitude of the baby separated from the tutelary being he knows, and representatives of subtle communication, albeit lured.[17]

Further, as Dolto stresses, it is not the object per se that restores unconscious security, but rather that the invested object restores the securing presence, the return to the archaic triangular situation—i.e., the "third" returns the "second": "It is the words of a third that presentifies, for a subject, an absent person."[18] Thus, all infants are "welcomed into language."[19]

A. Phonemes

The "umbilical castration" inaugurating the oral stage of psychosexual development represents a formidable environmental upheaval for the infant. Faced with such rapid changes, the wish for self-preservation drives him, from birth, to secure unconscious continuity between his archaic environment and his reality. Given the relative longevity and strength of precocious audition in the womb, as Dolto narrates it, relations in language will be crucial to elaborating separation[20] as the infant transitions to "aerial life."[21] From the flow of words that greet his arrival, to the sudden awareness of communication all around, the infant finds himself in a veritable stream of voices from every direction.

In this wild new topography, the infant searches for a "road of a listening,"[22] using what Dolto poignantly calls "phantasmatic archaic languaged landmarks"[23]—unconsciously seeking to follow associative pathways from his dream-work. By this, "what he perceives of the interior … is articulated with what is perceived as coming from the exterior world."[24] In sum, his affective securitization is established through unconscious continuity, which then enables his affective investments in real objects: "Mediating lures permit the restitution of symbolic continuity … by persons whose voice is known to the child."[25] Dolto elaborates:

> Language repetitively hits the baby's hearing as an effect of his being in the emotional impact of his parents, at the discretion of sonar syllables, modulations and affects he perceives intuitively … It is as if all affects accompanied by phonemes incarnated a primary narcissistic mode of being.[26]

The phoneme matters because that is the sound unit that reoccurs repetitively in varied combinations (e.g., Monday, daydream, daisy, foundation, etc.). Dolto describes how precocious audition during gestation lures affective investments in reality: "The voices they hear from the age of four months are really what attracts then to be born to be in relation with them."[27] Phonemes infuse words with a "biological, affective truth"[28] that echoes the infant's archaic security in the "language bath that is [his] body."[29] And this, in turn, inscribes the "affective roots of language."[30] Some recent research on priming supports what Dolto uncovers: "Priming occurs passively and automatically,"[31] while "a single prime can produce many different downstream consequences";[32] and priming entails "spreading activation through a semantic network of associations."[33] As Dolto puts it, "language on the 'outside' lures us into relations with the sources of those voices."[34] So doing, "language humanizes the world" for the neonate.[35]

Contemporary scientific findings by Rita B. Eisenberg, the respected researcher on early auditory development, also richly support Dolto's assertions about precocious audition. Eisenberg writes that "cochlear function is demonstrable as early as the fifth fetal month,"[36] and "the fetus has been shown responsive to pure tones and other sounds."[37] She also notes that "most newborns, including premature infants … can discriminate sound on the basis of numerous acoustic variables";[38] and that "differential 'tuning' to the carrier frequencies of language may be built in during intrauterine life."[39] Eisenberg observes that infants have a "preferential responsivity to human voice, as opposed to noisemakers … [with] many patterns … detectable within the first five days of life."[40] Furthermore, infants as young as six weeks of age "could differentiate pairs of foreign language contrasts … to which they never had been exposed."[41] Eisenberg upholds "the existence of a rudimentary 'affective' system even in earliest life,"[42] and that "speechlike signals are prepotent in early life."[43]

Freud was first to discover that "language is a privileged setting for transference."[44] Dolto concurs, declaring that "the word is the best transitional object for the transference."[45] The phoneme serves a "mediating object's role in bringing affect to consciousness,"[46] as the infant experiences affective continuity in reality via familiar, pre-invested phonemes. Dolto describes how "the word is a transitional object that the child acquires to never be separated from it."[47] For the child needs compensations in language for the loss of «jouissance»[48]—i.e., consolations for his separation from the self-securing dream-work of the archaic. And in serving the transference of affect to reality, "phonemes bring narcissistic joy,"[49] being a "souvenir of the inter-relational language that is at the origin of the psychical structure."[50] Familiar voices offer "a dialectic expressed … by the phantasms subtending speech"[51]—and for the infant, the affect invested in archaic phonemes is "experienceable in transference."[52] Dolto adds:

> Each child develops his autonomy as a function of words—from phonemes, their sonority, the timbre of a voice that is tense or amused, worried or joyous … It is this interior audition, interiorized, that puts the child in security or insecurity.[53]

The phoneme is a mediating object for the transference that scaffolds the infant's transition to reality. And the invested objects of dream-work are "objects liminarily indispensable,"[54] precisely because of the archaic foundations of the oral stage.[55] For the infant cannot abandon the unconscious security on which his self-preservation depends. As ever, Dolto emphasizes that the phoneme serves as a mediating object by returning the indissociable securing presence rooted in the archaic triangular situation. As she astutely infers, then, "emotional resonance is the operational fact of the transference."[56]

Clearly, the crucial role of the phoneme in securing the infant's mental and emotional transition from the archaic stage to the oral stage endows the mother tongue with staggering importance. As Dolto explains it, "phantasms subtending speech are expressible only in the mother tongue."[57] For the child is at first open to everything, passively waiting for lures, looking for that road of listening: "Phonemes of the mother tongue and even foreign languages are heard before nine months of age."[58] But what he needs are familiar phonemes, so that he can unconsciously follow the pathways of his prior affective investments, for this is what will unconsciously secure reality as archaic phonemes are taken up, or not, in the mother tongue.[59] Slowly, then, affect becomes more attached (i.e., readily transferred) to some phonemes over others, for the archaic affect they hold and/or echo (i.e., by association). Thus the child effectively becomes enlisted in his own mother's tongue over another.

The phoneme is the infant's sustenance, enabling him to presentify without undue anxiety. That is why Dolto declares that "audition is like eating"[60]—and that babies need to "breastfeed words."[61] At issue is that the infant is not only a physiological being but also a symbolizing being—one whose rich mental and emotional life is just as critical to sustain. In other words, insofar as the infant's milk, "the gift of food[,] is proof of love,"[62] as Dolto says, then infants also need to be «alimenter en vocabulaire»[63]—i.e., fed words. In turn, the vital role played by phonemes in the infant's securitization returns Freud's insight on how words are treated as things in dream-work. For as Dolto comments, infants and young children experience language "in metaphoric, metonymic ways"[64]—playing with words, living words, and rooting truth in them.[65] This means that phonemes will be "heavy with phantasms for intelligent children."[66] And the result is readily observable among parents and educators: youngsters take words literally, almost visually, as if phonemes suggest things in themselves, rooting some archaic truth.

Dolto stresses the individual nature of every infant's experience with phonemes. Two infants may share the same mother tongue (and mother), but each one—even identical twins—will have a different unconscious archaic affective history with phonemes due to small variations in audition, wakefulness, proprioception, etc. So Dolto is very clear that phonemes are "idiosyncratic for individual human capital."[67] In short, we cannot generalize from one person to another. Therefore, "under the same words, people have different [affective, unconscious] experiences."[68]

The role of phonemes as mediating objects for unconscious affective circulation is also why Dolto insists that a "mother can only be maternal in her mother tongue."[69] The implications are highly significant for anyone materning in a second language; for language migration (the mother's and/or the infant's); and for mother tongue attrition. Dolto describes how losing an unconscious affective investment before it can be displaced to another object causes an enclave[70]—hidden, trapped affect—which she qualifies as an "infirmation at the oral stage."[71] The result is a loss of the potential for affective investments in reality, along with a reinvestment of old pathways—i.e., regression. Dolto refers to such problems as "illnesses of language."[72] For the neonate entering the oral stage is still entirely passive and needs his environment to offer phonemes that are continuous with the invested phonemes of the archaic stage, so as to lure his engagement by conferring unconscious security. In their absence, the infant withdraws his affect in the unceasing drive for self-preservation. Thus, the incapacity to be secured in language "provokes disinterest in the exterior world,"[73] Dolto states, leading to the "oral autistic type."[74] I believe Dolto is compelling:

> The autistic child, for example, that is the child who looks at nothing, hears everything. He only seems to be elsewhere … We must never believe that the subject is not in full lucidity, even when the individual who is there, present, seems besotted, sleepy or even comatose.[75]

The child is unceasingly symbolizing while trying to unconsciously secure his progression towards consciousness. And yet, he finds himself unable to circulate affect to secure continuity between his dreams and his reality. Whatever the cause, Dolto concludes that "it is this impossibility of symbolizing a disappeared link … that is the case with autism."[76] His primary roads of listening are effectively impassable.

B. Traces

The archaic stage offers rich returns to literacy. For the infant is born symbolizing, with affect invested in repetitive phonemes encountered in dream-work during gestation. He scaffolds consciousness through associative networks circulating affect from archaic objects to objects of reality to maintain his unconscious security. And as audition offers countless liquid objects for dream-work prenatally, the infant is primed to be lured postnatally by language: to displace affect onto the words heard around him and the voices that issue them.

The infant's unconscious security gradually spreads over a wider landscape as loved ones of loved ones inherit affect by association, and the mother tongue offers innumerable pathways for circulation. As Dolto notes, he has "hearing available to all significant traces"[77] because the "archaic affect of the fetal epoch leaves its living traces"[78]—and in "speech and hearing, a trace of archaic security remains."[79] Dolto puts the phoneme at the heart of a vital theoretical construct, the "unconscious image of the body,"[80] as "the structural trace of the emotional history of a human being … [in] the emission and reception of interhuman languaged affects."[81] Dolto further defines how the infant's archaic history with phonemes means that he experiences "sensory elements in resonance with vocabulary words."[82]

Dolto believes reading effects a return of archaic affects as "communication through a silence inhabited by a pulsional tension."[83] As she emphasizes, "desire which, at its origin, is always unconscious … demands, too, the appeasement of its tension in an accomplishment, in a consumption for the sake of pleasure."[84] Further, since archaic affects remain unconsciously potent lifelong—even at great associative distances—we always retain a "trace of the first lost link"[85] during the upheaval of birth. So if indispensable phonemes are no longer audible—risking regression—Dolto believes recovery is always possible through other sources of invested phonemes: "Nothing is to repair, nor replace. It is to effect a relay all along."[86] Unsurprisingly, then, young children decipher the alphabet and other repetitive signs far earlier than they are officially deemed to read simply because they are compelled to locate landmarks for their unconscious continuity in reality, to sustain their archaic security.

Freud specifies that reading "entails a frequent shift of the direction of the association,"[87] and he notes that misreading is often a "disturbance in reading … utilizing a 'switch-word.'"[88] He is emphasizing how words are embedded in associative networks that can move affect in either direction—back towards the archaic, or forwards towards reality, so to speak. Further, Freud is explicating how conscious thought can be disrupted by the unconscious affect in some words. In turn, words read become objects for dreaming just as easily as words heard: "Reading … provid[es] an abundant and not easily traceable source for … dreams."[89] So reading enables the retrieval of archaic landmarks, what Freud calls "unconscious psychical trace[s],"[90] since dream-work is at the origin of our mental and emotional development, and "phantasy carries traces of its origin."[91]

The renowned psychologist, Daniel Kahneman, writing on the influence of "System 1" (unconscious, involuntary) in decision-making, states that "associative memory is at the heart of System 1,"[92] and System 1 values "associative coherence."[93] As Kahneman describes it, "associative activation … [a] complex constellation of responses occurs quickly, automatically, and effortlessly,"[94] for "associative thinking is silent, hidden from our conscious selves."[95] Kahneman concludes that "experiments have confirmed Freudian insights about the role of symbols and metaphors in unconscious associations,"[96] and that humans "unconsciously detect associative coherence."[97]

The phoneme's legacy is evident in the first stories read to children, for example, as Dolto notes that they "use fairy tales to construct themselves in reality."[98] The haphazard (re)finding of archaically invested phonemes happens unconsciously—and the book can be found by accident, too. But unconscious circulation happens nonetheless, as the infant's archaic past secures his present: "Quantities of synchronous external and internal encounters take on the value of language signs."[99] As a result, Dolto believes that "epistolary relations are sufficient for the function of the symbolic father."[100] She is affirming that associative pathways trace their affect to the archaic triangular situation. And as "traces are … differed and diffracted in language,"[101] the "human being draws from the force that filters through words."[102] The experience is highly idiosyncratic, Dolto observes, for "under the same words, each put[s] his personal experience that [is] different from that of the other."[103] Needless to say, this makes foremost the liberty of free reading—i.e., of selecting what one reads for oneself. For Dolto is unequivocal that by enabling the circulation of unconscious affect—as phonemes resonate in archaic echoes—reading is reparative.

Any text represents a sizable provision of phonemes, then, of which some may echo (or not) archaic affective investments. We cannot know which phonemes matter, but we infer that there will be greater quanta in texts in the mother tongue (or in a phonetically similar second language).[104] So doing, a text becomes an environment—just as the mother was an environment in the womb—for the arrival of liquid objects. And in this way, a text might deliver sufficient quantity (weight) of "thirds," so to speak, to return the "second"—the unconsciously securing presence of the indissociable other on which survival depends. Logically, this would be especially true if an author produced many texts. Freud discovers that "condensation is everywhere,"[105] and the "need of the unconscious for liberation."[106] The result is a self-preserving drive to sustain circulation, and an instinctive resonance to condensations of archaic affects. And as the respected psychiatrist and pediatrician, Stanley Greenspan, declares:

> Models which have attempted to ignore Freud's theory of instincts have had difficulty finding a useful way of accounting for the phenomena Freud was trying to understand … [i.e.,] precognitive somatic levels of excitation and other neurophysiologic events … [and] the pre-representational aspects of early development in the first years of life.[107]

Further, we recall that unconscious processes operate outside of time and space—returning the past as if present, and stratifying people, places and events in dream-work. So it is inconsequential if the author is not actually present. This experience of "the transference in texts"[108] happens unconsciously via "messages coming from persons alive in another space, another time."[109] Dolto stresses the importance of familiars reading fables without adding explanations,[110] to enable the author's own presence.[111] For a text (even more so, an author's corpus), harbours the potential for condensation—i.e., for offering abundant phonemes that are older and heavily invested, at higher nodes along affective pathways, deep in dream-work. So, enigmatically, reading can deliver the unconscious reanimation of the archaic triangular situation.

The result is (potentially) an unconscious engagement with the author (or main character as "speaker").[112] Freud elucidates: "The original form of emotional tie with the object ... may arise with any new perception of a common quality shared ... The more important this common quality is, the more successful may this partial identification become."[113] So it is that a condensation—a phoneme drenched in archaic affect and/or repeated, encountered randomly while reading—serves as a "common quality" and an identification forms. The notion of accidental finding is crucial. For any deliberate attempt (e.g., by an author) to include specific phonemes will not restore the archaic triangular situation, since every child unconsciously "intuits his history,"[114] Dolto insists. He must find his own road instinctively, and instincts are resistant to conscious manipulation.

Freud believes that "identification is the earliest ... form of emotional tie ... where the mechanisms of the unconscious are dominant, [and] object-choice is turned back into identification."[115] Freud is stressing how the first experiences with objects happen in the fluidity of dream-work. As he puts it, then, we are dealing with the "infantile roots of love,"[116] with a "prehistoric, unforgettable other person."[117] And as Dolto attests, invested phonemes are first experienced with an indissociable "like-me" with whom the infant is so profoundly identified as to consider himself not only *with her*, but *her*.

Dolto states that "a message can travel many centuries before touching another,"[118] and messages invite unconscious "slides of identifications."[119] The implication is that reading can achieve a "putting into resonance of his affectivity, by the similitude of being, of feeling or of thinking evoked in him by this witnessing of the author."[120] In brief, reading is an "intercommunication with similars,"[121] one sufficient to deliver evidence of an unconscious presence. Thus, reading recalls the archaic condition of indissociability with a "like-me" through a powerful opportunity for the circulation of unconscious affect which Dolto calls "fusional transference."[122] This condition naturally facilitates "reversibility"[123]—shifting "positions" (as in the archaic triangular situation). And since such "alternating affects of emotional participation and of projection ... characterize personal rapports beginning at the oral stage,"[124] identifications in reading not only repair but support every child's mental and emotional development.

Thanks to her theorization of traces,[125] Dolto considers autism to be a regression to the archaic. Perhaps there was some unnarratable suffering during gestation (archaic stage). Or, perhaps suffering occurred in the first months of the oral stage, when the infant was still dominantly passive and (from an emotional and mental standpoint) still in that state of indissociability:

> It is often an absence of only a few days of the mother that is not explicated ... he felt himself to be no longer be existing ... She returns, he hesitates to re-graft

> himself. That is how we can explain … autism in little ones … [he] restarts with a trace that remains all his life … in a search for communication with an imaginary world that will permit him, perhaps, to be an exceptional inventor.[126]

In fact, Dolto—who had a difficult childhood history of her own[127]—was an avid reader who openly wondered how anyone can live if they don't read.[128] For as language effects a "transference of things past, archaic things,"[129] reading is a ready vehicle for the return of archaic security. And since anxiety is always lessened when affect circulates freely, we easily predict that the autist—regressed but unceasingly symbolizing—will read precociously, instinctively. He will read whatever presents itself as a possible code of calls, a potential pathway for interhuman affective circulation. Investing dream-work, he will form imaginative interpretations of those signs, developing a creative (and very private) interior life. For the indisputable fact about instincts is unchanged from Freud's brilliant exposition over a century ago: "The universal and indispensable attribute of all instincts…[is] their capacity for initiating movement."[130] Hence the autist's need to read will be unstoppable.[131] The autist reads to save his life.

C. Witness

In legating to literacy, the archaic stage offers startling proposals for writing. To start with, we can understand writing as a phantasy of self-feeding—of putting phonemes into one's mouth by one's own hand. It is also a means of creating matter in which the transference in texts can happen. As such, writing can serve an auto-recovery as "auto-materning,"[132] to use Dolto's powerful term. For the writer creates an environment for the arrival of invested objects (as the mother did *in utero*)—and, as Freud describes it, the "wish-fulfilment's power of representation is diffused over a certain sphere."[133] So doing, any text might serve up "thirds"—some deeply invested phonemes with the affective reserve to return the indissociable "second" on which unconscious survival depends. Enigmatically, then, the writer re-presents his own "second" in reality, thus serving as a witness to his own survival in a kind of "othering" that returns vital unconscious affect. And all this is possible simply because our mental and emotional life begins unconsciously in an idiosyncratic archaic triangular situation.

Archaic security necessarily involves an indissociable other—a blurry "second" of dream-work, the "me-mymother" on which the infant was reversible—a "like-me" with which he was so deeply identified as to feel himself to be this other. Together, they experienced "thirds" (objects) in archaic dream-work, including the deepest, the symbolic father, when two blurred into a nebulous three, forming the archaic triangular situation where the continuous circulation of unconscious affect begins. Dolto considers that every "subject experiencing discontinuity in reality exhausts himself from not having any encounter that echoes to give him coherence,"[134] because he needs "the echo of an archaic peace [wherein] one's being resonates, peace prior to the time of appearances."[135] In short, he desires to find the "echo and ricochet effects"[136] of his archaic investments in his new landscape. “Language is made to bounce,”[137] Dolto quips, evoking a dream play of echoes. And because “instinct and its physiological substratum characterize all that is life,”[138] the infant is driven to seek in language the continuity of his securing dream-work. Dolto refers to the recovery of affective circulation in reality simply as «la solution de la continuité.»[139]

The archaic triangular situation predisposes a potential unconscious reversibility—a blurring of “positions”—whenever one is with a similar-enough witness (upon whom archaic affect is conferred by association) while experiencing invested objects. It is a sense of being both self and other that restores unconscious security. Freud detected the “dream-work’s preference for reversal,”[140] and Dolto elaborates:

> The human being is made such that he feels himself to be the prolonging of the being he loves, or else the being he loves is his prolonging. If he is at a distance, he believes himself to be the being he loves; he is not at his place, he is at the place of the other.[141]

And since we unconsciously retain the archaic triangular situation lifelong, it is perpetually retrievable via the transference. It is that to which writing—and art—testify. At issue is that affective investments are inscribed that, when (re)read, may deliver the reconnaissance of unconscious similitude.

Dolto saw children in her clinics for years and viewed millions of their drawings.[142] But even with art, she specifies that the “listener is foremost a witness.”[143] That is why she encouraged children to draw (or model with clay) only if they could not or would not speak—and she relied on the child’s description of his own art, the phonemes used, rather than preset symbols for her interpretations. Always, she sought “what is said in drawing.”[144] Continuity matters so much to the child that she noticed how “the most authentic drawings are drawn on a surface already valorized by lived experience [i.e., used].”[145] For both writing and art, she believes, “relay archaic material as a means of de-muting the subject.”[146] Creative work thus serves as “a vehicle for the transference of latent content,”[147] Dolto says, that “opens … the path of actual unconscious affects to latent souvenirs.”[148] She elaborates:

> This witnessing, he gives it as a result of gestures that each deposits by leaving his trace in matter without volume … It is provoked by the need to express that which cannot be said otherwise and which, if it is not said, would choke its author in a solitude of sterilizing thought, in an emotional magma that would congeal him … that would not leave him his own identity.[149]

Like Freud, Dolto considers that art, like a dream, is a witness of the unconscious.[150] In this notion of witness, Dolto is stressing that a creative work, as a common object, achieves a “putting into resonance of affect by a witnessing.”[151] Her word, “resonance,” again evokes archaic echoes, as an invested object that is experienced with a similar-enough other. She emphasizes that it is the witnessing of the invested object that returns affect: “Drawing or painting is a witnessing that can become a language, if it happens to be understood, heard by the eyes of oneself or of others."[152] And Freud sums up the solution of continuity like this: "If a person who is at loggerheads with reality possesses an artistic gift ... he can transform his phantasies into artistic creations instead of symptoms ... [to] regain his contact with reality."[153]

In effect, the archaic triangular situation that endures lifelong provides of means of externalizing unconscious affect given two conditions: a common means and a witness experienced as unconsciously similar. In turn, the unconscious triangulation of invested object and witness enables the transference through what Dolto qualifies as "a similitude of being, of the affect or thought evoked in him by this witnessing of the author."[154] She narrates this unconscious process as "a witness to suffering or joy ... as proofs of the [author's] affect ... making us feel a similar emotional constitution."[155] And she emphasizes that every child wants to be witnessed.[156]

As Dolto puts it, "writing leaves traces,"[157] and "communication can be deposited in traces on paper ... as differed and diffracted portions[,] ... this unconscious language underlying consciously communicated language."[158] We recall that audition is prior to vision in the archaic stage. So we predict that a greater quanta of affect can potentially circulate via phonemes (texts) than art. That is why Dolto believes in a "duty of testimony,"[159] as she calls it—the obligation each of us has to produce texts as common means for unconscious witnessing—by whomever, whenever—so we can incidentally relieve each other's suffering by liberating affect for one another. She is decisive: "The very fact of writing is for leaving a witnessing. The one who has written or has created, to witness his passage, does so for others."[160]

As writing diffuses unconscious transits beneath conscious communication, our texts are inevitably inscribed with our affectively invested phonemes. Enigmatically, then, the similar-enough other witnessing an invested object might be oneself, given sufficient "distance" (time) for conscious forgetting—since consciousness is antithetical to unconscious processes. The recirculation of affect via one's own words stems from the reversibility, in dream-work, inhering in the "me-mymother." In turn, this capacity for self-triangulation on invested objects (by being one's own witness) becomes a means for assuming responsibility for one's own security in reality. Dolto describes it as becoming a "subject of desire not only as a witness, but as an actor in his own history by the intermediary of the body."[161]

Dolto noticed this phenomenon with her patients, as they made rapid progress because she copiously noted all their words (she was famously quick), then reread these to them: "The role of script-girl seems lowly but is *après-coup* of very great critical interest."[162] Dolto also noticed this phenomenon with herself, following extensive hospital work during her training when she experienced the transference upon rereading her patients' words: "What I received ... it was not at that moment [i.e. when working with them] that I made the connection. I made the connection writing my thesis."[163] I believe we can all imagine rereading a diary or poem from decades back—or, finding a signed scribble by our three-year-old self. The deep suffering or joy experienced in those early years returns instantly to the present as affect floods back powerfully. Such a witnessing of oneself enables affect to be "realized"—i.e., made real.

It seems evident that the archaic triangular situation is the unconscious precursor of conscious joint attention. Researchers attest that joint attention is "fundamental to learning language, developing collaborative and cooperative behavior, and advances in social-cognitive development ... [and] our sense of social relatedness and intersubjectivity."[164] Unsurprisingly, we find a relationship to autism:

> Since 1979, an uninterrupted line of 500 studies has attested to the importance of joint attention in autism syndrome development ... Understanding joint attention will not completely explain autism, but it is very likely that no explanation of autism will be complete without a definitive understanding of joint attention's role.[165]

We also obtain evidence of the indissociable other ("me-mymother"), that two that feels like one, plus an invested object: "Up through 8–10 months, sharing [positive] affect may be primarily a dyadic process."[166] And we detect the infant's gradual individuation from the "me-mymother": "After 10 months, sharing affect increasingly becomes a triadic process."[167] We further confirm the importance of encountering common objects of affective investment for securing reality from the start of the oral stage: "Evidence indicates that the behavioral development of joint attention is underway by 2–4 months of age."[168] Finally, we affirm that triangulation is prepared in the archaic stage: "Data suggest that some aspects of joint attention may be under development in the first days of life."[169] In sum, new findings on joint attention corroborate Dolto's view of autism as a regression to the archaic.

To put affect into circulation in reality, there must be a securing of continuity through the co-witnessing of invested objects—that is, unconscious experiences of joint affective investments, just as happened abundantly in the archaic stage. And because this reparative process is elaborated in dream-work, it is inconsequential if the witness is real (alive or dead), or a beloved storybook character. As the autist is regressed, he needs to find a witness to a prior time in his prehistory—back far enough to find another "sufficiently similar to feel secure in his presence."[170] At issue is that the transition between the archaic and oral stages could not quite be completed due to the infant's regression(s) during either (or both) these stages. But some recovery can happen if the autist can be supported in "living out slowly [that] out-of-date phase."[171] The result, Dolto insists, is that "the [affective] energy put back in play is irreversible. It is like a source."[172] If she is right, then one letter or one word at a time—with a witness to share and echo his words back to him—the autist could slowly write his way out of his withdrawal.

D. Exteriorization

The continuity of affective circulation in reality assures the infant's unconscious security by perpetuating his self-securing dream-work. Circulation flows along associative pathways, dispersing and diffusing affect, liberating it, onto increasingly greater fields of objects—or, as Dolto puts it, from "a short circuit of desire, immediate, to a longer circuit that mediatizes pulses."[173] Freud considers that "venting is essential to regulating excitation"[174] as, "the subjective translation of a quantity of pulsional energy."[175] And in pioneering the "talking cure," he discovered that words liberate affect too: "Language is a substitute for action … whereby affect is abreacted almost as effectively."[176]

As Dolto articulates it, "communication ventilates everything,"[177] because it is "exteriorization that discharges anxiety";[178] and "anxiety is released by using phonemes."[179] Talking exteriorizes affect, then, and if that talk is in the presence of someone felt to be a witness (in affective similitude), this unconsciously resonates with the archaic triangular situation. That is why Dolto affirms that humans have an inherent "reversibility of subject positions upon the one to whom we speak"[180]—in whom we "recognize sameness."[181] When we talk (our spoken words being as infused with traces as our writing), we are unconsciously susceptible—thanks to the enduring influence of the archaic triangular situation—to automatic reversals in which we alternate "positions" with one in whom we recognize sameness. In this unconscious identification at the origin of projective identification, I believe we can locate another important relation between the archaic stage and the phenomenon of priming: "Behavioral priming is a natural and ecological phenomenon, as imitation and mimicry effects of perceiving another's behavior on one's own behavioral tendencies are clear manifestations of behavioral priming effects in the real world."[182]

The circulation of unconscious affect is driven by the instinct of conservation. By definition, then, unconscious capacities for auto-recovery—self-preservation—will abound. Dolto has already delineated how reading and writing can support an auto-recovery—and our dream-filled sleep is a daily means of recovery, too. The drive for self-preservation also explains why the infant is compelled to find a witness—wherever and however he can—for he simply cannot live securely in his present reality without the continuity with dream-work that returns the "presence" of his indissociable other.

Dolto observes in the clinic, for example, that human beings are naturally inclined to "phantasizing trees, birds, nature and even anthropomorphized objects as witnesses."[183] As she elaborates it, "archaic desires remain lifelong so the child unconsciously projects them into vegetation, animals and nature, as security is unconsciously represented by refuges in nature."[184] This projective identification—this alternation of "positions"—becomes possible because a witness returns (i.e., re-animates) archaic triangulation. In fact, Dolto found many cases, even in older patients, that "indicated a projection of their narcissism in representations of flowers or vegetal forms."[185]

Dolto believed so profoundly in the self-securing, reparative capacities of these representations in nature that she designed a "flower doll" with the head of a daisy.[186] She was very specific that it should lack hands and a face so it might concord—in affective similitude, as a witness—with the child's passivity. She explained how "a flower has life but no movement or speech"[187] and it is, free of "digestive dependence"[188]—so it is "in resonance" with this stage.[189] For decades, Dolto confirmed the formidable effectiveness of this doll[190] in liberating affects[191] for patients "stuck in profound regressive symptoms."[192] The flower-doll was instrumental in reviving libidinal history;[193] returning dreams and useful aggression[194] (i.e., activity beyond passivity); and enabling "the projection of "illogical affects"[195] (i.e., pre-conscious affects). For the flower-doll, as she theorizes it so originally, "symbolizes the libido of someone who is not yet conscious."[196] She astutely notes the signature of this unconscious reparation when she explains that her therapeutic innovation "secure[s] abreaction even if it is found accidentally."[197] It is likewise for the securing role of nature, wherein random "objects of transference"[198] arrive within a benevolent environment, accidentally and unexpectedly.

Given that affective circulation is beneficial for our mental and emotional health, and that words liberate affect, why (how) does psychogenic mutism[199] ever happen? Dolto offers the following explanation: "The question of language [is] close to the problem of identification because when we speak, we do so because we can project part of ourselves."[200] The implication is that the child needs a witness (in affective similitude) to co-experience his invested objects because this secures the unconscious reversibility that enables projective identification. Therefore, "recovering a child requires helping him to find a similar to liberate his expression,"[201] Dolto relates. And she clarifies the vital role of the witness: "Speech is unconsciously mediated by the first humans who welcome him."[202] So it is not a given that a child will talk, she concludes, for "speech demands to be awakened."[203]

In truth, the child has been unconsciously secure in dream-work from the start of his life. But speech requires a shift between passivity and activity—a trade of archaic pleasures for real ones, for the "fruit" of speech exchanged,[204] as Dolto puts it. And the transition is not necessarily easy:

> In this phenomenon of the cry, incompatible with attention … is inscribed an endogenic necessity to repress to obtain a certain pleasure. The pre-subject himself represses a pulsion of passive expression … to focus his energy on an active pulsion, the cry.[205]

Perhaps the child is simply too regressed to be able to make that trade, economically speaking, because he cannot give up his self-securing dream-work without risking his self-preservation.

Dolto elaborates how, by "pronouncing the phonemes of the mother tongue … [the infant] sublimates orality."[206] In effect, he puts affect into new investments as "similes, onomatopoeia [and] speech … [mark] the start of the exchanges, of the commerce issued from the functional transference."[207] If all goes well, then, "a selection of cries valorizes mother tongue,"[208] as a result of which the mother tongue offers securing motherification.[209] Thus, speaking becomes another form of auto-materning (as writing is)—a "putting into his (own) mouth what is needed."[210] Furthermore, hearing his own voice provides an echo of his symbolization—his thoughts. So doing, talking expedites unconscious securitization in reality by enabling a ready-access to a similar-enough other who is actually oneself. For speaking secures a witness, as Dolto suggests: "[Primary] narcissism is reversible on whom we speak to."[211] From here, learning to speak will involve a "vocal and auditory selection coupled with mimicry … of the tongue said to be maternal."[212] And to make this transition from passivity to activity possible, the witness (in affective similitude) will need to be not in one's dreams but in the here and now, somewhere.

The trouble is that while it is possible to relive an out-of-date stage in our mental and emotional lives, as Dolto expounds (and psychoanalytic therapy amply demonstrates), the body is not at all flexible in this way. Physiological progression continues in the regressed child, and there are mechanisms for the onset and refinement of motor abilities (speech included) that develop incredibly rapidly during gestation and the first months postpartum. On the one hand, it may be that these motor skills somehow require greater conscious involvement than the regressed infant can manage due to his dominantly passive disposition. On the other hand, it is also extremely likely that these motor skills have a fixed developmental timeline that, once missed, cannot easily (or ever) be recouped—for, "'critical periods' for specific kinds of learning are common in the animal kingdom"[213] and, "the discovery of the critical period became one of the most famous in biology in the second half of the twentieth century."[214] In practical terms, both suppositions amount to the same thing—for truly, as Freud once famously stated, instinct is at "the frontier of biology and psychology."[215] So the regressed child will still be symbolizing (thinking)—because that never stops, even when circulation is relatively constricted to archaic objects and their close associates—but he will be unable to consciously initiate speech. Freud himself notes the devastating irony that "withdrawal from reality is the main purpose of the illness but also the main damage caused by it."[216] As it turns out, then, perpetuating our dreams is indispensable—whereas coming to reality is contingent.

The inability to speak means that the mute child (e.g., the nonverbal autist) will be deprived of an immensely powerful means for ventilating affect in the social, as "a dialectic expressed … by speech and by the phantasms subtending speech."[217] With her feet deeply on archaic ground, Dolto sums up the problem succinctly: "sudden weaning causes mutism,"[218] as does suffering.[219] It is a suffering prior to words, as she makes clear—an unnarratable, unnameable suffering.[220] Perhaps the "sudden weaning" he suffers from is the abrupt loss of his invested object(s), as "mutes lack semiotic elements for their alimentation."[221] Or, perhaps the "sudden weaning" means the loss of a witness in reality, which he can no longer locate. Then again, perhaps he suffers both losses due to being so deeply regressed. But whatever the cause or extent of his regression, surges of anxiety result from his incapacity for exteriorizing affect. Paradoxically—in a vicious circle inhibiting further exteriorization—the only solution is a (further) regression to an "organizing silence,"[222] as "mutism offers a passive defence"[223]—i.e., the entrenchment of regression. His solitude is assuaged only by his resourcing in dream-work. Such is the passive withdrawal to mutism of the nonverbal autist:

> Beings in language … but misguided in(to) a mode of receptivity and expression that makes them difficult to understand … Precocious children who were not recognized as such in the first weeks of their life, and who became definitely discouraged from searching to communicate with an entourage that did not understand them.[224]

When Dolto says that the entourage did not understand the child, she does not mean that words or behaviours were misconstrued by well-intentioned parents. Rather, Dolto is speaking as she always does, in a much deeper register, and she is alluding to a far more egregious problem: the child's inability to find in his entourage a witness with whom to co-experience his unconsciously invested objects. Crucially, Dolto never blames parents for precocious regressions: "It's never their fault, but it happens to be their fact."[225] It has simply happened. And as Dolto teaches us, every mute child can still find ways to vent affect through writing (however limited it may be, especially at first)—infused as it is with traces of his own unconscious investments. And he can still find, via dream-work, other entourages in reading and in nature[226]—environments which might randomly, unpredictably, offer witnesses to secure him in reality and enable his affective (re)circulation. For the unconscious provides lifelines for all beings in language.

Notes

1 For example, see Dolto 1984, 35 & 278.
2 Assuming some hearing capacity beyond profound congenital deafness.
3 Dolto 1981, 277.
4 In Djéribi-Valentin 2005, 239.
5 Dolto 1981, 277.
6 In Halmos 1994, 350; Halmos & C. Dolto 1994, 178.
7 In Djéribi-Valentin & Kouki 1998, 73.
8 In Manier & Kouki 2003, 185.
9 In Caldaguès 1982.
10 Dolto 1984, 276.
11 Freud 1908b, 231; also, e.g., Dolto 1986b, 21.
12 1913, 171; also 1900b, 566–568; 1901a, 647.
13 1908a, 145.
14 1900b, 553; 1909b, 53.
15 In Djéribi-Valentin 2005, 329.
16 Ibid; also Dolto 1981, 277.
17 In Kouki 2005, 21–22. While the word "reconnaissance" has been assimilated into English, its phonemes in French, as uttered by Dolto, are portentous: *re* [again], *co* [with] and *naissance* [birth]—effectively, to be born again with an other. And decomposing the last word further yields the following (homonymically): *n'est* [isn't], *sans* [without] and *ce* [that/this]—effectively, that being without this is impossible. This sort of phonemic play happens throughout her corpus, as suggestions on phonemes provide a curious sort of direction for thinking and/or a confirmation of what matters most. I explore abundant examples (and implications for translation) in greater detail in my previous work on Dolto.
18 In De Sauverzac 1987, 203.
19 In Djéribi-Valentin & Kouki 1998, 207.
20 In Guillerault 1997, 244.
21 Dolto 1988, 9–10; Djéribi-Valentin 2005, 728.
22 In Halmos 1994, 17; Manier & Kouki 2003, 154.
23 Dolto 1986a, 117; also Guillerault 1997, 41.
24 Dolto 1982, 146–147.
25 In Guillerault 1997, 146–147.
26 Dolto 1984, 93.
27 Dolto 1987, 16.

28 In Halmos 1994, 41.
29 Ibid, 16.
30 In De Sauverzac 1988, 192–194.
31 Doyen et al. 2014, 19.
32 Loersch & Payne 2014, 152.
33 Molden 2014, 8.
34 Dolto 1987, 15.
35 Dolto 1981, 273.
36 Eisenberg 1976, 11.
37 Ibid.
38 Ibid, 116.
39 Ibid, 121–122.
40 Ibid, xxv.
41 Ibid, 133.
42 Ibid, 146.
43 Ibid, 107.
44 As described in Laplanche & Pontalis 1967/2004, 497.
45 In Caldaguès 1982, 136; Dolto 1987, 109; De Sauverzac 1987, 195–196; De Sauverzac 1988, 133.
46 Dolto 1956, 37.
47 Dolto & Nasio 1987, 24.
48 In Dolto & Winter 1986, 36; Percheminier 1991, 542.
49 In De Sauverzac 1985, 177.
50 In Djéribi-Valentin & Kouki 1996, 216.
51 Dolto 1977/1984, 249.
52 In Djéribi-Valentin & Kouki 1998, 103; also Lévy 2002, 92.
53 Dolto 1984, 260.
54 In Guillerault 1997, 113.
55 Ibid, 68.
56 Ibid, 79.
57 Dolto 1977/1984, 249; also Lévy 2002, 95.
58 In Halmos 1994, 16; also Dolto 1981, 250.
59 In Guillerault 1997, 37; also Caldaguès 1982, 121.
60 Dolto 1981, 275–277; Manier & Kouki 2003, 234.
61 In Caldaguès 1982, 83.
62 In Halmos 1994, 316.
63 In Guillerault 1997, 194.
64 Ibid, 181.
65 Dolto 1986b, 64; Halmos 1994, 41; Djéribi-Valentin & Kouki 1998, 283; Lévy 2002, 14; Djéribi-Valentin 2005, 808 & 844.
66 In Djéribi-Valentin 2005, 876.
67 Dolto 1979, 170; Dolto 1977/1984, 205; De Sauverzac 1985, 151.
68 In Dolto & Winter 1986, 22; also Djéribi-Valentin 2005, 844.
69 Dolto 1977a, 130.
70 In Guillerault 1997, 143; also Marette 1940, 29; Dolto 1988, 9; Guillerault 1997, 143; Halmos & C. Dolto 1994, 280.
71 In Djéribi-Valentin & Kouki 1996, 140.
72 Dolto 1987/1998, 61; also Dolto 1984, 85.
73 In Marette 1940, 29.
74 Ibid.
75 In Caldaguès 1982, 118.
76 Dolto 1984, 84.
77 Dolto 1971, 193f.
78 In Djéribi-Valentin & Kouki 1998, 90.

79 In Guillerault 1997, 26.
80 Dolto 1984, 48.
81 Ibid; there is rich secondary literature (in French) about Dolto's "unconscious image of the body."
82 Ibid, 44.
83 In Nasio 1987/1998, 210.
84 Dolto 1981, 269.
85 In Guillerault 1997, 113; also Dolto 1986a, 51.
86 Malandrin & Schauder 2009, 252.
87 1891/2011, 75–76.
88 1901b, 274.
89 1900b, 419 & 495; 1901a, 668.
90 1896d, 154.
91 1908a, 149.
92 Kahneman 2011a, 26.
93 Ibid.
94 Kahneman 2011b, 51.
95 Ibid, 52.
96 Ibid, 56.
97 Ibid, 73.
98 In De Sauverzac 1987, 123; also Dolto 1979, 37.
99 Dolto 1987, 27.
100 Dolto 1988, 36.
101 Dolto 1971, 206–207.
102 In Caldaguès 1982, 136.
103 In Dolto & Winter 1986, 22.
104 In this, I believe Dolto offers consequential insights for translation theory.
105 1913, 174.
106 1907/1962, 102 [Meeting of 30 January 1907].
107 1989, 125.
108 I propose this phrase in my prior work on Dolto.
109 F. Dolto 1989, 13.
110 In Halmos 1994, 324.
111 Dolto 1956, 27; also Dolto 1979, 41; Caldaguès 1982, 79; F. Dolto 1989, 107–108.
112 In non-fiction texts, the author and main character are identical; whereas in fiction (e.g., children's books), they differ. This is not without relevance to the quanta of condensations predicted to be experienceable in a work and/or corpus.
113 1921, 107–108.
114 In Halmos 1994, 242; Djéribi-Valentin 2005, 770.
115 Freud 1921, 107.
116 1915a, 166.
117 1896/1954, 180.
118 Dolto 1987, 78.
119 Dolto 1971, 63.
120 Dolto 1956, 27.
121 In Kouki 2005, 86.
122 Dolto 1985c, 197; also De Sauverzac 1988, 175.
123 Dolto 1986b, 96.
124 In Guillerault 1997, 21.
125 I consider the value of traces in psychobiography in my prior work on Dolto.
126 In Dolto & Winter 1986, 111.
127 I discuss her infantile suffering in my previous work on Dolto.
128 In Potin 2008, 116; also Dolto 1986b, 81.

129 In Djéribi-Valentin & Kouki 1998, 304; also Caldaguès 1982, 31.
130 1909a, 140–141.
131 This valuable self-securing capacity is widely misunderstood and thus regarded as a negative trait in autism: hyperlexia.
132 In De Sauverzac 1988, 26–29; Manier & Kouki 2003, 162.
133 1900b, 562; see also 1900a, 35.
134 In De Sauverzac 1988, 129.
135 In Kouki 2005, 80.
136 Hamelin & Rabaté 2011.
137 F. Dolto 1989, 107.
138 In Marette 1940, 24.
139 In Faure-Poirée & Djéribi-Valentin 1999, 24.
140 1900a, 326–327.
141 In Halmos 1994, 262–263.
142 In Nobécourt & Simonetta 1978.
143 Dolto 1987, 16.
144 In Dolto & Roudinesco 1986/1988, 37; also Dolto & Nasio 1987, 14; Caldaguès 1982, 26; De Sauverzac 1985, 207.
145 Dolto 1956, 31.
146 In Potin 2008, 217; also Dolto 1956, 38.
147 In Djéribi-Valentin 2005, 447.
148 Dolto 1956, 34.
149 Ibid, 27.
150 In Guillerault 1997, 116.
151 In Potin 2008, 192; also Dolto 1956, 27.
152 Dolto 1956, 27.
153 1909b, 50.
154 In Potin 2008, 192.
155 In Djéribi-Valentin & Kouki 1996, 209.
156 In Hamelin & Rabaté 2011.
157 In De Sauverzac 1988, 236.
158 Dolto 1971, 195–196 & 206–207.
159 In Manier & Kouki 2003, 193.
160 Ibid, 193–194.
161 Dolto 1984, 370.
162 Dolto 1971, 6.
163 Dolto 1986b, 119.
164 Mundy 2016, viii.
165 Ibid, ix.
166 Ibid, 73.
167 Ibid.
168 Ibid, 150–151.
169 Ibid, 151.
170 In Guillerault 1997, 24.
171 In Marette 1940, 217.
172 In Djéribi-Valentin 2005, 859.
173 Dolto 1981, 286; also Dolto 1984, 83; Kouki 2005, 29–30.
174 As described in Laplanche & Pontalis 1967/2004, 12, 325, 329, 333 & 340.
175 Ibid, 12.
176 Breuer & Freud 1893b, 8.
177 Dolto 1981, 22; Dolto 1986a, 66; Dolto & Roudinesco 1986/1988, 39; Dolto 1988, 22; Lévy 2002, 23.
178 Dolto 1981, 189.

179 Dolto 1984, 328; Guillerault 1997, 37.
180 In Dolto & Winter 1986, 124.
181 Dolto 1981, 256.
182 Bargh 2014, 218.
183 Dolto 1971, 53f; Guillerault 1997, 39; Potin 2008, 204.
184 In Halmos 1994, 351; Guillerault 1997, 59.
185 In Djéribi-Valentin 2005, 176f.
186 Dolto-Marette 1949, 546; Dolto 1981, 158–159; Guillerault 1997, 21; Faure-Poirée & Djéribi-Valentin 1999, 8, 40 & 46; Djéribi-Valentin 2005, 257 & 259; Potin 2008, 54–57.
187 In Faure-Poirée & Djéribi-Valentin 1999, 40–42.
188 Ibid.
189 Dolto 1981, 104; Halmos & C. Dolto 1994, 149; Faure-Poirée & Djéribi-Valentin 1999, 40–42.
190 In Faure-Poirée & Djéribi-Valentin 1999, 42.
191 Ibid, 47–48.
192 Ibid, 11.
193 Dolto 1981, 191.
194 Ibid, 193.
195 In Faure-Poirée & Djéribi-Valentin 1999, 39.
196 Ibid, 45.
197 Ibid, 37.
198 In Guillerault 1997, 72.
199 I.e., mutism with a physical or physiological causality.
200 In Faure-Poirée & Djéribi-Valentin 1999, 29.
201 In Nobécourt 2008a.
202 In Guillerault 1997, 117.
203 In De Sauverzac 1988, 129.
204 Ibid, 142.
205 Dolto 1981, 284.
206 In Djéribi-Valentin & Kouki 1998, 108.
207 In Guillerault 1997, 34.
208 Dolto 1981, 251.
209 Dolto 1979, 48.
210 Dolto 1987, 51.
211 In Dolto & Winter 1986, 124; Charial, Eliacheff & Valentin 1999, 53.
212 Dolto 1981, 251; Djéribi-Valentin & Kouki 1998, 112.
213 Pinker 1994, 298.
214 Doidge 2015, 52.
215 1913, 182.
216 1909b, 49.
217 Dolto 1977/1984, 249.
218 Dolto 1984, 215.
219 In Guillerault 1997, 216; Djéribi-Valentin 2001, 47.
220 In Guillerault 1997, 167.
221 In Djéribi-Valentin 2005, 701.
222 In Caldaguès 1982, 163.
223 In Halmos 1994, 21.
224 Dolto 1984, 325.
225 In Dolto & Winter 1986, 109; Nobécourt 2008b.
226 In this context, we expect animal characters, or those based on trees and vegetation, to have special value.

Summary for Part One

For readers outside France or those not fluent in French, I suspect Françoise Dolto is one of the most important people they've never heard of (as the saying goes). Her work is not easy reading, that is for sure. In truth, her ideas about the time in our development before thought are at the limit of rational intelligibility. And her notions about the tension between regression and anxiety are, in transference, regressing and anxiogenic for the reader/listener. I am in Year 12 with Dolto now and I still need breathers, to keep coming up for air. I admit that I'm also a paddler by nature, not a diver. Then again, most of us are walkers on land and surface-travellers on water. And yet, there is no way to grasp the indispensable material Dolto uncovers about the earliest mental and emotional life of the human infant—our first learning—without diving deep into the archaic. And while she herself—like Freud—is a product of the 20th century, I believe that comprehending the archaic stage is crucial for 21st-century interventions that better address the condition we call "nonverbal autism."

Dolto works backwards in time from Freud's elaboration of the Oedipal Complex to its precursor: the archaic triangular situation. And by leveraging Freud's opening onto the unconscious—including his invaluable contribution to our understanding of dream-work and regression—she effectively adds an earlier, archaic, stage of psychosexual maturation. The archaic stage is marked by dream-work, the dominance of precocious audition, a passive disposition towards objects, and a reliance on regression—the infant's only defence.

The continuous affective circulation that begins in the "archaic triangular situation"—i.e., archaic triangulation—can be said to characterize human survival since it only stops when we die. Archaic triangulation is fluid—it is a relation, not a structure. Archaic triangulation comprises a pre-self that is indissociably fused with an other in continuous engagements with objects arriving on the sensory horizon of perception and proprioception—more so as unconscious activity yields to preconscious activity closer to the infant's due date. Dream-work is seeded by objects, the most ubiquitous of which are phonemes because of the precocious dominance of audition *in utero*. Phonemes are syllable-type units that are audible in repetitions and permutations within strings of speech in every mother tongue.

DOI: 10.4324/9781032655123-7

Dolto discovers the formative role of phonemes in transporting unconscious affect during the archaic stage, which destines language to be the best means of disseminating unconscious affect—i.e., for keeping it circulating to achieve unconscious security. At issue is that any triangulation, by definition, enables a continuous circulation from one "position" in the relation to another. So affect flows from the pre-self and indissociable other to objects (e.g., phonemes). And through triangulation, affect also returns to the pre-self from the indissociable other (and her invested objects). Effectively, then, archaic triangulation enables the diffusion of affect by associations in a proliferation of triangulations on each "position," and triangulations upon triangulations, etc. Meanwhile, along those same pathways—sometimes at great associative distances—it also crucially enables the pre-self to (re)experience affect by unconsciously reanimating that first condition of sustaining, securing nourishment. And this return of affect (along associations) to the self delivers a proof of life.

In sum, during the archaic stage, the infant is dreaming—and dreaming is our first experience of existence. While dreaming, the infant unconsciously co-experiences objects in an environment of provision—i.e., in a relation with an all-providing, indissociable other who delivers security (survival). This indissociable other is so blurred with the pre-self unconsciously as to be taken *as/for* the pre-self. From here, affect is diffused (displaced) to new objects in the proliferation of associations to pre-invested phonemes and that highly invested other. Archaic triangulation thus becomes richer and more complex. For associative proliferations enable the pre-self to co-experience any object—any "third"—when he is unconsciously secure, in the dreamed presence of an associatively linked other that is intuitively similar to himself—the "witness-in-similitude." In turn, the object ("third") is most often a phoneme. This means that archaic triangulation—as the means for affective circulation installed in gestation—leaves a formidable living legacy in the unconscious register of language, which can triangulate a pre-self, witness-in-similitude and phoneme as a perpetual source of unconscious security.

The infant hears while he is physically dormant—entirely passive. And this passive disposition—his dependence on an other for his objects—remains until he is able to dissociate himself mentally and emotionally from the indissociable, all-providing other responsible for his objects. For it is not enough to be born, which only achieves a physical separation. The infant will also need to dissociate himself mentally and emotionally—to individuate—from the other without whom he cannot co-experience objects, in order to keep affect continuously flowing in reality. In short, he needs to become affectively independent to be able to self-secure. However, archaic triangulation is a permanent inscription, meaning that we can never abandon the unconscious other. As a result, there will be a natural regression to dream-work to refind security in the absence of affective continuity—i.e., when insufficient objects of reality can be recognized as unconsciously associated (however distant) with our invested, archaic objects. Put another way, unconscious triangulation is needed in reality for individuation to proceed.

To stress, the circulation of affect is achieved through elaborate pathways formed as associations become branches for liberation (displacement); conversely, affect can be withdrawn (condensed) along those same pathways. And any future relations that are capable of sustaining the circulation of unconscious affect will need to harbour associative connections to archaic objects, regardless of associative distances. These unconscious investments in words—traces of our archaic investments—remain hidden from view in the latent register of language and in our associative thinking. And in order to experience pleasure in our lives—in our loves and work—while being relatively free of anxiety, we will need a sufficient proportion of our interhuman relations to transit unconscious affect. For affect always seeks, for the health of the individual—his self-regulation—to be exteriorized. In fact, no message of Dolto's is clearer: language is the best means of transferring unconscious affect.

On the other hand, if conditions are adverse, affect is resorbed along those same associative pathways, conserved—reinvesting pre-existing objects and pathways. This is because unconscious self-regulation is governed by the instinct of conservation. For years, then, the infant's presentification—his coming to reality—is two steps forward, one step back. He is lured to investing affect in/by objects that bear associative relations (in enigmatic, non-rational ways) to his prior objects of unconscious investment. At the same time, any setback or suffering can cause stalls. And since affect circulates unceasingly no matter what, affect that can't be invested forward is reinvested backward, so to speak—in objects of dream-work. Affect then circulates in over-charged smaller loops, generating the experience of anxiety. Dolto is clear: anxiety is the result, not the cause, of regression.

Regression can happen anytime during progression—including *in utero*. If the gestational infant survives, then he is strong enough and his history of prenatal suffering will likely be unobservable. We cannot know why—nor do we seek or need to know at this point—but based on comprehending the conditions of the archaic stage, we can easily infer that an infant might be born regressed. If so, his most invested objects will be deep in dream-work, so they will find few correlates in reality. In other words, it will be difficult for his unconscious affect to be lured when associations are few. As a result, his unconscious affect will tend to remain withdrawn. And while the infant will meet his basic needs for physical progression, his mental and emotional regression will remain largely unnoticed for as long as it is considered normative for him to be passive. It is only when expectations change and he is expected to self-initiate activities requiring conscious intention—typically, at the moment when the onset of speech (as a motor act) is expected—that his regression will become observable.

In terms of a conclusion for Part One, then, Dolto's elaboration of archaic triangulation, including the lifelong unconscious role of phonemes in circulating affect, provides compelling support for rethinking autism as a regression to the archaic. As such, evidence from individuals with nonverbal (severe) autism should provide an indispensable confirmation of her theorization; reciprocally, her unprecedented articulation of the archaic stage of psychosexual maturation should serve as an invaluable guide to a better understanding of nonverbal autism. This is what we now undertake to consider in Part Two.

Part Two

Evidence

Preamble for Part Two

When I first read Dolto in 2011, I was struck by the strangeness of her language. French was not the problem—I'm a native speaker. But something about her style seemed so peculiar. She writes as if she were speaking, and she speaks in a fast-paced blur of personal anecdotes and clinical insights. It's frankly not at all comfortable to encounter Dolto, as hundreds of pages turn into many thousands; articles reappear over the decades with added insights; and examples enchain one another across conferences and collections edited by a wide variety of peers. It's as if time and space are entirely moot in her corpus. Yet I was also immediately alerted to Dolto's humility, sincerity and incredible respect for children: "If you speak to a baby as an equal, then you will have an equal with you."[1] On film, her candid humour cuts through the palpable tension of interviewers confronted by her compelling genius and the regressing material she brings to the table. Those new to Dolto might feel the same after reading Part One. For as Dolto herself pointed out, "listening about regression regresses listeners and incites defences."[2] I admit that I would often put her books down because of a massive headache or shortness of breath. But then I would notice hours or days later, in an effortless moment as I walked, cooked or did dishes, that I would suddenly comprehend something she said in new way, with unexpected depth. Her material works its way in somehow. I am not the first to notice this.[3]

As my second decade with Dolto begins with the present project, I wish to focus on one specific aspect of her immense legacy: Dolto's notion, from the start of her career, that autism is a regression to the archaic.[4] I believe Dolto is correct that nonverbal autists can think critically and creatively, and that the incapacity to speak does not entail an incapacity to think. Needless to say, Dolto's stance represents a seismic shift in the field of autism. For contrary to the generally low public estimation of the intellectual capacities of nonverbal autists, Dolto presumes competence. In fact, she predicts precisely what nonverbal autists will confirm. Then again, as she put it, "the unconscious never stops teaching us there where it most surprises us."[5]

In first recalling Part One to some extent, human mental and emotional development begins in the womb during the archaic stage of psychosexual maturation. The archaic stage lasts until birth—the umbilical castration, as Dolto called it—when the oral stage begins. The first form of mental and emotional life is entirely

DOI: 10.4324/9781032655123-9

unconscious, and unconscious processes are driven by the instinct of conservation. The two unconscious processes of particular relevance for our study, as charted by Freud and Dolto, are dream-work (i.e., condensation and displacement); and the continuous circulation of unconscious affect.

Dream-work always has the capacity to take in (i.e., use) objects of perception or proprioception; and as the infant develops, more objects from the environment (i.e., from his mother and her environment) are susceptible to becoming objects of dream-work. Among the most likely are those most accessible in the womb: sounds, including words and voices—particularly repetitive ones. Notably, there is evidence that precocious audition is operational by the 24th week *in utero*; and since the infant has no concept (yet) of a word, what is audible are long strings without definable boundaries. This gives phonemes—i.e., syllable-type units that repeat in diverse combinations in any language—a determinative role as objects of dream-work.

Objects of dream-work enable two critical processes that commence in the archaic stage. First is the ontogeny of thought, in that dreaming is the precursor of pre-conscious symbolization; as such, early thought is associative and influenced by the primary mechanisms of dream-work—displacement (outward movement) and condensation (inward movement). Second is the securitization of reality, insofar as objects with affect attached during the archaic will influence which objects can be most readily invested after birth to assure the continued circulation of unconscious affect.

The continuous circulation of affect begins early during gestation in a fluid relation that is effectively an "archaic triangular situation." We can infer that it is the archaic precursor of the Oedipal Complex that is so crucial to explaining psychosexual maturation. The archaic triangular situation is an unconscious relation of three in dream-work, though the "positions" are fluid. The three are the pre-self; the indissociable "like-me" on whom life depends (i.e., the mother, unconsciously blurred with the pre-self); and a "third" (i.e., any object co-experienced with the indissociable "like-me," including the highly invested father—or most significant other of the mother—who blurs with both in the liquid environment of dream-work). In sum, this triangular situation consists of dreamed (i.e., archaic) versions of his parents and himself in a habitus of unconscious security and endless provision. As the continuous circulation of affect represents survival, it endures unconsciously for as long as we live.

Affect circulates from the start through this relation of three in dream-work—this powerful, fluid condensation—at the onset of human mental and emotional life. From here, through displacements by association (i.e., triangulations from triangulations), affect transfers to other objects associated with priorly invested objects. Thus, gradually, affect is diffused over wider fields of objects. Simultaneously, unconscious life yields to preconscious life as perception and proprioception augment moving towards the infant's due date. Objects that are affectively invested in the archaic are vitally important because objects of reality in association with them inherit affect more easily—i.e., they lure forward displacements of affect. By this mechanism, new objects are inscribed with unconscious affect, scaffolding the infant's sense of security in reality—i.e., his capacity for investing new objects of world, including his familiars.

The labile displacement of unconscious affect onto larger circuits represents a liberation of affect (i.e., venting) that is beneficial to healthy progression. On the other hand, if objects are lost or experienced as absent, affect is withdrawn along those same pathways through condensation; this resorption reinvests prior objects in a circulation through smaller circuits. This is regression. Regression effectively achieves a conservation of resources as unconscious affect is preserved. And yet, because affect is difficult to liberate (and may get trapped for years, or indefinitely) if diffusion is impeded, regression generates anxiety. Anxiety signals an existential threat because some of the affective resources needed for success during the subsequent stages of psychosexual maturation have been withdrawn.

Objects engaged during early mental and emotional development must remain continuous with the archaic triangular situation, though they will naturally do so with increasing associative distance, through increasingly complex circulatory pathways, while involving an increasingly large number of objects. In turn, the capacity for flexibly displacing affect to the abundant objects of reality is critical to feeling secure in it. If, instead, the circulation of affect is restrained, then regression ensues. When a child is in the archaic stage or early (passive) oral stage, any regression is necessarily a regression to the archaic, since no other stage has been surpassed. We recall that regression during gestation is theorized as being due to some unnarratable suffering—such as the infant's or mother's illness, his mother's extreme anxiety, etc.—which he nonetheless survived. As the regressed newborn grows, he still manages many interactions with his environment because his physiological development progresses regardless, including perception and proprioception, and his basic needs will manifest. But regression leaves him with an invisible affective deficit at the entry to reality which makes his presentification challenging.

At issue is that regression makes it harder for objects of the infant's new reality to lure his affective investments to securitize the evolving conditions for his mental and emotional life—conditions that must be experienced as unconsciously continuous with the dream-work of the archaic. Depending on the extent, timing, and severity of his regression(s), he may keep one foot in the archaic for months—like a hot air balloon ready to float but still tethered to the ground. This will then limit the quanta of unconscious affect that can be put into circulation on the objects of reality, resulting in an insufficient investment of unconscious affect in real objects (including phonemes) during an oral-stage window for the development of speech (as a conscious, motor movement). We also need to keep in mind that during the archaic stage (and the first weeks of the oral stage), the child is entirely passive, thus he is incapable of initiating action. Functionally, he is dreaming and waiting for objects to arrive. So the child who is regressed continues symbolizing nonetheless, moving affect through associative pathways, but with somewhat of a perseverative (repetitive) quality—cycling affect on restricted objects and objects narrowly associated with them. There is a thick proliferation at great depth, but within relatively restricted fields for dispersal in reality.

In a nutshell, the archaic triangular situation enables our first encounters with objects, including the phonemes of our mother tongue. A phoneme that is often repeated and/or affectively invested by the mother has a high likelihood of penetrating the womb auditorily as a liquid object for dream-work. In turn, objects of dream-work are affectively invested; and this affect transfers easily to other objects in association with it (irrespective of the time or space of the encounter), animating the circulation of unconscious affect. So the mother tongue potentially offers innumerable objects with associative relations to pre-invested, archaic objects, thereby contributing substantially to the infant's securitization in reality. The phoneme (like all objects experienced during gestation) is supplied by the indissociable "like-me"—that all-providing environment. And any phoneme thus encountered can become an object of dream-work—i.e., be dreamt upon as a common object while the pre-self is with the indissociable "like-me." Therefore, due to the dominance of the archaic triangular situation in the ontogeny of human mental and emotional development, all objects encountered in the archaic are unconsciously co-experienced with another that is deemed similar, with whom affect on archaic objects is necessarily shared.

As gestation advances, enhancing both the infant's perception (e.g., of the mother's heartbeat and voice, and ambient sounds) and proprioception (i.e., of his own body), he slowly begins unconsciously preparing for individuation—that is, for becoming dissociated from the indissociable "like-me." In actual fact, that individuation can only happen in dream-work at this early juncture because he will still be indissociable in reality (i.e., physically) for weeks longer, normatively until his birth. But as his due date approaches and he becomes more (self-)aware, the infant commences experiencing the archaic triangular situation a bit differently. He slowly and partially becomes aware of the "like-me" as being somewhat other than himself. Through this natural maturation, and the concurrent development of his mental and emotional capacities, the infant starts to experience the archaic triangular situation as a pre-self (i.e., himself) with a "symbolic father"[6] (i.e., the hyper-invested other of the mother who is normatively, but not necessarily, the biological father)—who, together with him, co-experiences this (m)other that is with them both yet "other" than them.

At this crucial pivot, in a determinative preparation for individuation, the mother enigmatically shifts "positions" from being an indissociable "like-me," to being an "other"—and the symbolic father becomes a (more generalized) witness-in-similitude,[7] with whom objects are co-experienced in the infant's migration to reality. This progression—whereby the symbolic father is the one the pre-self unconsciously co-experiences objects with—is such a crucial one for individuation that Dolto believes that (re)locating the symbolic father (through associative pathways in dream-work, usually but not only through psychoanalytic therapy) is sufficient for recuperating the continuity of affect: "What heals them, is to refind the symbolic father of their early childhood, and to be able to establish the [unconscious affective] relay with their actual symbolic father."[8]

From here, progressing towards birth, triangulation involves the pre-self affectively experiencing an object—i.e., any "third," including the (m)other—while unconsciously in the secure (dreamed) presence of the symbolic father. Pre-conscious learning, then, involves an encounter with an object that is affectively invested because it is unconsciously experienced as being shared with a witness that is blurred with the self in archaic dream-work—i.e., a witness-in-similitude. In sum, during the mental and emotional maturation of the gestational infant towards his due date, the archaic triangular situation inscribes the means of learning as an unconscious relation of three: the pre-self; an object (that comes from the outside but acquires affect through dream-work, and/or through associations with other invested objects); and a witness-in-similitude.

The continuous circulation of affect is maintained because new objects are triangulated based on associations with prior objects. So the invested object returns the witness-in-similitude—and the witness-in-similitude returns affect to the (pre-)self. That is why (and how) the unconscious experience of the witness-in-similitude returns powerful quanta of unconscious affect from archaic reserves to restore the potential for progression. Recovery happens because invested phonemes recall the witness-in-similitude—what Dolto calls "'the other' similar enough to himself to be in security with him."[9] I believe there is also a suggestion here about the ontogeny of projective identification. For while triangulating on phonemes ("thirds"), the pre-self and witness-in-similitude keep blurring "positions" in dream-work; and it speaks further to the crucial role of the phoneme in the infant's transition from his dreams to his reality.

The witness-in-similitude effectively becomes the guarantor of reality, delivering the unconscious experience of a securitizing endorsement—a conferring of trust and safety upon any object. So archaically invested phonemes "recall" the unconscious experience of the witness-in-similitude in the truest sense of an echo. The reason is that affectively invested phonemes, even when encountered haphazardly years later (because time and space are irrelevant to the unconscious), return the witness-in-similitude, thus automatically conferring unconscious security on the objects of reality—including language. This is the sheer power of the phoneme, as Dolto discovers it through her unprecedented elaboration of the archaic—and by which the mother tongue is revealed as a source of archaic echoes that can return the witness-in-similitude that, in turn, unconsciously securitizes reality and makes newly accessible (i.e., labile) the oldest reserves of archaic affect. As it turns out, language acquisition is dominated by unconscious processes that are entirely driven by the instinct of conservation and commence *in utero*. And language is an intersubjective engagement from its inception, whereby every word can offer unconscious echoes that return the witness-in-similitude with whom we first shared it, from whom we begin learning our mother's tongue.

To stress, regression in the infant does not have a physical appearance. It is, instead, a disposition which may pass unnoticed in one too young to be expected to initiate action. In other words, as long as the infant's relative passivity is taken as normal and routine, his regression is almost certain to be entirely overlooked.

However, because he is regressed, he will be anxious. This anxiety may be relatively minor at first—and it may be passed off as ordinary behaviour. But the longer regression is entrenched, the greater the anxiety because the unconscious is a powerful reserve of affect. In fact, psychosexual maturation is set to progress along a normative course, so huge quanta of affect are automatically coming online, so to speak, to fuel the affective transfers needed for the mental and emotional growth of a human being who will need to integrate with others to optimize his chances for success.

Simply put, it is part of the developmental agenda of our species to have and use unconscious processes in our maturation. However, the increasing quantity of affect needs somewhere to go. So if there is a surplus of affect and a regressed position (i.e., small circuits and few new objects for diffusion), there will be relatively constrained pathways—that is, insufficient associative relations to lure sufficient investments of affect. The result will be a constantly increasing quanta of affect moving in relatively restricted affective loops. The child's symbolization will thus be vibrant—he will be thinking brilliantly, creatively and unceasingly—but his thinking will rely on a relatively small number of objects, many of which may be intimate objects of dream-work with relatively few associations in reality.

Predictably, the situation with regression is akin to a dysregulation between physiological progression and mental/emotional progression. The gravest impacts will be observed with respect to conscious intentional activity: in difficulties impacting the ability to interact readily with new objects (including investing common objects); to autonomously seek new objects and experiences; to move affect easily and quickly from one object to another (rather than persevering with, and repeating, relations with long-invested, preferred objects); to demonstrate affective investments in real others versus others of dream-work (including characters from literature, movies, etc.); and to independently set and work towards goals (including small and large motor movements). Also seriously impacted will be the child's capacity to "feel himself" as "I," we could say: to be an individuated self instead of being a "you" or "s/he" who understands speech better when it is spoken to an other (or to a group of which he is a part, or in proximity to), rather than being addressed to him directly; and to speak intentionally by actively and flexibly using the abundant phonemes of his mother tongue in his relations and responses in (to) reality.

Since the archaic triangular situation in which affective circulation begins is its fountainhead, then restarting (i.e., resuming) progression requires restoring continuity with it. And what is especially critical about the unconscious processes that drive mental and emotional maturation during the archaic stage is that time and space are moot. This means, first and foremost, that every mother tongue carries random phonemes that were idiosyncratically invested during the infant's time in the womb—and encountering these haphazardly (at any time) can return unconscious affect. Second, reading freely in the mother tongue—or perhaps in a phonemically close language, or in another familiarly invested language, such as a liturgical one—can be unconsciously restorative since books offer abundant phonemes, some of which (as in speech) will be idiosyncratically invested with affect.

So a book—better still an author's corpus, or a library—can provide archaic continents rich with associative pathways to follow instinctively, traces of affect. And a beloved author might even serve as a witness-in-similitude, as that author's texts become an environment for the return of invested phonemes. Third, writing can be a means for becoming one's own witness-in-similitude, as our words cannot help but carry unconscious echoes of our history of invested phonemes. Effectively, we leave traces in our texts. Thus, affect is disseminated accidentally in writing that can unconsciously be experienced by readers (including ourselves) through the transference in texts. In this way, writing can be a substitute for speech as a means of unconscious securitization by offering (as speech does) the necessary scaffolding for individuation.[10]

Furthermore, if autism is a regression to the archaic—as Dolto maintains—we would naturally expect a phenomenon that is, in fact, widely observable in the autism community: precocious reading. For while other theories about severe autism cast doubt on the veracity of this vital skill, Dolto predicts it assuredly. At issue is that anxiety is automatically lessened if there are longer and more diffuse pathways for affect to circulate (thanks to objects being available for new associations). So as the infant moves into toddlerhood, he will be driven by nothing less than the instinct of conservation—which works unendingly, by definition, to regulate the system for optimal survival—to being passively lured by phonemes as objects for affective investment and security since the archaic stage. He will instinctively find words anywhere and everywhere in the environment, unobtrusively (very likely, undetected): reading labels, lists, product guides, packages, menus, mail, book covers, calendars, and whatever else he comes upon. And because he is amply capable of symbolizing (i.e., thinking)—and also because he is highly receptive to audition and long-skilled in symbolizing on what he hears—he will manage to teach himself to read early on. For in a very real way, his life depends on it. Yet this ability, too, may pass unnoticed (or be disbelieved), though it is one of the most predictable traits of nonverbal autism, following Dolto's elaboration of the archaic—as clinically certain as mutism.

This is not to deny that there may be evidence of the regressed infant's babbling in the early oral stage—his trying to use some phonemes, to issue them from his own mouth. But the "cathexis" (i.e., the affective charge or load) of the oral stage, including the oral motor apparatus, will be insufficient due to affect being stalled in small circulatory loops as a result of regression. The insufficient cathexis of the oral stage and its apparatus will thereby impede progression during a crucial developmental window that, we infer, permanently closes within months simply because neurological and physiological maturation presses on as part of the normative physical growth of the young human being. Therefore, if as an older child or adult, he is capable of producing any speech at all, it will almost invariably be perseverative utterances of a handful of hyper-invested phonemes due to the relative incapacity for wider diffusion; these will be used in a few combinations that exactly repeat what has been heard in over-determination (repetition).[11] But self-initiated speech—including talking and responding orally in real-time to conscious current events and to relations in reality—will be largely or entirely foreclosed.

With Dolto, we can further predict that two interventions will bring substantial relief from anxiety—though the tendency to rely on regression as a defence (and the passive disposition that ensues) will remain with the autist lifelong, necessitating the security of daydreaming. For as impractical as regression may be—in that it constricts our capacity to invest in our lives and loves in reality—it is the oldest and strongest human defence. It is, in fact, indestructible and formidable in comparison to that other (much later, much more fragile) defence: the ego. Further, regression (by definition) assures a return to the archaic safety of that earliest age when we were alone, yet not. In terms of relief, we can therefore predict that the natural world will reduce anxiety in being an all-providing environment (recalling the mother),[12] that presents—randomly, without any conscious effort on our part—witnesses (in similitude) for dream-work. So doing, it returns the unconscious security of the archaic triangular situation. Even the relative silence of the wild outdoors is more conducive to daydreaming than human chatter or media. And anytime affect can be exteriorized (i.e., displaced to objects of reality), there is relief from anxiety.

Another powerful form of relief is traceable to our unconscious investments in phonemes during the archaic stage and the associative thinking that informs our earliest mental and emotional development. If the autist can somehow begin to write—through whatever physical and/or emotional scaffolding is needed, for however long it is needed[13]—then we can predict that he will eventually learn to write independently[14] because this recovery (like reading) facilitates the self-regulation of affect. So skills progression will be naturally driven (i.e., expedited) by the instinct of conservation. And through writing independently, we can predict that the nonverbal autist will begin a slow reparation as both a reduction in anxiety and a capacity to individuate—a return of agency. However, he will not recover the ability to initiate speech. For by the end of the oral stage—as the result of a process that remains unspecified yet inferable—it seems that this developmental window will have closed. But he will be as-if speaking: he will be communicating. And critically, this relief is available lifelong—it is never too late to start. For the window for recuperation through writing remains open in perpetuity, as long as we live, since it leverages unconscious processes that are entirely immune to time and space, and that inhere in our very survival.

In Part Two, equipped with Dolto's formulation that autism is a regression to the archaic, we will seek the signature of unconscious (primary) processes in the invaluable evidence so generously shared by four authors with nonverbal severe autism, whose rich mental and emotional lives are communicated through the reparation of writing. It is, I believe, extremely strong verification for what Dolto is saying. But the goal is not to prove a theory—Dolto's or anyone else's. Rather, the objective is to take Dolto's opening onto the archaic stage of psychosexual maturation as a wide doorway to a better understanding and education for nonverbal autistic individuals who are, in fact, mute but thinking.

In Chapter 4, the focus is on regression as a primary, unconscious defence that has become entrenched, and the anxiety that naturally ensues—along with the challenges of individuation. In Chapter 5, the emphasis is on audition as the primary influence in associative thinking during the formative, enduring condition of passivity—and the restorative role of free reading in unconscious securitization. And in Chapter 6, the stress is on the primary reservoir of the unconscious, by which recovering pathways to the archaic triangular situation through writing practices can reduce anxiety and support a gradual progression.

Ultimately, Part Two is perhaps best understood as a prosopography—an examination of the shared characteristics of a group of people, nonverbal autists, at a particular historical moment wherein public favour is heavily (and most unfortunately) weighed towards behaviourism. Some critics will say that relying on only four authors provides insufficient data in support of Dolto. But we might recall that Piaget's own watershed insights were founded on observations of his own three children. I am very thankful indeed to each of these authors (none of whom I have met) because their works can contribute so significantly to our understanding. They have been selected judiciously from my collection of autism memoirs, which currently takes up almost as much real estate in my personal library as Dolto's works. It includes texts by autists who can speak; some works largely created by parents; some fine compilations of short pieces by autistic authors; and an extraordinary movie, *Wretches and Jabberers*,[15] which offers a compelling presentation of nonverbal individuals typing independently in Finland, Japan, Sri Lanka and the US. With all due respect to all these commendable initiatives, I am choosing to focus on four authors who have uncontestedly and independently produced a sufficiently large corpus of writing.

Indeed, the effort to demonstrate that nonverbal autists are highly intelligent, intellectually competent individuals is difficult work that is dangerously at cross-current with the times and imperils virtually everyone who enters the field of battle. However, what is conclusive from Dolto's project is that while the so-called spectrum entails tremendous variations in performance and appearance, everyone on the spectrum can think. And while nonverbal autists cannot speak (and this seems unfixable), they can learn to write. In fact, it is the raw force of Dolto's theorization to predict that for nonverbal autists, not only is writing possible but it is reparative. Thus equipped with Dolto's road map to the archaic, we will now journey with four fellow travellers in the hopes of discovering unexpected gains through our adventure, as we strive to learn more about nonverbal autism from nonverbal autists. As one of these esteemed writers puts it so perfectly, "no more talking about us without us."[16]

Notes

1 In Halmos 1994, 255.
2 Dolto 1981, 49–50 & 124–126; Guillerault 1997, 13.
3 For example, see Halmos 2000.
4 In Marette 1940, 30; this text was her self-published doctoral dissertation.
5 In De Sauverzac 1985, 55.
6 Any religious connotations are unintended and should not be considered an element of Dolto's theorization; Dolto is referring to the continuing and dominant role of *instinct* in

the development (through archaic triangulation) of the gestational infant's pre-conscious symbolization of the affectively hyper-invested other-of-the-mother.

7 Dolto uses either «témoin» [witness] or «semblable» [similar]; I combine both to convey her meaning as closely and uniquely as possible. It is a witness in that its presence is necessary to co-experiences that continue affective circulation; it is "in similitude" in that it must be unconsciously recognized as being affectively similar to/by the (pre-)self.

8 In De Sauverzac 1988, 204.

9 In Guillerault 1997, 24.

10 Speech is not the subject of the present project. However, I believe the discussion herein allows us to reasonably infer that speech is a natural expeditor of securitization in reality. For speech produces countless echoes much more easily and quickly than writing, at an earlier developmental stage—without the need for tools, materials or training. I believe it is quite reasonable to suggest, then, that hearing our own spoken words is crucial to establishing the ego as the human defence that normatively supplants the reliance on regression, thereby enabling economic efficiencies.

11 I believe this allows us to predict that it is possible for a nonverbal autist, later in life, to acquire new set phrases for repetition, through over-determination, from any witness-in-similitude in dream-work—e.g., from a favourite character in a book or other media.

12 Coincidental to Dolto's theorization, we come upon the commonplace notion of "mother nature."

13 To stress, in order to be beneficial, this scaffolding must never be forceful or coercive since fear will necessarily trigger the customary defensive response (the only one available to the child at this developmental "point")—i.e., regression.

14 Barring grave difficulties with graphomotor skills that cannot be overcome with diverse technologies.

15 Higashida is one of the individuals featured in this movie.

16 Kedar 2019.

Chapter 4

Primary Defence

Preliminary Words

It's a common idiom and belief that defences in the face of threats come down to "flight or fight."[1] The choice is said to originate in an automatic response generated somewhere deep within the system, where physiology and psychology (behaviour) are entwined, as an adaptive response developed in a species through the course of evolution. The existential threat is palpable through a physical response that includes rapid breathing, a racing heart, changes in blood flow (e.g., facial flush or pallor), hyperactive digestion, light-headedness, etc. In truth, the experience of facing a threat is (unfortunately) in the range of customary human experiences, for it is difficult to survive in our complex world of relations without ever being or feeling threatened. The two main psychological responses are just as familiar: perseverative thinking about the problem (i.e., the target or issue); and acuteness of proprioception (e.g., awareness of one's own anxiety, etc.). The ever-expanding nomenclature for defensive reactions enters our daily conversations: catastrophizing, dissociation, generalized anxiety, intrusive thoughts, OCD, panic, paranoia, phobia, PTSD, social anxiety, etc. Meanwhile, the phrase "flight or fight" has stood its ground for almost a century. And yet, it cannot account for the threat response of an individual who cannot engage in flight or fight because he is incapable of either. In brief, it cannot account for the human infant's responses to threats. This, even though humans are driven by the instinct of conservation—and even though humans have the longest period of dependency of any primate, the most prolonged altriciality. So an older and more primary defence in humans is being missed in this reductive notion of "flight or fight."

A significant psychological study on dissociation following trauma, carried out in 2010, reworked the classic defensive schema to add "freeze" as the first step in the "defence cascade,"[2] defining "freeze" as "attentive immobility: [an] orienting response."[3] In the adult population studied, researchers noted that the "freeze" reaction is very short, "only a few seconds after onset of fear of the threatening stimulus."[4] Most notably, "freeze" is characterized by a paradoxical surplus of alertness—i.e., by "heightened sensory perception and processing of contextual details";[5] this capacity is deemed crucial to "achieve concentrated attentiveness to

DOI: 10.4324/9781032655123-10

focus on the signs of threat."[6] In sum, "freeze" entails a hyper-vigilance in regards to the surroundings—a high degree of passive receptivity, we could say. Researchers attribute the "freeze" response to evolutionary forces: "Ethological research has demonstrated that prey that remain frozen during [a] potential threat are more likely to avoid detection … and shift[] resources to perceptual and executive functions to better locate the predator and plan escape."[7] The notion of conserving and reallocating resources is a vital one. These scientists further consider many provocations for the "freeze" response in adults, of which two seem most pertinent to the interdependent infant during gestation: "total helplessness … [and] being contaminated, contact to [sic] infectious material."[8]

It seems, then, that scientific work in our times confirms Freud's and Dolto's psychoanalytic findings of the previous century. For the infant wholly lacks the capacity for either "flight" or "fight." In fact, he can only "freeze." Understandably, these fine researchers sought alliteration to make their schema memorable: "freeze, flight, fight, fright, flag, faint."[9] And yet, with respect, there is not much that is frozen about it. The infant may be immobile, but his internal resources are hyperactive, (re)deployed to "locate" (i.e., find) objects in the environment, and "plan" (i.e., think about objects). Assuredly, he also enjoys the return of unconsciously securitizing dream-work which is, as always, moot for time and space. And while this defence may not be entirely practical (in entailing a withdrawal from reality), it is entirely reliable. Further, we should note that the attentive immobility and orienting will last far longer than seconds in the infant, simply because of the lack of any other defences. It may last for indeterminate periods of time. Not coincidentally, then, we can recognize in the behavioural presentation of many (if not all) autists multiple signs of anxiety—such as panic, phobias, PTSD (re triggers) and OCD. We will also discover that a life grounded in regression necessarily entails a form of dissociation that challenges individuation.

Alliteration aside, this primary defence is most properly named "regression." And returning to the infant, we infer that he somehow temporarily (or significantly) suffered during gestation, and that this suffering stalled and/or slowed the infant's normative progression: that is, his ability to nourish associative pathways for affective circulation through the displacement of affect onto an increasingly wider field of objects. He was strong enough to survive and, as a fact of what is unknowable during gestation, his suffering and the ensuing regression(s) remain unnarratable. The cause may have been the gestational infant's illness or his mother's. It may have been the gestational mother's accidental exposure to a negative environmental or nutritional event, perhaps unnoticed by all. It may even have been his mother's anxiety, to which the gestational infant, in being indissociable from her, was inevitably exposed. In other words, she herself might have suffered a temporary regression (e.g., due to a threat to her life or the loss during gestation of her archaic objects, such as a parent or secure environment); as a result, the infant could not help but experience a regression "by contamination,"[10] as Dolto puts it—a kind of contagion of anxiety. Dolto's firm belief is that events affecting the infant's earliest life (even during gestation) must be explained at the soonest—even though he "appears" unable (i.e., too young) to listen. For while no life (or pregnancy) can ever be secured from every problem, prevention comes down to an unconscious reparation via interhuman communication:

> Prevention … is not to spare a child from suffering … It is to put words on that from which he suffers, and recognize his right to suffer from it, and that we recognize with compassion that he suffers from it. But not to spare him from it, making a zone of shadow on his suffering. This will provoke a trauma that will leave a trace.[11]

Ultimately, whatever the causality in reality (known or not), the ultimate cause for the gestational infant is that he is helpless. There is simply no other response possible for him other than hiding: regression.

We recall—from Freud, Dolto and modern research—that the primary defence of regression (driven as it is by the instinct of conservation), necessarily involves a conservation of energy: energy is withheld within the system. And the routinized reliance on regression as a defence—that is, the "fixation" on a regressed developmental position, and the accompanying fixation on prior objects of affective investment—means that, along with a preference for sameness (i.e., repetitive objects), someone with such a dependence will always have a share of self that is regressed, securely tethered to the past. The challenge will be for reality to offer an exchange of unconscious pleasure against the guarantee of security which regression offers, in order to make abandoning the fixation to that "libidinal position" possible.

Crucially, this will not be about offering foods, games or other common, quick rewards. Instead, the proper lures to reality (i.e., the incentives needed to enable new affective transfers) will be found in unconscious "rewards": in what is valued as unconscious security. This means what it always means, in that unconscious pleasure translates the wish to survive, which in turn requires the continuity of unconscious affect. So luring the regressed to reality will require offering the path-means for securing the continuity of unconscious affect: first, interhuman language—i.e., phonemes with possible associations to affectively, idiosyncratically, pre-invested phonemes; and second, the opportunity for free, passive, random encounters in the environment with a witness-in-similitude—one similar enough in dream-work to confer security. These two unconscious vehicles are what will enable reparation.

The gestational infant's regression may have been short or long; it may have happened once or several times; and it may have happened early in gestation or closer to his due date. We cannot know. But his recovery (i.e., his re-progression) will require offers to his dream-work that unconsciously lure him, coaxing him out of hiding, if you will. And his progress is just as likely to be affected by his constitutional endowments (e.g., the acuity of his hearing) as his environment (e.g., the ambient prevalence of his mother's tongue). In any event, while he will typically present without physical signs of his regression, he will nonetheless be greeting the world as any regressed individual ever does: withdrawn yet hypervigilant. As the months pass, his body will develop and he will be thrust into diverse relations in reality, though invisibly he will remain at least somewhat withdrawn affectively. I believe many adults with PTSD know well this experience of being in a crowd, at work or at a gathering, yet feeling quite apart.

Regression is an extremely powerful, highly effective defence that leaves anyone who relies on it with a vulnerability to perpetually depending on it: triggers easily multiply (by association), and withdrawal from the social can become a way of life. Furthermore, regression is experienced in/with/as a kind of silence, a soothing hushing of the world in the (re)finding of private solitude. For, by definition, regression signals an insufficient transference of unconscious affect onto new objects, including the phonemes of language, leading to a withdrawal from communication in favour of one's own securing words, stories and dreams. It is a refuge. It is too good of a one, perhaps, but one that nonetheless assures survival through the conservation of affect as a resource.

But what happens to an infant who is regressed during a crucial window for the development of speech as a motor action (i.e., necessitating a large share of consciousness), so that he ends up with the inability to speak—he is nonverbal? For if speech is foreclosed, are not "flight" and "fight" gravely restricted too? Consider: what defence is left, other than regression, if one cannot verbally defend oneself, orally choose between options, or talk one's way out of things? In fact, when we invoke the notion of "flight or fight," we mostly mean through speech, do we not? After all, we don't normally see people throw a punch in the initial moments of a confrontation—they usually argue first, then escalate. And we don't see too many people in a showdown run out of a room immediately without saying a word (though nonverbal autists may)—they usually argue first, then storm out. In fact, we should pause to reflect on what defences are left to the mute human being, given that life is not survivable without defences.

And what might an entrenched reliance on regression feel like? At issue, first, is that unconscious affect increases throughout the infant's development as a natural resource needed to fuel his pending psychosexual maturation. So the sheer quanta of unconscious affect in the system augments during early life. Second, also at issue, is that the unconscious circulation of affect never ceases while an individual is alive—but regression exerts limitations on the labile diffusion of unconscious affect because of the difficulty of investing in new objects. This results in an increasing quantity of unconscious affect moving in relatively restricted associative pathways (loops) of limited, pre-invested objects. Some of the affect is effectively being impeded in its natural drive for liberation, and this is what triggers existential anxiety. Anxiety is a symptom of regression, not its cause. Further, deeper (older, more archaic) and/or enduring regressions mean that fewer of the child's invested objects are likely to have relevance (i.e., associations) to reality, meaning that few objects in reality will invite/suggest associative pathways along which to lure these objects of dream-work. Thus, it becomes harder to displace the trapped affect, by which regression—the dissociative withdrawal to solitude—can become firmly engrained.

This alone seems to issue powerful new directions for interventions. For we can predict that it will not be easy for anxious individuals to relax or calm down, since anxiety is an automatically generated, unconscious response to an existential threat. It is thus not readily amenable to conscious control. In fact, reducing anxiety will require something different: it calls for an emergence, however partial, from regression. If progression can resume to any degree whatsoever, anxiety will begin to decrease. Dolto once joked that, "Psychotherapy begins in the morning, when you live alone, when you speak to the news seller."[12] But her point is extremely serious. As defines our species, we are inherently communicative, "languaged"[13] beings who need one another to maintain the continuous circulation of unconscious affect necessary for our optimal success as individuals. And as it turns out, our words carry an inevitable trace—an unconscious current of affect—that is experienceable by the listener/reader. Dolto elaborates:

> At the same time as we live our relation to the other, logic, referring us to the meaning of words, we also live on another register a relation to which we do not pay attention, from the domain of the unconscious … Clear language carries, when it is spontaneous, at the same time as what is manifest of its speech, a latent speech, the language of the unconscious.[14]

So the infant needs the words of others, formative in human speciation, to enable him to transition from his dreams to his reality by investing unconscious affect in the objects of his world—including his familiars. In the regressed child, this crucial transition in infancy (from the archaic stage to the oral stage) has been impeded somehow, somewhat—and this is what needs to be repaired. Reparation will thus require someone beyond himself to draw him out through language, insofar as this is always the natural means of the transition from unconscious to conscious mental and emotional life in our species.

I believe Dolto is alerting us very clearly to the fact that language has a vital function in human self-regulation right from gestation. But the child cannot do it alone—no human can. And yet sadly, as Dolto comments, all too often, the severely autistic child appears not to be (capable of) listening, "and it is that which is troubling and that results, finally, in our speaking about them without addressing ourselves to their person."[15] So the regressed child, who desperately needs others to interact directly with him through authentic language[16]—to repair gaps, lapses and stalls in progression during very early maturation, by which he has been left with a huge burden of anxiety—ironically becomes the very child to whom others stop talking, effectively further disengaging him from language. His solitude becomes more entrenched and his anxiety builds.

In this chapter, we will now explore the lived experience of reliance on regression as a defence, leading to a kind of dissociated mental and emotional space as a place (way) to hide (freeze). As the years go by, this routinized means of withdrawing affect becomes familiar to autists (as it does to any individual with PTSD), as the assurance of security that comes from pulling in resources and battening down the hatches, so to speak. We will also investigate what it means for nonverbal autists to live with existential anxiety, insofar as regression has become the go-to defence given the incapacity for speech. We predict that, even more than mutism, chronic anxiety is likely to feel like the most problematic comorbidity.

A. Regression

On the Humber River these days, there are countless indicators of the seasons changing—and not only in the bold red and yellow palettes of the leaves. Paddling well after sunrise now, I need waterproof gloves and a warm hat, and I can see my breath. The geese are almost all gone and the herons are starting to leave, while squirrels and groundhogs are frantically busy under the brush. Only the ducks seem unbothered, sleeping on the chilly banks even though coyotes are roaming in force close by—scraggly-looking pups trying to bulk up for winter. Everywhere in the natural world, there are signs of preparation for the cold that is encroaching. Some animals will hibernate—decreasing their body temperature, heart rate and breathing to enter a deep sleep for months. Some animals will brumate, as they stop eating and slow their metabolism but periodically wake up for water. Others will begin torpor, lowering their heart rate and breathing to save energy in the bitter cold, but resuming activities when the day is warm. In fact, human sleep is a kind of torpor. And at issue in all these energy-saving mechanisms of living beings is a defence: the environment is changing to limit access to external resources, so internal resources must be carefully allocated to secure long-term survival. In fact, regression in humans achieves a similar goal: the conservation of internal resources through a withdrawal to a refuge (of sorts), and the minimization of new energy expenditures while external resources (objects) are limited.

We will now study regression with four nonverbal autistic authors through three approaches: first, through verbal descriptors that characterize the experience of feeling withdrawn and/or of relying on an internal refuge or retreat; second, by examining their particular self-awareness of the encounter with reality through their considerations of time-space; and third, by surveying the problem of individuation that is palpable for them as something other than a unitary self. In terms of an initial overview, in describing withdrawal, Sellin speaks of "drowning in loneliness,"[17] and Kedar states that "during these years [prior to learning to write] I felt so trapped."[18] Higashida reports, "My brain has this habit of getting lost inside things,"[19] while Mukhopadhyay, writing in the third person about himself, reveals a boy who always attempted to hide.[20] In turn, in noticing the difficulty of encountering reality, Kedar admits, "I spent so many years not fully present"[21]—while Mukhopadhyay discloses, "I feel trapped in the continuous flow of happenings."[22] Sellin boldly calls himself an "opponent of reality,"[23] while Higashida concludes, "I am connected to neither the past nor the future."[24] As for the problem of individuation, Sellin frequently qualifies himself as "a withoutme person"[25]—and Mukhopadhyay describes "the helplessness of a scattered self."[26] Provocatively, Kedar's character,

Anthony,[27] wonders what a child can do if his mind and body won't comply with his wishes.[28] And in lamenting the efforts directed at controlling the manifestations of a (difficult) self, Higashida says, "They make us feel like robots, with each and every action pre-programmed."[29] We will learn through this new journey in thought that—as is the case for any living being who sleeps for months while the environment warms and new developments encroach on his habitus of security—the world keeps changing. Time goes on while one is withdrawn. Slowly, then, the world becomes unrecognizable, making it very difficult indeed for anyone to emerge from their retreat. A safe refuge is a hard place to leave.[30]

First, we consider the **retreat or withdrawal**. Autists feel withdrawn from others and describe this internal sense of separateness. They also reveal a paradox: their refuge delivers security and isolation. Sellin states: "I want to contribute to research into autism … to get more and more people out of their boxed in lives."[31] On the one hand, as Sellin declares, "I love my own reality too[,] it offers me protection and refuge and gives me dignity."[32] On the other hand, he adds, "There's a muddle going on inside words sentences ideas get all torn apart and torn up … a thought is really difficult like being boxed up in the inside world."[33] The refuge shields the autist from suffering, as Sellin elaborates: "It is as if a stone being is holding me a prisoner and it thinks sorrow is a security risk."[34] Also inhering in this separation is the notion of a refuge for thinking—in fact, of refuge *as* thinking. For example, Kedar explains (in the third person) that his character, Anthony, was able to escape in his mind in anticipation of extensive dental work;[35] and (also in the third person) Mukhopadhyay reveals the deep pleasure of withdrawing to thought, for when he is prevented from doing so [by noise], this is experienced as a lost opportunity: "There was no chance for the boy to get lost in his thoughts."[36]

There is inherent loneliness in nonverbal autism stemming not only from the challenge of mutism but more, it seems, from relying on an internal withdrawal to safety. Thus, Sellin believes that "every autistic is lonely."[37] He adds poignantly (in a poem) that he frequently wishes he were dead because of the sheer depth of his loneliness.[38] Yet here again is the paradox: "They [autists] … give other people an impression of the unusual world of the lonely"[39]—yet he admits, "I particularly like the island of loneliness."[40] At issue is that withdrawal has become a way of life and there is pleasure in a refuge in/as/to thought—in intense mental activity *as* activity, as Sellin describes it: "A lonely person is always replacing important experiences of poor humanity on this Earth by constant talking mostly in his lonely mind."[41] And (yet) he titles one of his books, *I Don't Want to Be Inside Me Anymore*.

There is also a self-awareness of the power of silence—a respect, one might even say—that prevails in these authors' texts. Sellin refers to it as a "retreat into the silence and peace of our dignified and honest autistic world."[42] It is a condition fraught with tension, however, because talking is valued, as Sellin explains: "Talking is too precious and … I can't learn how because I'd only talk nonsense."[43] Yet the autist also has a sense that an enigmatic tether prevents his speech: "a power forces me to keep quiet about it."[44] So coming out of silence is a struggle.

Mukhopadhyay even titles one of his books, *Beyond the Silence*. And Higashida seems acutely aware that this silent retreat is a withdrawal into thinking: "I'm fascinated by some things that other people have no interest in whatsoever."[45] Mukhopadhyay conveys the persevering enticement of silence and the autist's desire to sustain his imaginative dream-work and personal thoughts; for example, he considered what he calls "mirror travel" to be a perfect means of detaching from a noisy environment.[46]

Thus, Mukhopadhyay resents interruptions:

> He tried to think of the staircase and the wonderful world of silence, which he used to imagine. But he could not concentrate as he used to. This was because of education, which had opened a new world for him. He was frustrated for not being able to be on the imagined staircases.[47]

And he offers another example: "I would finally reach the mirror in hope of seeing a story and in the hope of some silence. But with Mother standing behind me, I could only hear her voice."[48] Here is a desire to defend the safe space of his inner world of thought, his personal stories. And tellingly, within a story, Mukhopadhyay's character, Emma,[49] reveals that she can never appear to him when there are too many people (i.e., voices).[50] So a silent space for thinking both enables and marks his restorative, securing retreat.

Second, we contemplate the entry to **reality and the problem of time-space** it engenders. I offer that it is as if these four nonverbal autists are singularly able to narrate the transition from dream-work to reality, from the vantage point of someone with a mature capacity for thought. Mukhopadhyay also ponders the problem of time extensively through his storytelling; for example, his character, Emma, explains that time is one of those things that is infinite.[51] And Mukhopadhyay himself relates the following:

> He got lost in a situation that was unreal or super real. The chairs and tables were still there, but a book or a magazine or some eatables were seen in places where they were kept previously. "I can see in the past," thought the boy … In fact he could actually "feel" the previous incidents around him.[52]

And he further philosophizes about time:

> Nothing in the world is stable. It is very painful to see that what we love most, and consider as our own sometime or the other, is to be given up and is taken over by time. Then we sigh and tell ourselves, "Ah, that was once mine and I still miss it. I wonder whether it misses me too!"[53]

Mukhopadhyay even finds certain times of day difficult, stating he "wants 'no evening day,' the time between the afternoon and dusk."[54] He attests that, "The boy of my story in the past two years has a finite position watching the hands of the clock move and the pages of the calendar turn."[55] He further confesses, "I love calendars. I collect them."[56] Sellin also records some critical musings about time: "Like everything else a date happens to be a matter of rotating events, it's a fact time serves the purpose of a little of the total eternal centrifugal one-dimensional framework in which we humans live."[57] Higashida seems to concur:

> I'm not so conscious of the flow of time, a holiday of a month is merely one more scene embedded in the past. People who can remember the events of their lives in the correct order, on the other hand, need time to realign their pre-holiday selves with their post-holiday selves.[58]

He also seems to connect the problem of time in reality to the non-time of early audition, as he adds, "I very quickly forget what it is I've just heard. Inside my head there really isn't such a big difference between what I was told just now, and what I heard a long, long time ago."[59] Higashida adds that, "for us, time is as difficult to grasp as picturing a country we've never been to."[60]

The notion of space invites questions for reflection as well. Higashida considers how space impacts time and individuation:

> By the illusion that unless we can find a place to belong, we are going to be alone in this world. Then eventually we get lost, and have to be escorted back to the place we were at, or the person we were with before.[61]

And Mukhopadhyay contemplates the intersection between space and individuation: "My body feels more grounded indoors"[62]—as does Kedar, whose character, Anthony, craves freedom and space yet declares that he does not quite feel ready for it.[63] And in viewing the space he inhabits as "other," we could say, Kedar actually titles one of his books, *Ido in Autismland.*

Mukhopadhyay extends his reflections on space to pondering the relation between cause and effect:

> One experience diffused into the next. And every experience settled in my mind as an example of a natural phenomenon, which laid down the rules of the world. For instance, if I saw a bird on a tree, and, at that very moment, I saw someone walking across the street in front of our gate, I concluded that every time a bird sits on a tree, someone needs to walk across the street.[64]

Reality presents as something to be encountered, confronted even. Kedar explains: "My parents and aides have different strategies to pull me back to reality."[65] And he considers the problem of trying to find interventions to address his actual needs as principally being one of attempting—as his character, Anthony, puts it—his integration with a real world that is both sensorily overwhelming and incredibly boring.[66] Sellin believes his own life takes place from "second-class reality … [from which he sends] messages from worlds below to the people of the straightforward world above."[67] Among the four, Mukhopadhyay has the most to say about this—and he is bitingly cynical:

> Unmattered intellect and consciousness within its puzzle brain; talk about "theory of mind," talk about a spectrum of explanations—all can be found in the famous research papers funded by the yearly walkathons and runathons and singathons ... If they cannot explain something, then it doesn't matter. It remains un mattered.[68]

Mukhopadhyay further elaborates how "he refused everything that belonged to 'the world.'"[69] And he explains how intense intellectual acuity serves as a coping strategy, describing the "mental maps" he creates to mitigate his anxiety: "I have a mental map of how things should happen around me. When they do not take place as expected, the anxiety is no less than any physical pain. It produces an amplified sensation throughout my gut."[70] He provides more detail: "What is a mental map? A mental map is a mental picture I form, which I expect to face in the process of events, so that I am not surprised or shocked at any sudden situations."[71] For, as he confesses, "Sudden situations, which invade my mental map, are like meteors hitting a sublime corner of a peaceful planet."[72] This seems like clear evidence of intense defensive intellectual work. Thus it is impossible, I believe, to avoid the conclusion that autists give us a clear window onto the difficult human transition to reality—and further, that long before coming to reality, there is thought.

Third, we reflect on the **difficulty with individuation**. Needless to say, the problem of the encounter with reality, and of being withdrawn to an internal retreat of thinking, gravely impacts the (already considerable) challenge of individuation. This takes different forms in various people. One form is what we might consider calling a feeling of "no self." Sellin, for example, frequently refers to himself as a "withoutme figure"[73]—even as a "withoutme being from the kingdom of dark figures."[74] Sellin describes the sensation in greater detail:

> I felt the need to keep myself occupied all the time and did not know what to do with myself when I had no work to do. I was feeling lost without any activity ... in difficult moments of internal restlessness I always withdraw into me withoutme.[75]

For Kedar, this is about how, "New environments throw off the chance of success because the body isn't able to memorize the sequence. It isn't a lack of understanding. It is a horrible body control deficit."[76] I believe Mukhopadhyay describes a similar sensation: "The travel in the world of thoughts had increased. The imaginations took shape and form to a virtual existence of his self in that world."[77] This feeling even leads him to reflect how he "refused to accept the existence of his body and imagined himself to be a spirit."[78] The sense of being disembodied is palpable.

And while it may be of limited value to try to categorize the various manifestations of the difficulty with individuation, a substantially different experience seems to highlight the issue of anxiety as contagion for what we might call the "fused self." I believe that Sellin explains this perfectly:

> I do not distinguish between their [other people's] anxiety and mine[,]it smells unpleasant and it transfers itself to me[,]anxiety is the cause of loveless people the cause of harshness and terror[,]I can't live in peace and quiet with this anxiety[,]I must scream anxiety gives the boxed in feelings the upper hand and they stifle me[,]I am withoutme I am a slave to the vast force of anxiety.[79]

For his part, Kedar has observations of a similar phenomenon. For example, he divulges that his character, Anthony, when learning to type, felt less and less able to rely on his mother as a communication partner whenever she became more anxious or especially stressed.[80] Kedar is incredibly specific in describing how Anthony feels, stating that he (i.e., Anthony) wishes more than anything that he could tell his mother the truth about his own fragility, and the extent to which he so easily absorbs her anxiety that it starts to feel like the anxiety is his own.[81] He also reflects on how one of Anthony's aides was, in contrast to his mother, someone whose steadfast and peaceful disposition was critical to enabling his success, releasing his potential.[82] He concludes that, "in autism we get so affected by the moods of others."[83]

In turn, a third type of problematic individuation might be called the experience of "two selves." In this, we include the common phenomenon of autists communicating in the third person: for example, Mukhopadhyay writing as "he," "the boy," or even "Emma" (his recurring story character); Sellin alternating between "I" and "Birger" in his self-descriptions; and Kedar writing autobiographical fiction through "Anthony." But there are other instances of doubling, too. For instance, Mukhopadhyay states that, at one point, "My shadow, I believed, was my greatest companion";[84] and at a new school, he "misses the shadow."[85] He also shares this disclosure from when he was a teenager: "I believed that there was a parallel world behind any mirror which was as real as the world where I stood. I often wondered what mirrors thought of this world."[86] And in one poem, he beseeches his other self, which he knows to be a part of himself, to help guide his actions;[87] in that same work, he adds that, despite his entreaties, the two selves remained separate from one another.[88] The sense of dissociation seems evident. Mukhopadhyay also offers this astounding self-description of the challenges of dissociation:

> He saw himself as two different selves. One was the complete one—the thinking self, which was filled with learnings and feeling. It could feel the sorrows, joys and satisfaction. It could even create the abstractness in the surroundings. But "being in the abstract" had already faded away into a better awareness of the other self. The other self was the acting self that behaved and had no self-control.[89]

Closing this tentative—and perhaps moot—tangential project of categorizing the different experiences of problematic individuation is one we might call a "fragmented self." Here, we again rely on Mukhopadhyay's remarkable insights. He writes that "the fragmented world needed unification, fragmented world of fear and pieces, beyond 'our' understanding and reaches, broken into bits and parts";[90] and how, in a new house,

> the toys looked so different and frightening that the boy stopped playing with them. He could not find any association between things that changed places … It was a very fragmented world for the boy. He could recognize the places first and then related the objects to these places.[91]

We note his specific mention of how fragmentation occurred when associations were lost—and the phenomenal extent to which objects are associated (and able to be used) with(in) an environment.

As we might predict, there is a sense of disconnection between the body—which steadily grows—and the reflective self dwelling securely in its refuge. The result is a body that will not easily comply—a deficit of intention—and which feels almost entirely alien to that self. Kedar explains the feeling of fragmentation in practical terms. Pertaining to speech, for example, he states: "I talk in my mind but my mind doesn't talk to my mouth."[92] And he adds, "My thoughts get lost on the way to my mouth."[93] Kedar elaborates on the challenges of this disconnection: "I live in a world in which my brain is sort of only for thinking and my body needs guidance."[94] He also notes the stunning challenge of remembering that his body has two sides: "I have a habit of washing one hand. I often forget about my right hand and need to be reminded to wash it."[95] In a similar vein, Mukhopadhyay describes how "he felt that his body was scattered and it was difficult to collect it together." He adds that "he saw himself as a hand or as a leg and would turn around to assemble his parts to the whole."[96]

Mukhopadhyay extends his reflections on living as a disconnected self to include the high cost to social inclusion: "I can never play."[97] And he adds bluntly, "I loathed PE!"[98] He also has an incapacity to self-report pain, "to point the place where the pain was."[99] Even "pointing at objects was difficult too, as he pointed only at the letters on the board and could not generalize it with the other things."[100] As experienced, Mukhopadhyay (in alternating views from third to first) relates that "the main difficulty was that the boy was losing control over his body"[101]—because "my body parts do what they will."[102] And reflecting on learning to use his body, he comments, "So this is what they called trying … This wanting to do an activity by using your body."[103] Movingly he concludes, "I am the person, whose body is trapping the freedom that I seek, thought the boy."[104] Thus we can confirm that the problem of individuation and withdrawal are inseparable, as both are intrinsic to a lingering reliance on regression.

B. Anxiety

Paddling ahead of yesterday's chilling rain, I ventured into a small inlet that has all but dried up as winter advances in the Humber River watershed. Other than a narrow opening, the inlet is bounded by reeds about three metres high, stretching for a hundred metres or more. Two coyotes suddenly appeared in front of me, slinking forward on the mud. I was trying to spot the last herons of the season, and they were on the hunt for sleeping ducks. And here we were, with the length of a school gym between us. I've never seen a coyote swim but apparently, they're very skillful. And these were two adults, not scrawny little guys like I'd been seeing for weeks. They took a few more steps towards me and stopped, perhaps assessing me as a potential threat. And assessing them as a potential threat, I started quietly paddling backwards. They seemed to stare even more intently. I paddled harder. But in moving backwards nervously, I hit the shoreline behind me and got stuck in the muck. They resumed advancing steadily in lock-step. With frantic effort, my anxiety rising, I got myself unstuck and managed to paddle forwards again, exiting the inlet as fast as I could. They immediately lost interest in me and resumed pacing the perimeter, as if I had never been there. Apex predator meets apex predator?

On the one hand, these two sizeable coyotes had been cautious, staying close to where they could hide—though they were capable of a devastating attack. I, on the other hand, had lacked the due caution needed in the fall, when bulking up before winter means everything—though I was entirely incapable of a competent defence. Seeking herons, I had forgotten about coyotes. Or am I exaggerating the event? Were they just focused on the ducks, or actually threatened by me? Is withdrawal in the face of the unknown prudent for any living being? Does a measure of anxiety serve as a useful warning that all may not be well in the direction we are heading? And are all lifeforms perpetually walking this perimeter in mind—the fine line between advancing and retreating, in complex interactions wherein it is not always clear who threatens whom?

We will take now stock of anxiety through two considerations: first, as the self-awareness of an anxious disposition and the accompanying fearfulness and restlessness; second, through an exploration of "stims," since they offer a means of withdrawal and/or a way of relieving anxiety. In terms of an initial overview, through his character, Anthony, Kedar describes an anxiety so severe that it makes him unable to move or act;[105] while Mukhopadhyay explains (also in the third person) that "he would have a fear if they [he and his mother] tried a new route."[106] Higashida reveals that "from out of the blue, I get incredibly distressed, burst into tears or just start panicking."[107] And Sellin declares, "I'm just afraid of ordinary things … I'm always scared."[108] As to stims, Kedar identifies the functions of venting and withdrawal: "I need to move and to release energy kinaesthetically … If I'm on my own I retreat to stims";[109] while Higashida points to familiarity: "people with autism get quite a kick out of repetition."[110] For his part, Mukhopadhyay relates stims to the challenge of individuation: "He was not able to find his body. Only if he ran fast or flapped his hands he was able to find his presence."[111] And Sellin discloses the autist's awareness of his own inappropriate responses, his engaging in "kidstuff and lead[ing] a crazy person's life."[112] Overall, anxiety seems to be the crux of the gravest issues that need "management," but trying to consciously self-regulate anxiety is understandably difficult. Ironically, then, the primary obstacle—mutism—becomes relatively secondary.

First, we consider fearfulness and the overwhelming experience of **constantly being anxious**. Sellin describes the sensation vividly:

> Fear comes over me that's all[,] first I have a funny feeling in my stomach then the anxiety comes up on the sky to attack my whole body like a cunning beast … what they call Birger can't get the fear out of his mind.[113]

He also believes fear affects all nonverbal autists: "We are let's say so scared it's a fear like no other";[114] and he implores, "fear of the fear is really there all the time … I do urgently beg you to avoid anxiety situations."[115] The wish for freedom from fear is palpable in Sellin's work: "I would love to be free of the groundless fears[,] I wish for nothing more fervently."[116] There are also signs of catastrophizing in his writing: "I have eyes and I can see so I have been terribly scared and so I didn't want to say any more about that[,] I was afraid of the end of the road and the end of humanity."[117] Seemingly, he is also hinting at a fear of losing continuity.

For Kedar, fear is pervasive: "I still get frightened for nothing."[118] Like Sellin, Kedar also experiences fear as a threat against life itself. And he relates this fear directly to what is new: "I should do more. I always get scared to try."[119] We find a similar reflection in Mukhopadhyay: "It was already frightening to go to new places and see new roads."[120] And here again is a fear of losing continuity with what is known. Like Sellin, Kedar believes fear is an intrinsic component of autism: "Most autistic people have phobias."[121] And Higashida draws a remarkable relation between the defence of the intellectual retreat and fear: "There's also the dread that by being touched our thoughts will become visible … We put up a barricade around ourselves to keep people out."[122]

Living in fear and self-awareness of one's social missteps leads to sadness, shame and hypersensitivity to ridicule. Sellin says of himself (in the third person), "Birger is so sensitive that he can't stand anything that disturbs him."[123] For Kedar, this acute sensitivity tragically gives way to self-loathing: "Life is hard to predict. Even harder to count on … Inside I get sad and edgy and I know I must fight it. My limitations irritate me so much. I lose myself in rotten resentment";[124] elsewhere he adds, "Internally I'm so sad. I hate my situation in life."[125] In turn, Mukhopadhyay relates the tension that this fear evokes in relation to the need to protect the inner self: "The special needs heart tells the special needs mind to be careful, lest it smoke out its own emotions."[126] And Higashida conveys the devastating interaction between fear, anxiety and shame: "However tiny the mistake, for me it's a massive deal … the fact of it starts rushing towards me like a tsunami … To get away, I'll do anything … I hate myself. I just hate myself."[127] Higashida also relates the following: "My motive for running off when I was younger was that I hated myself so much that I didn't want anyone else even to see me."[128] And he concludes: "If I tried to describe what it's like to be non-verbal in the World of the Verbal in a single word, I'd choose this one: agony."[129]

There is considerable restlessness associated with this anxiety as well. Mukhopadhyay confesses: "When temptation grows big, my Titoistic field grows with it";[130] and in a story, he elaborates through his character, Emma, that wishes grow into expectations that generate impatience to have them fulfilled.[131] Mukhopadhyay reflects on how anxiety builds over time: "The body grew like a prison, trapping all the anxiety and heat within its own limits."[132] And Kedar explains how anxiety and shame intersect, increasing in time: "You need to show your skills, anxiety hides them. Then people conclude that we don't have them."[133] He adds, "I find it hard to speak, control my body or my anxiety. How else would people who can't control their body speak, initiate, and are consumed by anxiety act than like we do."[134] Adding to the issue, "some treatments make anxiety worse,"[135] states Kedar—even, some individuals: "I need to trust the person who helps me or I get very anxious."[136]

Uncannily, Kedar even offers a new direction for research that is compatible with the present project: "I just can't relate when my anxiety is overpowering me. So this is one request to all researchers: start looking into anxiety. I think it may be a key to solving the riddle of autism."[137] Kedar is clear that this is not his problem alone:

> It's obvious to anyone who spends time with an autistic kid that we are always anxious … I see kids flee and flap and cry and scream. They have no good outlet for strong tensions so anxiety is a symptom of autism … I'm anxious twenty-four hours a day.[138]

And he provides this remarkable summation that draws together fear, shame and anxiety: "The struggle for emotional control is always with me … the momentum keeps moving me onward. Once I stop I feel so embarrassed or sorry. The triggers can be silly to others. Inside, they are serious. I get nervous. It overflows."[139]

Sellin, too, is aware that he is "bursting with restlessness and impatience"[140]—and he refers to his "murderous exhausting anxiety";[141] "crazy total anxiety";[142] and "stereotypical anxiety."[143] Anxiety is actually predictable as the massive energy build-ups remain trapped, prevented from venting adequately through language. Sellin seems acutely cognisant that his own anxiety is rooted in "the agitation of not being able to reply to talking people."[144] And he asks: "Do you really know how deep-rooted anxiety can be in an individual, the way it eats away an individual, the way it works personally on a single person at the collapse of the first agonizing words"?[145] Sellin is truly remarkable in his insights. For example, he recalls the early origins of his anxiety in early childhood:[146] "The first thing to cause the anxiety was many years ago when I came home from the Wiesengrund Hospital then I was afraid of everything."[147]

Sellin draws the full landscape of regression, invoking the sense of being boxed-in (the retreat), the anxiety that ensues, and the resort to screaming (i.e., to some form of oral expression) for venting the tremendous surplus of energy that progressively builds up:

> Great depths of restless force … as long as I can remember the restlessness has been there a force like no one can imagine … when I was even smaller my

> stereotypical behaviour was a little help … [but] these mechanisms don't work so well any more[,] that is why I've been screaming so much recently … I can't live in peace and quiet with this anxiety[,] I must scream[,] anxiety gives the boxed in feelings the upper hand and they stifle me[,] I am a slave to the vast force of anxiety.[148]

In that thought is a refuge and an internal means of venting energy, Sellin finds solace in chasing questions—i.e., in a plan or phantasy of displacement:

> One anxiety I suffer from most of all is how to survive a day … I for my part protect against the icy times of day by setting up a socalled steely important list of questions[,] an idiot system as it were running away from anxiety.[149]

Second, we examine "**stims**" and their function for someone with a surplus of anxiety and a reduced capacity for venting due to mutism. As we will discover from the start, the word "stim" seems to be an unfortunate misnomer. For rather than "stimulate" the individual (as the word suggests), stims actually use up energy, dispersing it. We will thus find stims used for self-calming, making reality disappear and venting energy; we will also encounter, as predicted, the signature of the primary processes in the powerful component of repetition in stims.[150]

Kedar's character, Anthony, engages in stimming for self-calming[151]—primarily flapping.[152] And Kedar discloses that flapping is his own "most embedded stim."[153] Kedar describes how stims release energy: "I treat stims like a welcomed friend because they are really with me all the time … I feel forces like waves of sensory energy."[154] One of Higashida's book titles is actually inspired by his own favourite stim: *The Reason I Jump*. Like Kedar, Mukhopadhyay favours flapping: "I never quite understood why others did not find it as relaxing as I find while flapping my hands. Stresses and strains just start melting away leaving me light as air while I flap my hands."[155] And he is uncanny in assessing stimming as a substitute for venting, hinting at the share of dream-work at play:

> My risk-taking hands had nothing to do but flap until they had an opportunity to take more risks. Taking risks becomes a necessity when the world opens its eyes and yawns. The Earth can't be bored … I could at least keep it awake.[156]

Mukhopadhyay also draws a relation between stimming and the retreat to safety: "The hand had made a strange relationship with its shadow and he fluttered it and spent his hours, contented with the lone company of his shadow."[157] His insights invite the consideration of stims as a means of making reality disappear, so to speak, through a kind of daydreaming that remains accessible and prominent in mental life. For example, Mukhopadhyay stims to try to block out noise, to "flap away the sound with greater frequency."[158] While Kedar's character, Anthony, reacts to his ABA teacher by deploying a wild array of stims, trying to make her disappear from his reality.[159] Elsewhere, Kedar clearly expresses this very function of stims:

"I am so needy to escape reality and stims take me to another world."[160] For Kedar, stimming can even relieve the experience of suffering, for his character, Anthony, stims by whirling to get rid of his own pain.[161] I believe Kedar is also alluding to the critical relation between the need to vent and the need for defence, in stating that bolting can serve in the absence of speech. He puts things even more bluntly in a summation of the problem of the symbolizing human being who, due to regression, is unable to initiate: "I understood most things but I knew I was trapped and could not show I understood. It forced me to stim more because I had to live inwardly."[162]

Yet despite their salvific function in liberating energy, stims carry a highly problematic stigma. Kedar writes that his character, Anthony, was a social misfit who kept lining things up and constantly stimmed.[163] Kedar also calls stims "stupid and pointless and only a distraction from life, not a tool to live by."[164] At issue is that stims do not produce something useful—the activity does not easily lead to another that is valued by others and/or by the self. Further, the need for venting is driven by primary processes (to self-regulate the system), so stimming is not easily brought under conscious control. And insofar as primary processes hold sway, any stim involves a long string of repetitions. So, as Sellin reports, "It keeps making me repeat things all the time to hiss[,] do kidstuff and lead a crazy person's life[,] it's like an eternal battle."[165] The urge is understandably formidable, as Higashida says: "My impulse to recreate this sequence trumps the knowledge that I've been told not to do it, and I end up doing it again."[166]

Kedar elaborates: "I think the one challenge is the intense OCD aspect of these stimmy episodes. It is hard to resist";[167] and even his character, Anthony, finds himself unable to resist his compulsions.[168] Predictably, with age comes an increasing quantum of energy that is being withheld and seeks release, so as Kedar's Anthony describes it, the compulsions only rose in prominence as he got older.[169] Add to this the years of daily frustrations, as Kedar shares: "It's harder to stop stims when I am stressed";[170] he adds, "I'm overly stimmy if I'm nervous, like over-charged electrical energy."[171] Kedar is acutely aware that a tremendous force outside his conscious control drives the need for venting energy through stims. Kedar also reveals the following: "Stims are not predictable. They have internal drives I don't foresee. One day one stim is dominant. Soon another takes its place. I can't predict which will come but it's not hard to transfer to a new one."[172]

We detect here the signature of primary processes, as energy can be transferred from one mode of venting to another by association. I believe it also follows that stims will be predictably repetitive rather than innovative. That said, someone may have a set of preferred stims, and new stims can be introduced through creative thinking and/or daydreaming. For example, Mukhopadhyay reveals how he learned a new stim: "He got the idea of spinning from the fan as he saw that its blades that were otherwise separate joined together to a complete circle when they turned in speed."[173]

In brief, movement must be maintained to self-regulate massive amounts of internal energy. As Mukhopadhyay puts it, "movements are better than stagnation";[174] therefore, he says, "I needed … to keep myself on the move."[175] And Higashida draws a beautiful analogy that connects the need for venting with some classic outward manifestations of nonverbal autism:

> Most people look pretty relaxed when they're not doing anything in particular, but we're always zooming off madly … We're like cicadas who'll miss the summer unless we hurry, hurry, hurry … We cry our hearts out, shout our heads off, and never rest in our battle against time.[176]

Here is anxiety, then, right at the encounter with reality (i.e., time and space). In fact, the management of anxiety is a significant challenge for the nonverbal autist, while defences are limited by the inability to speak. Kedar's character, Anthony, provides an apt analysis of the confluence of retreat and anxiety that marks the nonverbal autist's necessary reliance on regression as a defence, as he explains that, in a moment of panic, this anxiety rises until it seems to crash over him—so he runs and stims, flapping wildly, and in such terrible moments, his ability for thinking rationally seems to leave him.[177]

In concluding this chapter on regression and anxiety, we confirm from these nonverbal autists the enduring power and presence of primary processes. It seems, then, that these become more apparent when the transition to conscious reality has somehow been impeded. For while we can reasonably infer that there is a time-limited window in which to transition to reality (normatively) to enable conscious volition (including the motor act of speech), unconscious processes always remain active, securing our self-regulation—survival. Equally compelling is the unarguable fact that the nonverbal autist is mute but thinking. Thus, Dolto's bold theorization is confirmed by their eloquent testimony: intelligent, creative thought is continuously vibrant beneath all appearances. In effect, thinking *is* the refuge.

Notes

1 This formulation is credited to the American physiologist, Walter Cannon, in 1932 (or as early as 1914–1915).
2 Schauer & Elbert 2010, 111.
3 Ibid.
4 Ibid, 112.
5 Ibid.
6 Ibid.
7 Ibid.
8 Ibid, 120; of particular concern and relevance here is the contagion of anxiety, as discussed by Dolto.
9 Ibid.
10 Dolto 1971, 214; Djéribi-Valentin & Kouki 1998, 219.
11 In De Mezamat 2008.
12 In De Sauverzac 1987, 109.
13 "Languaged" is a highly productive adjective for Dolto: e.g., "languaged affects" (Dolto 1984, 48); "languaged cloth [of a text]" (Dolto 1985d, 531); "languaged filiation" (in Halmos 1994, 44; Caldaguès 1982, 67); "languaged illnesses" (F. Dolto 1989,

61; Dolto 1984, 85); "languaged landmarks" (Dolto 1986a, 117; Guillerault 1997, 41); and "languaged means" (Dolto 1985d, 83–84).

14 Dolto 1985a, 283.

15 In Caldaguès 1982, 118.

16 Needless to say, commands to execute simple, routinized actions (e.g., as in ABA) do not constitute authentic language; it should be evident that Dolto means genuine words, creative and warm, that embed the individual in a nurturing social group.

17 1995, 25.

18 2012, 58.

19 2017, 61.

20 2000, 11.

21 2012, 97.

22 2000, 5.

23 1995, 193.

24 2017, 58

25 1995, 101.

26 2000, 20.

27 The preface to Kedar's novel includes a disclaimer that Anthony is not him but strongly draws from his own experiences and those of others. I respect Kedar's valuable insights, shared through Anthony, by identifying them as such in each case.

28 2018, 21.

29 2007/2013, 147.

30 In many of the citations from these autistic authors, there are atypical grammatical forms: for example, Sellin never capitalizes "I" and omits apostrophes. Rather than cluttering citations with the usual editorial marker (i.e., [sic]), I have opted to clean up capitals and punctuation (only). I hesitated on this point for some time, then concluded that dignity is better served without highlighting simple errors that might disturb readers' sensibilities during the conveyance of these authors' important content. Interested readers are encouraged to consult these writers' works for the original orthography. I keep untouched any new compounds suggested in their material (e.g., Sellin's "withoutme") and use [sic] only for misspellings; I have also added commas to overly long strings to enhance readability and I have indicated where I have done so as [,]. Admittedly, I also have practical considerations in that "autocorrect" keeps reversing these errors, risking further errors.

31 1995, 178.

32 Ibid, 25.

33 Ibid, 23.

34 Ibid, 26–27.

35 2018, 33.

36 2000, 19. When Mukhopadhyay uses the expression, "the boy," I strongly believe that he is speaking of himself in the third person—and that these are autobiographical reflections, not fiction (see also note below).

37 1995, 91.

38 Ibid, 50.

39 Ibid, 95.

40 Ibid, 101.

41 Ibid, 102.

42 Ibid, 26.

43 Ibid, 24

44 Ibid, 25.

45 2017, 264.

46 2000, 15.

47 Ibid, 28. To stress, when Mukhopadhyay uses "he" in these and other reflections, I strongly believe that he means himself; these are autobiographical rather than fictional expressions. In fact, throughout his writing, Mukhopadhyay seamlessly alternates viewpoints between "I," "he," and "the boy" (see also note above).
48 2008, 11.
49 I would respectfully like to suggest that Mukhopadhyay's character, Emma, is a familiar (recurrent) dream; his narratives are a melodic fusion of autobiography and phantasy, with hardly any line between—many recalling his childhood in India.
50 2005, 197.
51 Ibid, 203.
52 2000, 9.
53 Ibid, 9.
54 Ibid, 48.
55 Ibid, 59.
56 2005, 188.
57 1995, 80.
58 2017, 125.
59 2007/2013, 23.
60 Ibid, 95.
61 Ibid, 130.
62 2008, 139.
63 2018, 264.
64 2008, 7.
65 2012, 147.
66 2018, 17.
67 1995, 25.
68 2015b.
69 2000, 6.
70 2008, 210.
71 Ibid, 191.
72 Ibid, 191.
73 1995, 225.
74 Ibid, 25.
75 Ibid, 188.
76 2012, 160.
77 2000, 17.
78 Ibid, 15.
79 1995, 185.
80 2018, 230.
81 Ibid, 232.
82 Ibid, 202.
83 2012, 138.
84 2008, 20.
85 2000, 64.
86 2005, 150.
87 2000, 46.
88 Ibid, 50.
89 Ibid, 50.
90 Ibid, 56.
91 Ibid, 9.
92 2012, 47.
93 Ibid, 89.

94 Ibid, 101.
95 Ibid, 88.
96 2000, 20.
97 2005, 208.
98 2015a, 60.
99 2000, 17.
100 Ibid, 26.
101 Ibid, 17.
102 2015a, 57.
103 2000, 40.
104 Ibid, 14.
105 2018, 229.
106 2000, 7.
107 2007/2013, 63.
108 1995, 51.
109 2012, 45.
110 2007/2013, 109.
111 2000, 20.
112 1995, 26.
113 Ibid, 29.
114 Ibid, 57.
115 Ibid, 145.
116 Ibid, 218.
117 Ibid, 72.
118 2011c.
119 2011b.
120 2000, 6.
121 2012, 93.
122 2007/2013, 56.
123 1995, 52.
124 2011d.
125 2012, 44.
126 2015a, 82.
127 2007/2013, 65.
128 2017, 227.
129 Ibid, 89 (capitalization his).
130 2015a, 40.
131 2005, 211.
132 2008, 68.
133 2012, 59.
134 Ibid, 69.
135 Ibid, 60.
136 Ibid, 61.
137 Ibid, 60.
138 Ibid, 59.
139 2011a.
140 1995, 57.
141 Ibid, 149.
142 Ibid, 118.
143 Ibid, 118.
144 Ibid, 86.
145 Ibid, 80.

146 From the age of about 30 to 36 months, Sellin spent six months in the hospital (see ibid, 7–8).
147 Ibid, 106.
148 Ibid, 30.
149 Ibid, 29.
150 Related to stims are the autist's perseverative interests and repeated activities. As one researcher puts it, "every autist has a fixation or a ritualization" (Perrin 2015, 11); a new form of therapy for autism based on this assumption privileges, "affinity as a constructive solution" (R. Suskind in ibid, 18). The experiences of the renowned journalist and Pulitzer Prize winner, Ron Suskind, with his son, Owen, are chronicled in his beautifully written and highly informative autism memoir (2014).
151 2018, 146.
152 Ibid, 6.
153 2012, 43.
154 Ibid, 42.
155 2012, 44.
156 2015a, 59.
157 2000, 5.
158 Ibid, 11.
159 2018, 110.
160 2012, 42.
161 2018, 152.
162 2012, 57.
163 2018, 225.
164 2012, 101.
165 1995, 26.
166 2007/2013, 137.
167 2012, 147.
168 2018, 2.
169 Ibid, 114.
170 2012, 43.
171 Ibid, 139.
172 Ibid, 43–44.
173 2000, 20.
174 Ibid, 60.
175 Ibid, 68.
176 2007/2013, 100.
177 2018, 149.

Chapter 5

Auditory Influence

Preliminary Words

By adulthood, it's highly likely that most of us will have played a word association game at a social gathering. Out of curiosity, or even as part of an employment screening, many people may have also taken word-association tests. Such tools proliferate online these days, offering to help test-takers discover something hidden about their personalities. In effect, the idea that words are connected by associations has become commonly accepted knowledge. On the one hand, these games and tests are a long way from the careful analysis of word associations in dreams and therapy that Freud first devised. On the other hand, they are close in one vital respect because they require instantaneous responses. For word-association to "work," so to speak, it's important to avoid deliberate thinking and say what first comes to mind, without reflection. Interestingly, this means that a crucial fact about thought is already in wide public circulation: beneath rational thought—where ideas are linked logically—there is a deeper, much older, form of thought where words are linked associatively. And while associative thinking is enduring, it is often overridden by conscious filters that are, in every way, a secondary development in our mental and emotional lives.

As a result of needing a long apprenticeship to conscious social life, children lack such filters—as is well-known by all who care for them and work with them. And throughout the lengthy process whereby consciousness becomes reliably installed—i.e., for at least the first two years of life outside the womb, if not longer—a child's most accessible (and dominant) form of thought is under the managing influence of unconscious processes: it is associative thinking. Associative thinking, as we have already considered it with Freud and Dolto, is the result of two crucial developments, both of which begin during gestation. The first is precocious audition, by which phonemes become objects for dream-work and seed pre-conscious symbolization. The second is unconscious triangulation, by which affect circulates continuously through displacement and condensations, using associations as nodes or switch-points. The phonemes that make up words in any language are essential to establishing and proliferating associative thinking—through furnishing countless "objects"—and this vital process begins months before birth.

DOI: 10.4324/9781032655123-11

Therefore, associative thinking is defining of our intellectual life—it is formative. And even when, through maturation, conscious thought takes precedence, our capacity for associative thinking remains as a lifelong potential below consciousness, exerting its very powerful influence—sight unseen.

Understanding phonemes is crucial to a better appreciation of associative thinking. Thus, we will turn now to Edward Sapir, widely considered to be one of the most brilliant linguists in the history of the field.[1] Sapir is well-known for his theorization of the phoneme in the traditional linguistic sense, so we begin with his definition: "The concept of the 'phoneme' [is] a functionally significant unit in the rigidly defined pattern or configuration of sounds peculiar to a language."[2] He elaborates:

> Phonemes are built up into distinct and arbitrary sequences which are at once recognized by speakers as meaningful symbols of reference ... While the mechanical functional units of language are phonemes, the true units of language as symbolism are conventional groupings of such phonemes.[3]

We can hear in his words a significant relation between symbolism and phonemes. And we can also confirm that phonemes, while varying between languages, are in fact foundational to every language:

> The phonemes of a language are ... peculiar to the given language, and its words must be made up, in unconscious theory if not always in actualized behavior, of these phonemes. Languages differ very widely in their phonemic structure. But ... there is no known language which has not a perfectly definite phonemic system.[4]

The phoneme, as Sapir describes it, is not strictly a conscious entity but rather one with unconscious concomitants. And he offers this further insight: "In the physical world[,] the naïve speaker and hearer actualize and are sensitive to sounds, but what they feel themselves to be pronouncing and hearing are 'phonemes,'"[5] as members of a language group have "phonemic intuitiveness."[6] And it is precisely here, in this notion of what ordinary speakers feel themselves to be pronouncing—and what ordinary listeners feel themselves to be hearing—that we locate Dolto's highly productive interpretation and application of the phoneme.

Sapir clarifies: "Phonetic phenomena are not physical phenomena ... [it is] the intuitively felt and communicated forms which alone give significance to such expression."[7] In other words, right from the infant's first exposure, phonemes have an intuitive dimension that they retain even as the child acquires mature competencies. He elaborates:

> Language is not merely articulated sound; its significant structure is dependent upon the unconscious selection of a fixed number of "phonetic stations" or sound units ... Through the unconscious selection of sounds as phonemes,

> definite psychological barriers are erected between various phonetic stations, so that speech ceases to be an expressive flow of sound and becomes a symbolic composition.[8]

In addition, Sapir points decisively to the relation between phonemes and precocious audition:

> Auditory-motor associations are probably always latent at the least, that is, they are unconsciously brought into play. Even those who read and think without the slightest use of sound imagery are, at last analysis, dependent on it. They are merely handling the circulating medium … of the fundamental auditory symbols.[9]

I believe we can also find evidence that Sapir ascribes to phonemes a distinct role in the circulation of unconscious affect, in his emphasis on how unconscious associations antedate speech. For, like Dolto, Sapir reflects in his own way on the vibrant current of affect circulating beneath conscious speech:

> Volition and emotion are … never absent from normal speech, but their expression is not of a truly linguistic nature … There are socially accepted feeling-tones, or ranges of feeling-tone, for many words over and above the force of individual association, but they are exceedingly variable and elusive things.[10]

It is precisely because phonemes factor in our earliest mental and emotional life that they become so indispensable to pre-conscious symbolization. As Sapir puts it, "a truly deep symbolism, for instance, does not depend on the verbal associations of a particular language but rests securely on an intuitive basis that underlies all linguistic expression."[11] He extends his valuable considerations further:

> Most words, like practically all elements of consciousness, have an associated feeling-tone, a mild, yet none the less real and at times insidiously powerful, derivative of pleasure or pain. This feeling-tone, however, is not as a rule an inherent value in the word itself; it is rather a sentimental growth on the word's true body, on its conceptual kernel. Not only may the feeling-tone change from one age to another … but it varies remarkably from individual to individual according to the personal association of each, varies, indeed, from time to time in a single individual's consciousness as his experiences mold him and his moods change.[12]

I believe that Sapir is highlighting how our precocious experiences with phonemes charge them with affect. And by making a reference to the securing of pleasure, he is arguably sourcing this affect in instinctive drives. He also roots the word's conceptual kernel deep in the unconscious, while being specific that these affective roots are highly idiosyncratic, leading to elusive and variable associations in our individual experiences with words in conscious reality. Sapir also explains how he believes the unconscious roots of phonemes influence language acquisition and use:

> The symbolic expression of thought may in some cases run along outside the fringe of the conscious mind … the appropriate paths of association … are touched off so lightly during the process of thought as not to rise into consciousness … modern psychology has shown us how powerfully symbolism is at work in the unconscious mind.[13]

And as phonemes are unconsciously rooted, Sapir further reflects on the consequential role of words in associative thinking:

> That an association once established by historical causes will be felt as a direct and simple psychological association is quite obvious, also that it may become productive, by analogy, of further associations of a related sort … by virtue of the inherent associative value of the otherwise unconnected phenomena in the mind of a particular individual or group of individuals. Such an individual association, if given an outward expression, can become socialized.[14]

Sapir is speaking about the productivity of associations in proliferating further associations—and how associations that are idiosyncratic can nonetheless be impacted through usage in the social within specific language communities. I suggest that we have here the foundation of how familial influences nurture some associations over others—and we can infer some effects of changes in the familial environment. This concurs with Dolto's important suggestion that certain phonemes (as objects) can lure the infant's affective engagement—whereas some objects in which the infant has pre-invested affect may not be offered (i.e., findable) in the sonar landscape of his reality. Sapir shares the following from his abundant field work:

> In the case of certain individuals more than 50 distinct "words" were found to build up a constellated system in which the meanings were rather obviously the results of certain intuitively felt symbolic relations between the varied sounds. In the case of other individuals actual word associations tended to creep in, but on the whole there was surprisingly little evidence of this factor. The subjects were found to differ a great deal in their ability to hold on without effort to a constellation once formed and to fit new meanings into it consistently with the symbolisms expressed in previous responses. Some would give identically the same response for a stimulus word that had been—so it was claimed—forgotten … Others lost their moorings very rapidly … [in] variations of sensitivity to sound symbolism, i.e., to the potential meaningfulness of relations in sound sets.[15]

Through his detailed description, Sapir is offering a formidably valuable statement on how words, through their associations, comprise mental constellations that facilitate both memory (i.e., the retention of prior objects and relations)—and learning (i.e., the engagement with new objects). I believe it is also evident here that meaning is being ascribed to sounds due to "intuitively felt symbolic relations," as he puts it.

In other words, phonemes make unconscious suggestions to thinking, by which we can better understand their spectacular role in symbolism. Needless to say, the "suggestibility of a child,"[16] as Dolto herself observed, has profound implications. For children receive suggestions not just *on* but *from* phonemes, investing words with a truth that both exceeds and precedes rational thought.[17] The result is that, during early childhood, some core beliefs about one's world and familiars are formed by the natural suggestions of phonemes, as facilitated by associative thinking. Furthermore, unbeknownst to the adult, these illogical but highly potent memorials of childhood remain perpetually dormant below conscious thought.

Also noteworthy in Sapir's words is the sense of slippage from consciousness—i.e., the forgetting—of the source of such unconscious symbolism. Sapir offers a useful summation of this phenomenon:

> There is in all languages a certain randomness of association. Thus, the idea of "hide" may also be expressed by the word "conceal," the notion of "three times" also by "thrice" ... Sooner or later the less frequently occurring associations are ironed out at the expense of the more vital ones. In other words, all languages have an inherent tendency to economy of expression ... All grammars leak.[18]

Leaky grammars, to borrow Sapir's wonderful term, make it more challenging to try to rationalize or quantify language acquisition and usage. For what Sapir emphasized throughout his professional life is the intrinsically rogue, unquantifiable role of unconscious symbolization that inheres in the phonemes of anyone's mother tongue. This inscription invests a powerful legacy in the words comprising these phonemes. Thus, far below consciousness, the role of associations through phonemes—and suggestions on phonemes—is formative in the precocious development of symbolism that, once installed, is enduring.

What Dolto adds to these considerations around phonemes, crucially, is the archaic triangular situation. As discussed, the earliest objects are experienced when the infant is unconscious and indissociable from his "like-me," with whom he co-experiences all objects. So we can functionally describe an unconscious triangulation of the pre-self, the "like-me" and the phoneme. From the child's birth, even the phonemes of his name are triangulated between his pre-self and "like me," for affect is displaced and diffused through progressive triangulations—as associations scaffold affect from prior to new objects—during the process of coming to reality. In her inimitable style, Dolto describes this phenomenon in 1956:

> This permanent self that carries the reference of the phonemes of the name of the subject constitutes itself with the rapports, mass to mass with the mother ... then with the things in contact with the body and around the body, which brings perceptions of its cutaneous limits and which are associated, more or less, to the mother.[19]

Thus, the earliest affect circulating during gestation becomes intrinsically woven with words, as language becomes unconsciously formative in the gradual maturation of the human infant.

From here, the child engages increasingly wider fields in triangulation via the proliferation of associations to pre-invested objects. And as early as 1949, Dolto articulated how the child moves from the archaic to his full presentification in reality as a function of triangulation with this (m)other, from whom he remains indissociable mentally and emotionally, even as birth detaches his body from hers:

> The object of fixation is, at this stage, the maternal object—the only intermediary between the world and the child—in a mode of relation of the type participation experienced in totality ... It is the stage of unconscious identification, unconscious life. The child certainly exists, in fact, but does not feel himself to exist any more in reality than in phantasms.[20]

Dolto's emphasis on the continued influence of the unconscious—that is, on the securing dream-work of the archaic—reminds us that birth is only a transition for the body of the infant. In contrast, his mental and emotional transition will require more than the physical separation of birth. For just as the child remains dependent on his mother (or a near substitute) for his nutrition, he remains dependent on her—unconsciously indissociable—for the continuity of affective circulation that he needs but is not yet capable of providing for himself. Put another way, just as the infant is not yet physically self-sustaining, he is not yet affectively self-sustaining. This is precisely why Dolto refers to the need to provide the infant with an alimentation of words. For more than anything, a transition to reality will require the progressive offer of suitable objects (from his outer world, his new reality) that are continuous with the affectively pre-invested objects of his inner world.

Of course, the transition to reality will be easier to achieve if the newborn is already invested in the objects of his reality through his pre-conscious activity, as a result of a normative progression during gestation. If, instead, he is deeply or substantially regressed at birth, his affective investments will be tethered to the most archaic objects of dream-work and his progression will be delayed as a result, or at least somewhat (or substantially) impeded. So it will be harder for him to be lured to reality—to recognize objects in his new reality with sufficient unconscious associations to the objects in which he is already affectively invested in order to, in turn, invest in what is new. Yet until this transition is completed—i.e., the substantial shifting of affect from objects of dream-work to objects of reality—the child will necessarily live between two worlds. And insofar as phonemes are the most valuable to the transition to reality because of the prominence of precocious audition in furnishing objects for dream-work during the archaic stage of human maturation, then it will be interhuman language—with its interminable unconscious current—that will best ensure his unconscious security in his new environment.

The result is that language is far more than words. It is a deeply tethered force that acts within and through the social—our interhuman interactions. Language is impacted by our unconscious histories and, reciprocally, the unconscious roots of phonemes influence our conscious histories. That is why Dolto is adamant that the human species is foremost a languaged being. That is also why she stresses that unconscious interhuman exchanges nurture the continuous affective circulation that is so essential not only to our individual survival, but to our capacity to experience happiness through living.

Further, on Dolto's view, it is actually the alternation of the mother's presence and absence during the transition to reality that scaffolds the infant's slow individuation—and his speaking:

> He discovers what remains of his mother when she is not there ... He is the remainder of his mother, functioning and giving him security. The mother is thus present in all laryngeal movements that produce the phonemes concerning these objects ... perceptions associate themselves in language...[as] the mother tongue is integrated to the child.[21]

The logical inference is that if she never "leaves"—i.e., if he remains unconsciously indissociable with her due to his transition to reality being impeded because he was born somewhat or substantially regressed—then the alternation of presence and absence cannot readily happen. And because audition exists *in utero* but not sight, as Dolto firmly believes (as abundantly noted), the "conditions of presence and absence ... depend on audition only."[22] In sum, language has a truly formidable role. First, audition is what determines the presence or absence of the indissociable (m)other. Second, this rhythm is essential to the necessary transition from indissociability that enables speech. Dolto elaborates:

> The child is always one of the poles of a triangulation. If it is missing, he cannot have *connaissance*[23] of himself, nor knowledge of the other as such. Maternal security introjects itself in the child and becomes the "you" of that which is "me" ... If there is no "you" for this person thanks to which I am "me," the child cannot arrive at an Ego that expresses the sense of "me-I" ... The human being thus has his roots in his relation to the other, his first other, in the communication of unconciousnesses.[24]

Here in language, then, we can detect a difficult tension between being indissociable versus being unconsciously secure enough to individuate. We can also notice the telltale marking, in grammar, of incomplete individuation through problem pronouns: speaking as "he" or "you," instead of "I." I believe autists, their familiars and their educators will readily recognize this signature communication style in autists capable of some speech.[25]

Thus we arrive at the crux of the matter. The phoneme has a formative role in the ontogeny and continuity of associative thinking; every time we speak (or write), we cannot help but leave traces of our idiosyncratic history of unconsciously invested phonemes, disseminating affect through the accidental transference in texts of latent material; unconscious affect is therefore circulating wildly in human language, and it is experienceable through words by a listener (or reader); and we are driven by primary processes (for the purpose of sustaining the affective circulation ensuring our self-regulation) to being lured by the unconscious echoes of our invested phonemes. This provokes a paramount question about reading: might an author (or corpus) serve as a good-enough witness-in-similitude to scaffold individuation?

In this chapter, we continue exploring the texts of our four nonverbal autistic authors. First, we locate their deep affective investment in phonemes, as evidenced through a love of language and play with words and letters. We also observe—as predicted—a consuming passion for reading and stories, in that these offer a sense of security. Second, we consider the vibrancy of mental and emotional life under the jurisdiction of primary processes, wherein a human being is in a state of utter passivity. In this condition of fusion (i.e., indissociability), dream-work nourishes symbolization, leading to highly creative thought as "objects" from the environment—especially, words—are engaged. Thus, despite the grave difficulty with initiation, continuous learning happens through what we can call a "passive education." Yet in surviving a non-normative transition to conscious reality in infancy, it seems that the nonverbal autist is relegated to perpetually living in the liminal zone between dreams and reality—that is, in a thriving space for thinking replete with archaic echoes.

A. Phonemes

Last week, on one of the warmest October days in memory, I passed a lone Canada goose on the shores of the Humber River. It seemed strange that he was alone for geese are incredibly social. But I paddled away into the sunshine. As I got into my rhythm, dipping left then right, I found my thoughts drifting to Mother Goose, read in my mother('s) tongue, as Perrault's «Les Contes de ma mère l'Oye.» At some nebulous moment in this daydream, as soft waves lapped my kayak, Jemima Puddle-Duck came to mind. Was it in association with Mother Goose? Or because I passed some sleeping ducks? Aesop's "The Goose that Laid the Golden Egg" also "arrived" briefly. I then remembered countless times I have stopped my car for a mother goose and her goslings to cross—and that one time I came so close to hitting a lone swan waddling across the road. Then I was back to pondering what might be wrong with that lone goose. Moments later, I came upon a gaggle of 18–20. They seemed to be enjoying the weather as much as I was, whereas the other gaggles left about a week ago.

I carried on further before turning around, so that on my return two hours later, I passed the solitary goose again—same spot, same posture. I got almost close enough to touch him and he only took two steps. He did not try to fly or swim—and, most notable for a goose, he did not try to nip me. While he seemed fine physically, I noticed a band on his left leg. Had he just been released from tagging? On a Saturday? Had he been left behind by a departed gaggle? Or had the remaining gaggle banished him? Do geese do that? I was determined to Google it (the play with "gaggle" only hit me later)—and a search quickly suggested itself after

I typed just two words: "*Do geese* get ostracized?" I immediately felt swept up in a thousand people's stories. Who knew stranded geese were so common? It was my first—and the prognosis was not good. Ostensibly, it was likely injured or ill in ways I could not detect, or it had lost its mate. This second possibility sent me into a tailspin of resentment—what injustice to exclude an individual for having no mate! And off I went on another thought tangent. All this, thanks to a solitary goose.

Yet while that unfortunate bird stood idle on the mud, I had journeyed in mind through Perrault, Potter, ducks, Aesop, animal crossings, swans, waterfowl migration and socialization, conservation initiatives, goose health and group ethics. Such is the associative nature of thought. It is what happens naturally when we let our minds wander freely—for example, while we float, drive, or sit on trains and buses—disabling our conscious "override." It is a blur of daydreams, remembrances and reality that can be soothing and even playful (though, just as easily, a trauma can also enchain and return countless associations). Associative thinking weaves our experiences with deeply held stories—lived or read, even in infancy—with what we perceive through our senses. And it can offer formidable returns, leading us to provocative questions for investigation and new learnings about our world.

We will now interrogate the role of phonemes in associative thinking through three considerations: love of language; word and letter play; and a passion for stories/reading. In terms of an initial overview, Mukhopadhyay features prominently in this discussion since he is the most prolific, titling one of his books, *Plankton Dreams*, and even conceiving a "plankton language."[26] For his part, Sellin, is bold and blunt: "without language I am a poor madman."[27] Letter and word play—along with pondering words deeply—is evident in all their works, as typified by Higashida: "Words are bridges that connect me with others."[28] And Mukhopadhyay provides many examples of how letters offer pleasure, as daydreams invite questions: "Why should A be better than Z? When will we adopt a democracy of letters?"[29] We also confirm the early acquisition of literacy, as attested by Kedar: "When I was very young, I taught myself to read."[30] And each author maintains a lifelong passion for stories, as Mukhopadhyay expresses in an evocation of creativity and memory: "Stories, stories back and forth, come again as memories swing."[31] Without a doubt, associative thinking is alive and well in nonverbal autism—and it enables boundless internal play in the wild world of words.

First, we contemplate **love of language** as an attachment to—and pleasure from—not only letters, words and stories, but also multilingualism. It may seem paradoxical that a mute individual would be passionate about language—but that is only if we focus on language production: i.e., speech. If, instead, we prioritize language comprehension, then it makes perfect sense. At issue is that the nonverbal autist is auditorily attuned and passively highly receptive. Sellin, for example, is interested in studying linguistics;[32] and he enjoys spending some of his time translating words given to him by his mother (in German) into English.[33] Higashida (whose mother tongue is Japanese) declares that, "English feels like an old friend to me."[34] Yet he has a deep love for his own language, too: "The letter that is special to me is の [pronounced 'no' as in 'not'] because of its beautiful curve";[35] and he adds, "My favourite word is … *kibou* [pronounced 'key-bor']—hope."[36]

In turn, Mukhopadhyay's family speaks Bengali and English, and he spells the words he writes in English.[37] Mukhopadhyay actually understands three other languages in addition to English.[38] And he values even ordinary moments of contact with varied tongues: "I heard pieces of conversations in different languages. I could understand some languages, while others I could not. The ones I could not made me wonder about their words. I formed my own translations just by guessing."[39] Furthermore, Mukhopadhyay regards human movement and expression as a language all its own: "I could understand the glances from the other body languages which the person carried."[40]

Higashida is also self-aware of his attraction for words: "I have an interest in letters and numbers."[41] It seems evident to him that memory—encoding the past—depends on words:

> What I took in with my eyes in New York, what I heard with my ears and felt with my skin, I wish to swap for words. Words I wish to write down. Words I wish to send on their way.[42]

Reciprocally, there is a sense that wishes and desires for the future are also effected through words.

With Kedar, I believe we can feel the security that a relationship with language delivers: "I loved letters and I stared at them any time I could."[43] Further, the nonverbal autist's receptive competency with language—and his deep valuation of words—should inform all interventions, according to Kedar: "If I could educate the specialists the first thing I'd recommend is to talk normally to autistic kids … Next, I would teach autistic kids grade-level lessons."[44] He also reveals that his thinking was "often in spelling," as he visualized the word in his head.[45] But perhaps Sellin best sums up this fondness for language: "I love language more than anything. It links people. A language gives us dignity and individuality. I am not without language."[46] In this love of words, we are following the natural course of the affective investment of phonemes and the pleasure this affect delivers. Not being able to speak does not mean being without language.

Second, we consider **word and letter play**. Sellin offers some instances of word play on his own name, calling himself "crazy Birger," "fantastic Birger," "pleasant Birger" and "fabulous Birger"[47]; or even, "refractory Birger" and "resistant Birger."[48] But the greatest number of instances of word play can be found in Mukhopadhyay's multiple texts. In fact, he seems to find some amusement and curiosity with letters even at the level of typography. Regarding how letters are rendered, for example, he feels that, "the alphabet of different books too looked different."[49] And reflecting on one of his educational experiences, he writes, tongue-in-cheek: "Who cares if the fill-in-the-blanks go hungry?"[50] Mukhopadhyay also eloquently relates his enjoyment of letters and words:

> The boy laughed imagining the letters that formed the word "goat" were in dispute, each one making its own phonetic sound—a resulting noise that was

> different from the way "goat" sounded. So the boy made a new game. He had learnt already how to read. He thought about different words and made the letters argue and talk.[51]

Mukhopadhyay is also acutely aware of how association plays a role in his early interactions with objects and words, as he shares the following: "When I was very little, I remember forming wrong associations between words and objects. For instance, when I heard the word banana while I was looking at a cloud, I labelled the cloud [in thought] 'banana.'"[52]

In an extended example of word play with "egg," Mukhopadhyay titles one of his essays, "A Bad Eggsample."[53] In it, he characterizes his male assistant (or teacher) as, "not even the mother hen kind,"[54] and himself as "my eggy self" (perhaps an association on his being a "bad egg" for disturbing the teacher). In this humorous story of a day in his special education classroom, Mukhopadhyay shares his hope of being a "liberated yolk."[55] Further word play includes creative coinage, such as "eggsactly"[56] and "eggsperience."[57] It also provides a stunning illustration of associative thinking because, over merely 500 words, Mukhopadhyay reflects freely on gravity, Humpty Dumpty, chicken coops, the primordial beginnings of language, letter permutations, "chirping" blanks on a worksheet calling for answers, Easter, hieroglyphics, and chicken scratch. Summarizing his adventure as an "eggsplorer eggstraordinaire,"[58] he admits that, "nothing fascinated me more that day than the thought of an egg."[59] What seems most evident in this "egg dream"[60] is the blur between associative thinking and creative daydreaming. And Mukhopadhyay shares another priceless example in his cynical reflections on special education, putting phonemes in play: "A hand without a green marker was like *Tuesday* without a *T* ... *Tuesday – T = useday. Useday – day = use. Use + less = useless.*"[61]

Third, we reflect on the **passion for reading**. Sellin reports reading since the age of five and greatly values the "objects" they offer: "I have read many extraordinarily impressive books since my fifth year of life and I hoard all their important contents in me like precious treasures."[62] And in his reflections on his history with literature, we detect how books (i.e., words) are associated to—and recall—an environment:

> I found reading so easy and so I looked in let's say important books for everything I could find[.] The books were all in that socalled room in that let's say study in Kreuzberg[,] but later there were also books from the study in lots of real apartments where we lived.[63]

In Sellin's writing, we also discover how objects from reading become objects for thinking: "I have read everything and very fast[,] I even read scientific books very quickly and I make up so much myself[,] even stories and poems."[64] And he is uncanny in his awareness that both sources of objects—reading and reality—blur together in a kind of associative play: "Birger puts everything he knows right in the middle of a heap of chaotic poetic nonsense he has read."[65]

Recounting his own experiences with reading, Kedar[66] critiques some interventions: "I love books and I would have enjoyed some age-appropriate stories, not baby picture books over and over."[67] He also discloses the passive receptivity of the nonverbal autist: "I am able to remember details in books, conversations, and other things too well."[68] And Kedar explains how, without support, he began reading: "My education has been a strange one. I taught myself to read when I was very young, but no one knew."[69] Further, he offers evidence of how words, as objects coming from reality, come up against the need to protect the silent retreat:

> Holding a book steady to read is simply out of reach. I am not able to hold it still for long and turning pages one at a time is awful. I prefer books on tape or read out loud to me for that reason. I am sad about this. I love to read but the words in my head compete with those on paper and I can't read the whole book that way. By that I mean that my head is full of written words all the time. I see every work spelled in my head in any language I know. Reading chapter books sends lots more letters into my system. It can be overwhelming sometimes.[70]

For Higashida, reading serves a securing function akin to that of the presence of real, trusted others: "When I hear the laughter of my family, I feel this bubble-like, evanescent sensation—it's like when I'm entranced by a really great picture book I love, set in a distant land, beyond borders."[71] His mention of distance is an interesting one, as safety seems findable in some imaginary elsewhere. Perhaps this suggests a continued reliance on the archaic landscape and its securing daydreams—or perhaps it reveals an intuition that, in fact, the border to reality still needs to be fully transitted.

In his own relationship with reading, Higashida also seems to convey the problem of an incomplete individuation. For he requires the scaffolding of the words of another—something that reading and song sheets offer: "I have no problem reading books aloud and singing, but as soon as I try to speak with someone, my words just vanish."[72] And he offers a unique perspective on the continued need for such a securing other (that is, yet is not, himself) in facilitating the full development of individuation:

> I showed zero response to any picture book of any kind, I caused my mother a great deal of worry—so I'm now told. One day, however, she noticed how often I was looking through old photographs. So Mum put together a photo book using our family pictures, and wrote short sentences alongside the images. It was thanks to this that the whole point of picture books "clicked" for me and from then on the number that I enjoyed steadily grew. Also, I could begin to relate my everyday self to the characters in the books.[73]

We should keep in mind the preference for non-fiction over fiction in this retelling. At issue is that the successful scaffolding of individuation, which brings relief, benefits from real others.

Also in regards to reading, I believe Mukhopadhyay relates something of this same experience of incomplete individuation when he shares that he learned to read, "in chorus" with mother.[74] Even today, as he says, "I can read my own books without facilitation. But I still feel good if someone reads with me as a motivating factor."[75] And like Higashida, Mukhopadhyay prefers literature with photographs of real people and objects, declaring his "love for magazines."[76] He is also keenly aware of his own reliance on reading and other informational texts (e.g., media) to help mediate his encounter with objects (including people) in reality: "Probably in some magazine, or somewhere on the TV, he saw a similar person and thus imagined him anywhere."[77] In addition, books are a source of security that seem to facilitate a sense of direction for Mukhopadhyay: "A woman [his mother's friend] with a world of books [that] whisper of hope in my ears, why do they echo yet so clear."[78] I believe we can also detect here a residual sense of otherness that is, yet is not, the self.

Furthermore, inherent in his passion for reading, Mukhopadhyay gives characters to objects in a frank and playful example of anthropomorphism—that innate human tendency that is so prevalent in the progression of mental and emotional life, and which in fact fuels children's literature: "I wanted to hear her [his mother's] reason-stories. Knots of all colours came alive once they each had a character."[79] For in being an abundant source of objects, not only are books (and/or their characters) felt to be real, but the reader can become profoundly identified with them, as an extension of himself—again, in a kind of otherness that is, yet is not, the self. For example, Mukhopadhyay explains how, "a torn page in a book may cause my whole body to itch."[80]

The result is the highly curious work of reading by which books can become instruments for presentification. On the one hand, reading non-fiction supports individuation through a kind of "me-notme"—the co-presence of what is, yet is not, the self in encounters with common objects in reality. On the other hand, fiction is blurred with reality under the influence of primary processes—daydreams and association—during the normative transition to reality. So even fairy tales are "real" for a child—and Dolto herself explains that for a child, a fairy tale "is not a story, it is true."[81] So storybooks, too, can offer secure scaffolds for transitioning to reality. Books truly inhabit a wide middle ground, and we leave the last word on this point to Mukhopadhyay, in this poignant description:

> Fools do not even know that there is so much to read and so little time. And so short a life. You try to look inside your bag to find something worth reading … But all your hands dig out is a two-month-old receipt. Next time you need to be more careful. Perhaps carry a bigger bag so that it can hold at least a paperback.[82]

B. Passivity

Water levels in the Humber River are currently at their lowest point in years. Its muddy banks are high and jagged, exposing what is normally submerged. Paddling close to the eastern bank, I spotted a frisbee-sized midland painted turtle—its front half on land, its back half hanging over the edge. It had probably landed there on a jet ski's wave, and now it was evidently stuck. I approached slowly to help, but that poor turtle (member of a threatened species) became even more frightened. So it tried to reverse and ended up falling backwards. Now it was lying on its back in five centimetres of water—entirely unable to move and shockingly vulnerable to all sorts of predators. One gentle paddle stroke at a time, I quietly manoeuvred my kayak alongside it and reached out my hand. The turtle let me make contact. I picked it up softly and, while keeping it submerged in the water as much as I could, I slowly turned it over. The instant it felt itself to be righted in the water, it swam off at an astonishingly high rate of speed and was gone. But how many other turtles might there be along the parched shoreline, I wondered? How many beavers might be losing their lodges to the receding waters this autumn? How many minks and groundhogs might be much more exposed—their coveted dens in the detritus now wide open to the air, and away from the water enabling their escapes?

And what about the trees? Huge maples boldly mark the river's winding in brilliant reds, oranges and yellows—but their roots are now boldly revealed. Instead of being securely under water, nourished abundantly, course weavings of cellulose protrude in the most suggestive shapes, at once aesthetic yet tortured. I worry about these beloved trees and whether they can outlast the receding river. I pass by some of my favourites—trusted willows who have sheltered me from unexpected rains, whose branches graze my head as I paddle beneath the soft arches they form along the river's edge, an archaic waterway. They are stuck, fixed in this place and unable—like that poor turtle—to initiate independent movement. And they are silent, incapable of relating if they are sufficiently secure—with deep-enough roots—or barely subsisting on their last drops. Will they make it to the spring rains? And even if they do, has their growth potential been irretrievably harmed? When they eventually fall, and conservationists assess the damage, will the story their rings tell reveal the suffering they incurred in 2022? Yet such is the plight of countless forms of organic life: they endure passively, fixed to place and unable to relocate, thus eminently vulnerable to the environment. Duress becomes an unnarratable suffering—and survival is not assured. And ultimately, what makes the difference between living and not living is the depth of roots reaching underground reserves.

We will examine passivity through four notions: fusion, passive education, non-initiation and daydreaming. In terms of an initial overview, the condition of fusion is evident, for example, in Mukhopadhyay's poignant testimony: "The lap of the mother should not be let off. The boy refused to walk."[83] And Sellin, like others, offers a window onto passive learning: "Collected thoughts totally dormant tremble with cold when they make their way to the outside light of Earth."[84] Daydreaming offers a smooth bridge between dreams and reality while also delivering pleasure, as Higashida relates: "I used to dream that I was able to speak."[85] And from Mukhopadhyay, for instance, we grasp the inventive thought this process enables: "He would change the environment around him, with the help of his imagination. He could go to places that did not exist, and they were like a beautiful dream."[86] Offsetting the tremendous creativity that inheres in passivity, however, is an incapacity for intentional activity.

Higashida admits, "My mind tends to go blank whenever I try to speak."[87] And Kedar discloses, "I am easily distracted from my goal."[88] Ultimately, passivity is a vibrant state of readiness and deep reserves of energy, and that insatiable receptivity—so often unnoticed—provokes an inherent desire and capacity for learning.

First, we reflect on **fusion**. Audition is the primary channel for engaging objects during our state of "fusion"—i.e., our non-individuated, inseparable life with an indissociable other who is, yet is not, felt to be the self. And if individuation is impeded somehow (because of a regressive position), then fusion (as a mental and emotional condition) will necessarily linger to deliver indispensable security.

Mukhopadhyay recalls that even as a child of five, he relied on his mother's continuous proximity: "Mother always made me feel that she was there";[89] and "he felt confident when she [his mother] was confident."[90] He poignantly describes a trip back to his home town as a young child (while playing between first and third person views):

> On the roads, he wanted to hold the hands of his parents in a particular way. I cannot recall why this was so, but he felt very insecure without the rituals as he felt his presence through them. It seemed impossible to stop.[91]

Thus, his sense of being present in reality depends on an other, and on repetitions of what cannot be abandoned.

Mukhopadhyay also reveals how, even as an adult, this need persists: "I still need mother or my class teacher ... to sit by my side not as facilitators, but as my environment which helps me to retain the flow with my language and communication."[92] His word choice is a potent one, recalling how every gestational mother is an all-providing environment. And with Kedar, we grasp how such a fusional dependence relates to non-initiation: "I need support to stay engaged, so if I'm doing a puzzle or a computer game when the person who is working with me leaves, I will stop trying."[93]

Mukhopadhyay also articulates the continuing dominance of audition, explaining that he "recognizes voices rather than people."[94] And he draws our attention to the notion of an echo—an auditory presence or return of that which is, yet is not, the self—that delivers a sense of security. For instance, while on a stressful outing, he reports that in repeating his mother's verse (she was reciting "Who has seen the wind"), "The boy was echoing it too and felt better."[95]

Furthermore, Mukhopadhyay engages in extensive musings about mirrors that are (oddly enough for a mirror) all about sound: "Some days I become like the mirror and I need to tell back all that is being told to me. It does not matter what is being told. As long as it is being told."[96] He also reveals the intimate relation between dream-work and this sustained reliance on audition:

> My dominant sensory channel is hearing. It dominates to such an extent that I dream in sounds most of the time, even when I sleep at night. So if anyone asks me, "What did you see in your dream?" I would answer, "I heard my dream."[97]

And in perhaps the most stunning reflection of all, Mukhopadhyay reveals the enigmatic tension between the dependence on hearing and the retreat to silence that marks regression as a defence: "Living in the past adds to the burden of disparity. So I have to continue my Voice of Silence with my own voice."[98]

Second, we consider the notion of a **passive education**. Beginning during gestation, objects engaged through audition nourish symbolization, becoming a veritable syllable soup. Thus, even the child with a passive disposition is guaranteed a secure access to continuous learning—a passive education. Sellin regrets how, "people didn't know I understand everything so they just said everything I wasn't supposed to be hearing."[99] The burden of pain is palpable, and Higashida concurs: "We're listening to everyone around us and we hear you, you know."[100] Furthermore, since the capacity for taking in objects through audition is governed by primary processes, the desire for engaging objects through audition is a powerful one. This is, in fact, why the passive child is so receptive. And Higashida confirms this prediction using an oral metaphor that precisely evokes that "soup": "It really gets me down that people just don't understand how hungry for knowledge people with autism actually are."[101]

Kedar is philosophical: "[Autism] gave me the ability to analyze and think things through in all my silent years [before writing]."[102] And he fully grasps the sharp contrast between his receptivity and productivity as, in the preface to his novel, Kedar explains his own deep frustrations: "I alone knew how much I knew—that I could read, spell, calculate, think and problem solve but remained trapped inside a non-obeying body."[103] And, through Anthony, Kedar elaborates in that novel the extent to which he was always listening to the conversations around him, despite not being given credit for doing so—and how much he understood of current events and the theories about autism being discussed around him.[104]

Kedar adds this powerful summation: "I know people don't believe that a little kid notices, but I did notice."[105] And due to the wide underestimation of passive capacities, Kedar reflects on the education he did receive:

> I could read from an early age. I could write too, only my fingers were too clumsy to show it. In school I sat through ABC tapes over and over and added 1+2=3 over and over. It was a nightmare. I was bored out of my wits. It made me die inside. I was like a zombie inside because I had no hope.[106]

Kedar concludes on the profound challenges of passivity: "Only you know that your mind is intact. This is a kind of hell, I am certain."[107] Yet he is not without hope: "It's the struggle of the silent to prove that still waters run deep and sometimes not the way that is assumed."[108]

Crucially, passivity enables not only objects but affect to be detected. Sellin describes the experience:

> A lonely and mute person depends on encouragement … a loving look does wonders without words … once on the subway I saw a woman looking at me kindly[,] I often think of it[,] I like to believe in it and I won't forget it[,] but many looks are hard to bear and bring dreadful suffering.[109]

Mukhopadhyay agrees: "I have a special instinct which allows me to know where I shall be welcomed."[110] And in Higashida, we find a related statement on the passive registration of affect. In it, along with asserting the continuing need for an other to engage objects, Higashida points to a critical turn in developing individuation wherein one might be one's own "like-me"—an auditory kind of other(ness)—through experiencing from two "views" in time:

> [Nonverbal autists] can unlock language by referencing common points between memory scenes and the moment they're in. This might take a great deal of practice, but their family, helpers and teachers mustn't give up on them. The person with special needs will sense that resignation.[111]

In Kedar, I believe we can even detect how the interrelationship between passivity, anxiety and audition might explain a common manifestation of nonverbal autism: "Eye contact is hard because the light reflecting off the eyes is not calming … I can listen better if I don't look at the person."[112] For the evidence is that the autist retains a preference for audition over vision. But the deeper suggestion is that triangulation—listening indirectly, with/through an other—is beneficial to experiencing objects. In fact, Dolto herself observed repeatedly that all children listen better while they are busy, as if they are not listening at all[113]—that is, when they are essentially passive while others talk.

Third, we contemplate the lived experience of **non-initiation**. Passivity, by definition, entails a grave difficulty with initiating motor movements, including speech. Sellin relates that "putting ideas into action is almost impossible for me."[114] In fact, his perspective is imbued with a fair measure of play: "I am living without knowing what I aim at again. Nonsense is an important aim."[115] For his part, Kedar elaborates on the cost of passivity to inclusion: "I'm not entertained by the ordinary things that most people enjoy. I endure what they love. I have no real reason to play games … I find them boring or almost like punishment."[116] Further, as he states flatly, "I'm not into games."[117] Kedar also provides a summation of the lived experience of passivity that almost seems to evoke its archaic moorings: "It's like a well. The autistic person is stuck at the bottom and needs to climb out. The trouble is how. The autistic person can't initiate the escape. It's not from a lack of desire. It's hard to explain."[118]

Kedar is highly analytical: "I have been thinking a lot about my non-responsiveness. It is almost like a form of paralysis, except, thank God, I'm not paralyzed, but I still think it's like a paralysis of intentional responses."[119] And in an indispensable anecdote, he reports that he can nonetheless initiate securing food, that most basic need for survival: "Sometimes my initiating problem is huge … How I wish someone would come and give me a blanket or take one off me. It's weird because I do react to my desire for food."[120] And Kedar identifies his need for an auditory other:

> I don't know why initiating is so hard. I may wish to say something or do something. I can't get myself to move on it … It is stupid passivity that makes me rely on input from others rather than myself … I don't have insight into this aspect of my illness. I just know it's there.[121]

In turn, Mukhopadhyay relates passivity experientially, as a state of waiting and thinking. For example, "he waited for some remarkable thing to happen and started to meditate for an answer";[122] thus, through much of life, he simply had to strive to develop patience.[123] He also describes a logical consequence for his artwork: "He could only copy designs, he could not be creative."[124]

But the boldest reflections on passivity come from Higashida, who confirms the power of the restraint against initiation while offering an uncanny narration of the transitional ground he inhabits: "To me, it's as if I'm standing at the fork in a road of a double life, seized by inertia."[125] Further, he relates passivity to non-individuation—i.e., to the persistent need for an other to initiate movement: "People with autism are sometimes unable to move on to their next action without a verbal prompt."[126] But most fascinating of all, Higashida feels the power of "lures" to reality, just as predicted: "My body moved because it was lured outside by something there."[127]

Fourth, we engage the rich value of **daydreaming**. Paradoxically, passivity enables a spectacular richness in daydreaming and creative thinking. Kedar puts it this way: "In the silence I lived in[,] I learned to think deeply about things."[128] And he arrives at a broader perspective on the human condition:

> The truth is that much of what people say is meaningless. They instantly say what comes into their head. Their lack of working on their thoughts makes their thoughts unfocused. It's not only a curse to be quiet, it's a blessing of thinking inside and saying what is important.[129]

Kedar also provides this comprehensive portrait of the nonverbal autist's vibrant mental and emotional life—despite all appearances:

> We, in Autismland, are socially isolated, and even if we have loving friends and families, it's not the same as a typical person due to our lonely illness that makes the outside world overwhelming and isolates people from us. Inside we are imagining our words and behavior and outside we are not able to do it the way we want. Frustrating lives. Sort of alone in company.[130]

Extending this notion, Higashida relates that, "A long time ago I used to dream that I was a neuro-typical child. In these dreams I was forever laughing."[131] Dreams and daydreams deliver pleasure—wishes as consolations for the disappointments of reality. Higashida also identifies dreams as a source of hope: "Tomorrow might be indistinguishable from yesterday, but on the far side of tomorrow the whole of our future is waiting, and it's our present selves who dream that future into being."[132] And he seems intensely self-aware that human pleasure originates in dream-work:

> Perhaps the dandelions can only dream, Someday I'll catch someone's eye and they'll turn around and notice me, and then I'll know for sure that the most beautiful flower is me. But I wonder whether it's actually the dreaming of this dream—rather than it ever coming true—that is where the real happiness lies.[133]

Mukhopadhyay, a prolific storyteller, explains how "imagination took shape to lead his mind to a world of fantasies"[134]—and he titles two of his books, *Plankton Dreams* and *The Mind Tree*. He describes the creative blur between daydreams and thinking as a liminal transitional space where the past (memories) and future (hope) remain in continuity, albeit undetermined:

> I wake and I dream with my mind in the permanence of some or the other kind of thought. There is a never-ending chain of some desire, some hope, some memories and some dreams. Some of them merge together to form a new kind of a twilight ahead which has the probabilities of "maybe's" and "ifs."[135]

Mukhopadhyay's texts also include many references to climbing staircases—arguably, a powerful symbol of emergence. In one example, "a staircase, which went high, higher and still higher [was] reaching somewhere—anywhere. But a great disappointment occurred if it took him to nowhere and he had to start elevating again."[136] He describes the staircase as "the first motivation he ever had,"[137] as dreams nourish his desires. And he clearly comprehends the boundary between dreams and reality, explaining that, "the obsession with staircases continued to exist even in the real world."[138] Yet whereas it might be natural to assume that the staircase would lead upward from a silent past to a speaking future, the reverse desire is disclosed:

> He sheltered in the unreal world[,] the staircases took him higher and higher away from the voices, into silence. The lonely self in a crowd. A contentment, aiming for liberation—a complete state of tranquility.[139]

Once more, we sense the pull of inertia and the lure of dream-work in this desire to retreat to passivity—i.e., in a dependence on regression as a defence. The powerful attraction of silence (withdrawal) actually seems to be a widely overlooked factor in nonverbal autism. For it is generally presumed that the nonverbal autist would talk if only he could. Yet as it turns out, provocatively, the archaic offers its own versions of pleasure and security against which reality's lures must compete.

Mukhopadhyay also offers a unique window on the enduring influence of triangulation as an engagement between the self; an echo of the self (i.e., an auditory other who is, yet is not, the self); and an object—whose value is in the stories it tells. For deep in the archaic stage, objects continuously spin stories in dream-work—and the origins of symbolization are to be found in the unconscious, prehistoric stor(y)ing of objects, including the idiosyncratic, unconscious storying of phonemes.

Thus, Mukhopadhyay explains how, "More than the reflections, I was interested in the essence of the reflected objects and the possible stories about them."[140] Daydreams on objects even spin stories from his stims: "stories passed in and out of the transparency of my flapping hands";[141] as well as from the surroundings he takes in passively: "I would seek out new stories in those shapes on the floor."[142]

Mukhopadhyay reveals that, "The story behind an object is far more important to me than the object."[143] And he provides an extended illustration of the work of association in linking objects, dreams, stories, thoughts and environments:

> I would remember a wall not by its flatness but because of a nail that had cast its shadow under the overhead light. And because of that nail, I would imagine and grow my probable stories around it. Stories of a clock or a picture hanging from that nail covering up the place where the shadow was cast. Or stories of a wall chandelier or perhaps a birthday balloon tied to that nail. And anything that would hang from that nail would mark the character on the wall and give my mind its wonder experience so that through it I would store the memory of that wall.[144]

And in a poem, he ultimately entrusts himself to dreams, as he explains how dreams, despite their unpredictable comings and goings, are what he always depends on.[145]

Closing this chapter on phonemes and passivity, the texts of nonverbal autistic authors reveal the continued influence of audition during the long transition from a passive dream life. In their works, we detect the vital importance of phonemes through a love of language and word play—and a passion for reading as a securing source of objects. On the one hand, we observe that the journey to reality crosses a wide middle ground during which individuation is not yet completed and initiation remains a challenge. On the other hand, passivity is revealed as a vibrant condition for creative thinking that ensures lifelong learning. Critically, we also confirm that language reception and language expression are entirely independent. For even when we are silent, audition feeds our dreams.

Notes

1 As a point of interest, Sapir was also a staunch defender of Indigenous languages and a polyglot.
2 1933, 45.
3 1933/1949, 9.
4 Ibid.
5 1933, 46.
6 Ibid.
7 1925/1949, 45.
8 1933/1949, 8.
9 1921/1971, 19–20.
10 Ibid, 38–40.
11 Ibid, 224.
12 Ibid, 40.
13 Ibid, 16.
14 1915/1949, 194–195.
15 1931/1949, 70.
16 1981, 58.
17 I explore the suggestibility of words in greater depth in my previous work on Dolto.

18 1921/1971, 37–38.
19 In Guillerault 1997, 139.
20 Dolto 1987, 41.
21 In Guillerault 1997, 210.
22 In Djéribi-Valentin 2005, 329; also Faure-Poirée & Djéribi-Valentin 1999, 277.
23 I.e., "knowledge"; but this loses the contribution Dolto's phonemes make to triangulation with the indissociable other: «co-naissance» [co-birth]; and the homonymic, «n'est sans ce» [is not without] (see also note above).
24 In Djéribi-Valentin & Kouki 1998, 63.
25 In his influential work on autism, Leo Kanner noted this hallmark trait and described it as "pronominal reversals which consist of the child's reference to himself as 'you' and to the person spoken as 'I'" (1946/1973, 46).
26 2015a, 81.
27 1995, 199.
28 2017, 215.
29 2015a, 21.
30 2012, 66.
31 2008, 69.
32 1995, 30.
33 Ibid, 65 & 65f.
34 2017, 241.
35 Ibid, 215; in Hiragana.
36 Ibid, 215.
37 2000, 2.
38 Ibid, 29.
39 2008, 101.
40 2000, 65.
41 2017, 264.
42 Ibid, 242.
43 2012, 66.
44 Ibid, 55.
45 Ibid, 66.
46 1995, 154.
47 Ibid, 126–127.
48 Ibid, 128.
49 2000, 9.
50 2015a, 66.
51 2000, 22; he was reading at around three years of age, inferring from dating provided on p. 20 of this text.
52 2008, 214.
53 2015a, 65.
54 Ibid.
55 Ibid.
56 Ibid, 66.
57 Ibid, 67.
58 Ibid, 64.
59 Ibid, 63.
60 Ibid.
61 Ibid, 77 (emphasis his).
62 1995, 24.
63 Ibid, 58.
64 Ibid, 64.

65 Ibid, 137.
66 I do not know these four authors personally. But I messaged Kedar (2020) through social media to ask him about his early history with reading. He helpfully replied: "I learned to read young, at two or three … I loved letters … I read license plates, captions, book titles, billboards, movie credits, whatever I could."
67 2012, 56.
68 Ibid, 88.
69 Ibid, 90.
70 Ibid, 98.
71 2017, 176.
72 2007/2013, 15.
73 2017, 248.
74 2000, 75.
75 Ibid, 75.
76 2008, 98.
77 2000, 8.
78 Ibid, 67.
79 2008, 90.
80 Ibid, 210.
81 In Lévy 2002, 15; also Dolto 1987, 36.
82 2005, 100.
83 2000, 6.
84 1995, 95.
85 2017, 89.
86 2000, 8.
87 2017, 48.
88 2012, 88.
89 2008, 91.
90 2000, 33.
91 Ibid, 35.
92 Ibid, 76.
93 2012, 45.
94 2000, 6.
95 Ibid, 45.
96 2005, 201.
97 2008, 196.
98 2000, 60 (capitalization his).
99 1995, 54.
100 2017, 87.
101 2007/2013, 115.
102 2012, 113.
103 2018, i.
104 Ibid, 109.
105 2012, 58.
106 Ibid, 50.
107 Ibid, 49.
108 Ibid, 118.
109 1995, 27.
110 2000, 66.
111 2017, 96.
112 2012, 49.

113 In De Sauverzac 1985, 219; Dolto 1987, 24; De Sauverzac 1987, 80; De Sauverzac 1988, 35, 144 & 146; Manier & Kouki 2003, 226; Djéribi-Valentin 2005, 728 & 808.
114 1995, 133.
115 Ibid, 171.
116 2012, 45.
117 Ibid, 96.
118 Ibid, 62.
119 Ibid, 101.
120 Ibid, 70.
121 Ibid, 63.
122 2000, 6.
123 2005, 204.
124 2000, 50.
125 2017, 179.
126 2007/2013, 143.
127 Ibid, 130.
128 2012, 104.
129 Ibid, 106.
130 Ibid, 133 (capitalization his).
131 2017, 179.
132 Ibid, 209.
133 Ibid, 178.
134 2000, 15.
135 Ibid, 97.
136 Ibid, 8.
137 Ibid, 18.
138 Ibid, 8.
139 Ibid, 11.
140 2008, 14.
141 Ibid, 23.
142 Ibid, 32.
143 Ibid, 54.
144 Ibid, 35.
145 2000, 76.

Chapter 6

Resonant Experience

Preliminary Words

CBC[1] Radio One (Toronto) recently reported that robots are being considered as carers for elders. The efficiencies are obvious—the costs, perhaps not so much. For while these non-organic entities are touted as a solution for labour shortages, their proposed use in the provision of care sparks obvious debates about the unique value of the "human touch." Then again, maybe that phrase is a misnomer, a form of speciesism. After all, anyone with a beloved pet will tell you that a caring "touch" is not strictly about (i.e., from) humans. Of course, a pet can't provide personal care. But it's a routinely reported fact, for example, that dogs may help elders live longer due to the unquantifiable benefits of that relationship. There are similar stories about prisoners and others in isolation forming life-sustaining engagements with rodents and even insects. Cat lovers are just as dedicated to their companions, and it isn't unusual to find people attached to rabbits and reptiles. It's also a frequent sight in cities to find many individuals committed to feeding the local pigeons. And for countless gardeners (and condo dwellers) around the world, the tender care of the organic life growing in even the smallest plots of land, or on balconies, gives them a sense of well-being—even purpose. The truth most humans will admit to is that we often speak to our dogs, cats, trees and plants. And while we are not always sure of understanding them, we are strangely convinced that they understand us—that they somehow recognize our true feelings, especially on difficult days. Fundamentally, then, in the very ordinary experience of sustaining the survival of another lifeform, we feel ourselves to be living. We receive an extraordinary proof of life.

What we intuitively grasp is that humans benefit from relations with organic life, through which we experience a return on our affective investments. Put another way, when we invest affect in organic life and it lives thanks to our care, we confirm what is good in ourselves. The relationship is ostensibly in the service of another lifeform—i.e., a pet, garden, elder, friend or child, for instance. But it is actually about ourselves because it returns affect to us—pleasure—to countermand our existential angst, our anhedonia. The reason is that the onset of our mental and emotional lives sets an enduring pattern for the circulation of affect. As a result, it's as if we always need affect to pass through an other to return it to ourselves. At

DOI: 10.4324/9781032655123-12

issue is that our own existence is made possible thanks to a relationship with an all-providing lifeform—an indissociable "like-me" whose identity is fused with ours for the decisive first months of our development as human beings.

In an unconscious blur of dream-work with the "like-me," every gestational infant believes himself not only to be *with* the (m)other but to *be* her. This is the beginning of the "archaic triangular situation" in which every human child unconsciously co-experiences liquid objects—most notably, phonemes, due to the prominence and precocity of audition *in utero*. In turn, objects of dream-work are invested with affect by association with this indissociable other. The triangulation is fluid—it is a relation, not a structure. It is an engagement with objects wherein the infant effectively represents two "positions," so to speak: a pre-self and an other who is, yet is not, himself. It is an associative mechanism by definition, as affect flows in triangulation to achieve continuous circulation. In turn, affect is displaced through associations with prior objects of investment to extend unconscious security to wider fields of objects.

As gestation advances, perception increases so that more objects can be experienced and dream-work facilitates pre-conscious symbolization. Through this normative process of maturation, objects that appear repeatedly, and/or in which the mother is highly invested herself, are automatically invested by the infant—most crucially, the other of the mother who is normatively (but not necessarily) the biological father. Dolto calls this fluid archaic entity a symbolic father. Simultaneously, proprioception is increasing, enhancing the child's awareness of his own body. This enables the pre-conscious experience of a subtle sense of difference, distance or dissociation from the indissociable other. So begins the gradual process of mental and emotional individuation in the gestational infant—even while he remains physically indissociable. And whereas the infant previously experienced himself as similar to his indissociable (m)other, he now considers himself similar to his symbolic father, since both are deeply associated with her, yet neither *is* her. She has become, in short, their common object.

From hereon, the gestational infant can co-experience myriad common objects with this symbolic father, as associations on all objects proliferate. That is why, as discussed, Dolto emphasizes that refinding the symbolic father is clinically determinative for restarting progression (following regression). As the archaic parents keep blurring with each other in dream-work, the role of this archaic other who is always felt as "present" and securing leads Dolto to speak more broadly of a witness recognized as similar being essential to all interhuman exchanges that are capable of securing the continuity of unconscious affect. It's as if this witness-in-similitude[2] confirms the truth of an object—its merits for protecting affective investments. In essence, then, inscribed in the process of individuation—and arising from the fact that individuation is a triangulated phenomenon—is a need to unconsciously co-experience objects with an enigmatic witness-in-similitude to sustain affective continuity.

Throughout her life, Dolto teased out this notion of the unconsciously securing other who is, yet is not, the self. For example, she explains that the self always feels like a «prolongement» of the one he loves.[3] Her word literally means an "elongation" or "prolongation," evoking the indissociable other as a tension, a "pulling" sort of relation that conveys a slow distantiation that is tenuous and never quite complete. And precisely because this other is, yet is not, the self, the unconscious recognition of affective similarity is essential. Dolto describes the "subtle recognition of similars [as] constantly and never totally knowable."[4] Her emphasis on not knowing is important, for we can never consciously anticipate such a relation. True to the primary processes driving that "recognition,"[5] the encounter will be haphazard, and the experience will be an entirely unconscious one. In addition, because of the dominance of precocious audition during the archaic stage, when triangulation begins, the subtle recognition of similars will most often take place through language. Dolto refers to this unconscious recognition of a "similar" that takes place through our texts—either spoken or written—as an "intercommunication between similars."[6]

In turn, the triangular pattern for circulating affect impacts all future relations and engagements with objects, as investments flow to new objects through displacements by association. Therefore, not only is infant learning driven by the need for affective self-regulation, but we find the affective roots of associative thinking in triangulation. As a result, Dolto is convinced of the permanent influence of the archaic triangular situation: "The specimen of the species is whole right from the rupture of the umbilical cord. The subject of desire, on the other hand, represents a third of the Oedipal triangle."[7] Furthermore, since all the affect circulating in triangulation necessarily has an associative relation with the original source of affect—the archaic triangular situation—somewhere deep, down along innumerable pathways, the continuous flow recirculates (i.e., returns) affect to the self. The result is self-securing. Meanwhile, the capacity to diffuse affect onto new objects through triangulation enables it to be externalized—vented, liberated, discharged—via larger loops for circulation, facilitating self-regulation by reducing anxiety. So (re)finding a witness-in-similitude in the world matters to our mental and emotional well-being.

In effect, it is our human nature to be as animated as possible by unconscious affect—that is what delivers pleasure. And what is required to sustain this circulation is language because it carries latent content—unconscious affect. Phonemes are affectively invested based on associations with prior phonemes, and so on, like wild current spreading unconsciously. And every such triangulation implicates three, as we have seen: the phoneme (auditory object) and two "listening positions"—i.e., the self and the indispensable witness-in-similitude. Now if we allow ourselves some associative play of our own, turning that triangle onto its "two feet" (i.e., base), we can infer that encounters with invested phonemes are experienced as echoes—that is, from two "positions" of the self. We first listen—and first learn—in echo.

It's worth taking a moment to hear the many nuances of the word, "echo," since this only adds to our understanding of triangulation. Every dictionary reveals that echoes are more than mere repetitions, reflections or reverberations of sound. First, a sense of identification and even trustworthiness inheres in the term, for someone we believe to be in allegiance with ourselves, on whom we depend, can be said to echo our thoughts, feelings or opinions; in parallel, our pre-invested phonemes, delivered through someone else's words, contribute to recognizing that other as similar. Second, an echo also invokes a sense of response—an echo-answer—such as found in the grammar of Finnish, Chinese, Latin and other languages, where polar questions are answered without "yes" or "no" by repeating (i.e., re-using) the verb: for example, "Did you eat yet?" "I did"; in the same vein, our pre-invested phonemes suggest affective investments in new phonemes (by association) as our new expressions build upon our existing ones—and we find safety in precarious environments (including intellectual ones) by repeating the phonemes of another.[8] Third, the notion of an echo implies a consequence or repercussion, in that a later stage of something, such as the world, may be considered an echo of what occurred in prior eras; so it is that our invested phonemes, which are inevitably inscribed in the unconscious register of our texts (spoken or written)—and to which we are susceptible through luring (when listening or reading)—are due to our idiosyncratic infantile histories. Fourth, in dreams and daydreams, echoes of our phonemes deliver comfort, a kind of consolation that we are not alone—a sense that someone similar to ourselves is with us, present. How many of us have called out to a mountain, or from deep within a cave, for the sheer pleasure of it—for the enigmatic sense of company, a presence?

Fifth, echoes can signify remembrances, in that when we speak of something echoing a moment in our lives, we evoke a remnant of history—a lingering of the past in the present; comparably, invested phonemes haphazardly revive unconscious history, making us realize that what seemed long gone remains. Sixth, echoes convey verification or confirmation, in the case where something is known not to be lost but we still want to reassure ourselves of its continued residence; similarly, echoes in our accidental encounters with pre-invested phonemes return the dream of all-securing provision. Seventh, echoes can convey a sense of the discovery of what is lost beneath the field of vision, like countless shipwrecks around the world, as nothing is visible on the surface but it remains findable through echo-location; likewise, the echoes experienced via the unconscious register of words return lost auditory objects of infancy—our invested phonemes. Finally, in a related sense, echoes can also signify a trace, in that recording devices can make what escapes our vision visible—for example, by displaying its acoustic signature; so perhaps publishing, as a record of words, is a comparable phenomenon—in giving echo to voice. Here, then, following multiple trains of thought about echoes, I believe that we arrive at a paramount question: might writing deliver echoes and, thereby, be a means of becoming one's own witness-in-similitude—triangulating phonemes (words) to scaffold individuation?

Moreover, following the distant echoes of our earliest development—in a most uncanny manner—triangulation relates to how our ears receive information. For it is familiar knowledge that an auditory object that is not exactly equidistant between our ears is received slightly differently by each. Abundant research is available, including the Canadian classic, *The Handbook for Acoustic Ecology*. In it, we confirm that even the most minute differences between our ears—those two auditory positions—are actually perceptible: "The ear can detect a time difference as slight as 30 microseconds [.03 milliseconds] and smaller differences through training." As it turns out, then, our ears perceive all auditory objects in echo due to the inevitability of interaural differences. In other words, every auditory object is experienced from two similar, but not identical, physical positions, delivering accuracy—just like every phoneme, as an auditory object, is experienced in echo from two similar, but not identical, unconscious "positions," delivering security.

Here, I respectfully suggest that we may be encountering the repetition of patterns in the natural world, in a manner not unlike how the Fibonacci sequence is detectable in everything from pineapples to pinecones—and by which hurricanes look like galaxies or seashells. So it is not unreasonable that the unconscious triangulation of affect which engages objects in echo—i.e., in a subtle unconscious doubling—would also follow a natural pattern. Besides, we humans betray a protective redundancy—from our two hemispheres to our two feet. Oddly enough too, unconscious triangulation overlaps with conscious triangulation. In geolocation, for example, the exact position of an object is detectable given two points of observation. Since the 17th century, applications of triangulation have proliferated in surveying, navigation, meteorology and astronomy. Then again, perhaps it is unsurprising that humans would invent a method for consciously locating physical objects that is informed by their intuition regarding their own unconsciously invested objects. For in following echoes, we can travel from our dreams to our thoughts.

But we return to our gestational infant now. Jump ahead a few months and he begins learning with an other through common objects that the learner (or caregiver) holds in his hand. Jump forward a few more months, and the learner can indicate an object by pointing. A few more jumps and the learner can locate an object from a gaze shared with a caregiver. A few further jumps and the learner can become the teacher in exchanges with his familiars—for example, by offering a beloved object (e.g., food) to his caregiver, stuffed animals or family pet—or even to a book character. All these are examples of the triangulation of self, similar and object. Jump ahead to somewhere around (or just after) his second birthday, and he can engage in an activity that is widely observable and documented: "parallel play."

Parallel play was officially first named in 1929, in the doctoral dissertation of the American sociologist, Mildred Parten. Parten considered it to be the fourth of six stages of children's play: unoccupied, solitary, onlooker, parallel, associative and co-operative.[9] It is impossible to overstate the importance of Parten's schema to daily programming and assessment in preschool settings. In parallel play, two children play next to each other but do not interfere with, or influence, each other. What makes this stage different from the preceding one—onlooker play (where the child simply watches others play)—is that a child engages the same (type of) object as an adjacent child. So they are both at the blocks table, or both at the crafts centre, etc. In effect, the child engaged in parallel play is in a relation with one similar to himself, due to the fact that they are both essentially investing in the same object. Conversely, the case of two adjacent children where one plays with blocks and one with modelling clay is not considered parallel play.

I believe that parallel play emerges as another example of triangulation, as two humans invest in a given object by which they (i.e., the players) are deemed similar. Through parallel play, a child occasionally changes his play (i.e., his use of an object) after becoming aware of what the adjacent child has done to/with it. That is, he adapts his use of the object in association to/with the adjacent child. Thus, parallel play reveals that identification is, in itself, a product of associative thinking—and also a derivative of triangulation. We should not be surprised, then, that the stage immediately following is called "associative play." In associative play—which is considered indispensable to belonging to a community—the child develops an interest in the adjacent child who is engaging the same object he is. For socialization naturally continues to follow the pattern of unconscious triangulation, in that an object of value holds the middle ground in a relation between two who are associated by their investment in that object.

That said, it is doubtful that the child adapting his use of an object from observing an adjacent child's play is using purely visual input. For we expect, based on our journey through theory, a powerful and more crucial auditory component—a listening to the adjacent child's long strings of verbalizations. For it is a known fact that young children talk to themselves as they play, narrating their actions and intentions in captivating scripts that are a pleasure to overhear (and are often noted by their teachers in anecdotal reporting). And while unconscious triangulation is hidden from view, parallel play arguably provides evidence that an invested object enables the recognition that another may be affectively similar enough, in association to that object. Parallel play is also pertinent to our discussion because it testifies to the continued dominance of associative thinking in the young child as the principal mechanism for new learning.

Following these lines of thought, loosely perhaps, I would like to advance the notion that the archaic triangular situation that commences during gestation marks the origin of what we might rightly call "play." It is unconscious play—and a source of pleasure—as affect circulates between co-living entities, in fusion, while they engage common objects. This pattern endures even as the pre-self begins to individuate, thereby gaining the capacity to engage objects with a trusted other that is enigmatically recognized as unconsciously, affectively similar. Furthermore, because phonemes are the most affectively invested objects in early life—due to the dominance and continuity of audition—the most common form of early play is an unconscious triangulation of pre-self, witness and phoneme. This uniquely human start in life leaves a permanent record far below consciousness that continues to be influential lifelong.

As a result, we can infer that when we write, we haphazardly enable our phonemes—as invested objects—to echo between two "positions" of the self, recalling the archaic transference situation, thus returning unconscious security. In this way, free writing seems to be a form of parallel play in itself—one that is inscribed deep in our archaic heritage and prescribed to deliver pleasure. Writing is a rich potential source of echoes because words conveyed on surfaces can accidentally evoke traces of our history with phonemes; writing enables a play of echoes between words on the outside (expressed) and words on the inside (thought)—and/or words set down at one time, but refound at a later time; and writing facilitates our words becoming common objects to be shared with trusted others (triangulation). And all that echoing gives silence a voice.

In this chapter, we complete our examination of the invaluable evidence that is findable in the texts of four nonverbal autistic authors. First, we review material attesting to the benefits of a relationship with nature—everything from trees to animals—as a source of security and a means of self-regulation, as well as being a form of parallel play. Second, we undertake an exploration of writing as the only means of expression given the prevailing condition of mutism, and its relationship to echoes. We consider the decreases in anxiety and increases in pleasure that are obtainable, including the feeling of freedom and hope. We also contemplate how the lingering state of partial fusion that is inherent in passivity compels a predictable transitional dependence on others that can be slowly diminished as echoes, experienceable through writing, deliver the security needed for the eventual progression of individuation. In sum, by leveraging unconscious processes, affective liberation is achieved through the right to write as a self-securing form of play.

A. Exteriorization

These days, the last heron to migrate surveys paddlers from a dead, hollow tree on the final big turn of the Humber River before it reaches an impasse of rocks and low water. He is perched some 15–20 metres up, with a view over the west, south and east. I love that heron and I look for him every time—but in truth, all herons seem special to me. With wings outstretched, great blues are larger than I am. They stand nobly and tread carefully on the muddy banks—and even at a distance, you can tell what they are looking at from the direction of their beaks, as if they were pointing. Herons are invariably solitary and dependably silent until they take off, when they call out as if saying "good-bye." Grey on grey, this one is a stunning symbol of the season as life itself goes into hiding in preparation for the winter ahead.

Almost daily, I come here to pause writing, seek clarity and feel calmer—to discharge my abundant anxiety. Over the months, I have observed beavers, carp, cormorants, coyotes, deer, ducks, eagles, egrets, geese, groundhogs, gulls, hawks, herons, jays, mink, ospreys, racoons, salmon, skunks, squirrels, swans, turtles, woodpeckers—and the first-ever nutria of my entire life. I admit that some of these animals spark word play I can't prevent, like a reflex that kicks in anytime I see them: dead carp floating are "carpe diem"—and those patently prehistoric-looking cormorants play homonymically in my mother's tongue: «corps mourant» [dying body]. I guess words are always good fodder for daydreams—easy pleasures. But more than any other creature, herons are what I seek—though I can't control where they are, or whether one will even appear.

At some risk to myself, I will disclose what I believe I receive from herons, wherever and whenever I come upon them. A heron feels like a gift—deep joy imbibed with benevolence, as if a kindly lifeform keeps watch over me, reappearing haphazardly when I need it most. A heron somehow confirms that I am on the right path, going in the right direction—and that I am good enough, or at least that what is best about me still lives. I always look where the heron is looking, as if there is something in that direction which I need to consider—as if the heron is speaking in silence, achieving a good-enough "point." But more than anything, a heron makes me feel that I am not alone and helps me realize that I am alive (against the odds)—that I am real, present in the world after all. So as the herons leave for warmer climes, paddling is still lovely but a bit lonely. Then again, I suppose I have no one to blame but myself if my best friends are herons whose names I will never know. But what is it about herons that makes them feel like witnesses in this strange life of mine? Why herons? Have they left a permanent record in my infantile history, in my dreams even, so that I see on the outside what was once on the inside?

I can't remember. But I can Google. Sure enough, Lafontaine—the 17th-century French poet—wrote a famous fable about a heron,[10] and his collection was in every 20th-century francophone household. As I (re)discover, the fable has a river and a carp, and it has a hard moral—be flexible, don't be difficult. I have not learned that lesson very well. Then again, Lafontaine is not my teacher—the heron is. And I need that heron—any heron—for, somehow, no other animal delivers what a heron can. Did I feel sorry then for the heron because he went hungry? Or because he was stuck in such a mean-spirited story? I have no idea. But herons remain my life-sustaining, securing and consoling witnesses. What in the world?

We will now study exteriorization through three components: revitalizing energy, self-calming and securitizing provision. In terms of an initial overview, Kedar states openly, "I love nature … I see beauty all around me, and I feel part of it."[11] And Sellin explains, "I feel this sincere trust as a spring which gives important so-called earthly energy."[12] For his part, Higashida conveys a far-reaching perspective with formidable implications: "Our fondness for nature is, I think, a little bit different to everyone else's … To us people with special needs, nature is as important as our own lives."[13] And in another of his powerful stories, Mukhopadhyay shares that while walking among rocks and stones on a hillside in the changing daylight, he discovered that he was lost, for he could no longer see the rock goat that served as his guide or the huge black rock that marked the path; but he believed that if he could refind a certain familiar cloud, then he would be able to find his way back to his dream.[14]

At issue is that interactions with nature provide countless opportunities to externalize affect through the deep pleasure, in daydreams, of a kind of play. In addition, the silence and beauty of the natural world makes possible the unconscious recognition on the outside what each one of us harbours on the inside—the presence of a witness-in-similitude. So sometimes a heron—or a goat—can be a good-enough other.

First, we consider the notion of **revitalizing energy**. Any passive individual, by definition, has difficulties executing intentional, deliberate actions. So he needs a lure, an impetus, an other to follow. This is the legacy of incomplete individuation. It leaves a person regressed, dependent on an other for movement and for the provision of objects. Referring himself to natural symbolism, Sellin conveys the experience of passivity with uncanny accuracy: "There is a surging hasty spirit working eagerly in me trying to keep the unripe fruits of a person like knowing lonely steely Birger from ripening."[15] What the passive individual requires is a kind of transport, a forwarding energy, something that pulls (lures) him to enable his movements (actions). This support, which the passive individual critically needs, follows an archaic, unconscious pattern wherein the provision of all objects comes from (through and with) an other—and an other is needed to lure affective investments. I believe this sense is palpable in Kedar's words: "I love the ocean … the salty smell is so nice … I am transported into a sense of nature."[16] And Mukhopadhyay makes many references to wanting to feel like a free bird.[17] What nature provides, then, is vibrant surroundings full of abundant sources of energy to follow securely.

Higashida, for his part, shares that just changing settings in favour of the outdoors is enough to obtain needed energy: "I encounter landscapes that I don't normally see and just by having a change of scene I sometimes feel that I've become a brand new me."[18] And elsewhere he adds that in contact with nature, "our entire bodies are recharged."[19] Higashida also explains how energy is associated with free lifeforms: "It's instinctual, like a wild animal running over a wide plain."[20] And he places stunning emphasis on how sound is what pulls (attracts) him:

> Sounds in nature—the chirping of crickets or a bush-warbler's song—attract me more than the sound of words. The fact that these creatures don't speak in words as such but send out messages using their whole bodies is a mystery to me, a mystery that human beings cannot duplicate.[21]

With Higashida, we grasp that non-human lifeforms in nature offer their (dreamed) messages and good-enough others to follow—whereas "imitating [human] others"[22] can be so challenging, as Mukhopadhyay relates. For unconscious security is rooted far earlier than the self. It is a dream originally nurtured by an all-providing archaic environment—and along this same pattern, nature as an all-providing environment nourishes a daydream that delivers unconscious security. Even a "semblance of wind"[23] is enough life to follow, as Dolto once famously said. Thus, even a tree has movement in this sense: in its fluttering or falling leaves; its bending branches; the organisms thriving in and on it; and its being an organic lifeform that grows and is subject to change.

Through key observations at an early childhood drop-in centre she founded,[24] Dolto noted that a child may grab an interesting toy another plays with only to discover that in his own hands, it won't move as it seemed to. She explains that every child ignores that he himself has the power to give "life" to a toy but accords that capacity to his similar.[25] At issue is that we are all passive during our early maturation—it is a normative, transitory human condition. And during that developmental passage, we need another to follow to have life.[26] The lure of another to follow originates in the experience of being fused with an other who provides everything, and with whom one's identity is indissociable and confounded. Mukhopadhyay expresses it perfectly: "When I see or think about the wind, I am the wind."[27] He also makes the connection between exterior objects of the world and interior objects of thought, as he muses on a glass of water: "[It] reflected the tree right behind the window. I saw those little leaves move slightly in their reflection. Like a little stray thought in the stillness."[28] And in one of his stories, Mukhopadhyay narrates how a hermit follows rock goats to avoid remaining trapped.[29]

Second, we contemplate **self-calming**. It might seem paradoxical that getting energized is calming. But passivity, as a symptom of regression, means that there are fewer new objects to facilitate looser, wider, longer paths for the circulation of affect. This generates anxiety as affect flows in smaller, more restrictive circuits. Affective continuity begins in infancy, in dream-work, when we co-experience every object with an other in an all-providing environment. From hereon, every new object is secured by its associative relation to this archaic dream in an unconscious triangulation of self, similar and object. And because primary processes are driven by the instinct of conservation, we all retain the capacity to be unconsciously secured by the return of this dream—even in daylight, as a daydream—thanks to the permanence of associative thinking. What nature offers is a return of this dream.

For nature is, by definition, an all-providing environment where lifeforms evoke the dreamed presence of an other with whom to co-experience its diverse objects. So new objects are engaged, new associations are formed, unconscious affect is circulated, and anxiety is reduced. It is a deeply restorative daydream of sharing a common object with a good-enough other. That is why Dolto states that diffusing affect far and wide enables a sense of calm—securitization—for it is "exteriorization that discharges anxiety."[30]

Our relationship with nature releases affect—what I believe Mukhopadhyay refers to as "fossilized hope."[31] For his part, Kedar explains the feeling of calm that is securable from nature as an experience of peace and beauty—emphasizing his audition of specific lifeforms:

> I love being in nature ... In nature it's just soothing sounds like birds or wind in the trees or ocean waves. It is like a reprieve from feeling haywire inside from noise and bustle. I also love the natural beauty of natural settings ... It's so lovely there with rolling hills, oak trees, and native grass blowing in the breeze.[32]

Here again is the semblance of wind to follow, for there is no clear line between what gives energy and what supports calm—both service self-regulation (i.e., reduced anxiety). Further, Kedar seems to intuitively sense the need for a good-enough other to secure the new objects he encounters: "Maybe my dogs helped me in some ways to deal with a changeable world."[33] And in Mukhopadhyay, we also locate the notion that a lifeform from nature can serve as a good-enough other to secure experiences with new objects, a changeable world, and even a growing self. For example, in another creative piece referenced to the environment, he writes that so much can happen in a day that can alter appearances permanently, such as how the jackfruit tree he observes changes when some of its branches are lost due to heavy rains.[34]

Further, exterior objects that are engaged through the senses become interior objects for thought that impact individuation, as Mukhopadhyay explains: "I came to know that I am a mind tree and I was just a tree before."[35] He also uses the tree in associations that open new paths for thinking, for example by asking how many trees a field might be able to hold.[36] And trees become living examples of calmness in the face of change, as Mukhopadhyay relates:

> The way some trees stand made me wonder how they could be so patient with the world. Day after day, month after month, year after year, they remained anchored to the same spot, saying nothing, accepting everything. Like stoical philosophers, they simply endured.[37]

Self-calming is also described as an experience of pleasure and delight by Higashida: "Every single thing has its own unique beauty. People with autism get to cherish this beauty, as if it's a kind of blessing given to us."[38] Gratitude is palpable in his words, as if he is intuitively aware of the relief made possible through interacting with nature. His appreciation is sincere and direct: "I love nature."[39] And he is just as clear about the reason: "It [nature] relaxes me and puts me at my ease."[40]

But the last comment on self-calming belongs to Mukhopadhyay:

> The field is in no hurry. It has seen the beginning of the Earth. It has seen the beginning and end of many lives around it. Perhaps it saw the rise and fall of many civilizations and kingdoms. Its measure of time is very different from what the clock tells us … Does it know that I want to plant a forest on it? And does it know that whenever I stare at it, they ask me what I look at so much, out over there?[41]

Third, we reflect on the notion of **securitizing provision**. Through many of the reflections cited up to now, I believe we have already discovered the relief that nature provides as a securing presence in confronting newness; in encountering the problem of reality (time–space) and the concomitant challenges to individuation; as well as in the continued influence of dream life in the silent retreat. Additionally, something of the archaic experience of security is directly expressed in a most uncanny way by Higashida, in his answer to a question posed to him, "Why do you like being in the water?":

> We just want to go back. To the distant, distant past. To a primeval era, in fact, before human beings ever existed. All people with autism feel the same about this one, I reckon. Aquatic life-forms came into being and evolved, but why did they have to emerge onto dry land, and turn into human beings who chose to lead lives ruled by time? These are real mysteries to me.[42]

In an evocation of nature and the archaic, an affinity for the colour green is also notable, as Higashida reports: "The greenness of nature is the lives of plants and trees. Green is life."[43] Mukhopadhyay concurs, remarking on how much he loves the green colour of some walls,[44] being his favourite colour; and on how green light is also the favourite colour of his recurrent character, Emma. He writes that Emma understands that green light issues from the trees and fields, but that she can only come back (to him) when the night—and its quiet—returns.[45] Arguably, then, in the withdrawal of daylight yielding to night—when nothing can be seen or felt but dreams, and voices are silenced—the colour green serves as an enigmatic symbol of nature. And nature is a wildly archaic—thus potentially securing—experience.

Archaic references also convey how nature is a place of belonging—even, of containing and provision. Kedar describes how "Nature isn't neat or orderly … plants grow in random places … I am so at home in the messy beauty of nature … I fit in with the path in the woods."[46] And Kedar admits (perhaps in a remarkable play on words), "I am into nature."[47] Higashida agrees: "Just by looking at nature, I feel as if I'm being swallowed up into it."[48]Along with this enveloping sense of security comes the pleasurable presence of a securing other. Higashida explains: "I'll always cherish the part of me that thinks of nature as a friend."[49] He adds, "Unfortunately, I'm less connected to nature than I used to be. If asked whether I miss that affinity, I'd say yes, I do."[50]

Further, I believe that Higashida makes an uncanny suggestion that the witness-in-similitude might even be oneself—that is, a different version of self—for example, as an echo in print or voice. For he seems to convey how it is nature that provides the context for (re)imagining oneself as safe in reality:

> Writing prose that I know will be read feels like discreetly placing a manuscript on a mountaintop and leaving it there. From a good vantage point at the foot of the mountain, I can look back up and watch travellers finding, crying or smiling over the pages I left up there. The mountaintop looks far away, but their voices echo down to where I'm listening.[51]

Kedar shares Higashida's passions for nature in a reflection that evokes my own:

> I also have a deep love of the mountains. I am hardly ever happier than when we are in the mountains, hiking or kayaking … It is spiritual to be in a lake, floating in a kayak, surrounded by beauty … I sleep well in the mountains.[52]

His suggestion of symbolic life, and of sleep, is also important, for unconscious securitization—our proof of life—is always sourced deep within a dreamscape. Yet no one could put it better than Higashida here: "The reason is that when we look at nature, we receive a sort of permission to be alive in this world."[53] Thus, in offering random living witnesses with which we can instinctively resonate—making us feel secure—nature scaffolds our affective (re)circulation.

B. Witness

Lately, my paddling on the Humber River happens closer to noon than sunrise. I am not a sun chaser by nature, but I am so easily cold to my bones. By lunchtime, it's wonderfully comfortable and my eyes track better than at dawn. Mind you, there's not as much to see. I can rarely spot a deer, and all the nocturnal creatures are hiding. There's hardly a heron either. Of course, geese still sun themselves in the marsh where coyotes are most often sighted in daylight. I count them—seven. Maybe six tomorrow?

Early morning paddles facilitate encounters with countless animals who prefer liminality to light. I tend to paddle more slowly then, to experience rather than exercise. And I often let the current carry me with it, instead of exerting my arms against it. I also notice what I ignore nowadays—like the sound my hull makes lapping the waves. At daybreak, invited by the natural muting of the surroundings, I become aware of the steady beat of my paddles and the gentle splashes each one makes as it pushes the water. I love that sound. It's inexplicably soothing to hear myself in this peaceful place—the echoes of my being in the "here and now."

And as I discern myself moving with this sound, I can't help but recall how my nonverbal autistic students enjoyed walking with clickers or noisy footwear. Clack-clacking on choppy water, slosh-sloshing on flat water—I can tell how the water looks just by listening. In marginal light, I take the time to hear the echoes of my displacements—ripples on either side of my bow, the soft wake from my stern, subtle eddies around each paddle as it dips, and tiny drops raining down from each raised paddle. It is a transient record, mind you. Within seconds, my path is erased by the continuous flow. For unlike footprints on the forest floor, water holds human signatures for only an instant. When I head back downriver later, there will be no sign on the water that I was even here—eyes will find no trace of my passage. Temporary echoes, in sounds and waves, are all that ever confirm my presence on water.

But now, instead of waking up to paddle as I used to, these noon paddles have become something I schedule after checking the hourly forecast. Rationally, everything makes sense. But intuitively, something feels wrong. Certainly, the work-out does me good—90 minutes at a steady pace. I scan the shoreline and skies for what I am missing. Evidently, a lot. I make an effort to relax, and yet I still come off the river planning my next errands and appointments. The dollar-store notebook I keep in my kayak for afterthoughts that often arrive following the morning's writing holds barely a few words, whereas I would often fill two pages. And on further reflection, even those brief notes appear redundant or ill-advised. Somehow, I have missed my train of thought on the way to midday. And looking, I can't find it. Perhaps there is something elemental about hearing our own movements, confirming our existence through audition. Yet now, coming later in the day, I busy myself deliberately looking for things and paddle so intentionally. Sure, I burn off the long morning's anxiety, but I am unintentionally entirely overlooking sound. It is not at all a good trade. My body is getting warmed, but "I" am getting lost.

We will now investigate the notion of the witness that is so crucial to safely presentifying by studying writing through three overlapping tensions: anxiety (versus pleasure); fusion (dependence); and individuation (awakening). In terms of an initial overview, the case for writing is made boldly by these authors, beginning with the provocative title of one of Mukhopadhyay's books: *How Can I Talk if My Lips Don't Move?* In turn, the capacity to write independently can scaffold the gradual progression of individuation, enabling self-reliance—so that, as Kedar puts it, "It's my job to free my soul."[54] This approach will also require thinking about writing as way to become one's own witness-in-similitude, as I believe Higashida explains perfectly: "When I'm writing a story, I try to inhabit it by becoming the main character."[55] Most poignantly, Sellin conveys the tremendous empowerment that is achievable:

> We will be a new generation of mute people[,] a whole crowd of us singing new songs[,] songs such as speaking people have never heard[,] of all the poets I don't know of one who was mute[,] so we will be the first ... I'm writing for my silent sisters[,] for my silent brothers[,] we want people to hear us and give us somewhere we can live among all of you[,] live a life in this society.[56]

First we consider the tension of **anxiety versus pleasure**. Without any doubt, the obtainment of pleasure from writing is the most dominant impression a reader gets from the corpus of each of the four nonverbal authors being engaged. Sellin explains: "I'm not a real person without the writing because it's the only means of expression I have."[57] And because he can now write, he considers himself an "able backward person."[58] He adds, "I really enjoy writing[,] I have so many questions."[59] And poignantly, he shares his conviction that, "If I weren't writing my lonely thoughts would die out."[60] Here is the vital notion that producing words on the outside keeps alive words on the inside. Mukhopadhyay shares this point of view: "With my physical and neurological limitations, I am unable to do certain kinds of work. But I can think. And I can write. I can write down my stories on paper with my pencil."[61] And Mukhopadhyay clearly alludes to the benefits writing provides: "I should be able to write, rather than just point on the alphabet chart, so that I could leave a record of my conversation."[62]

Kedar shares that he experiences a similar pleasure from writing. He explains that, "It's a telling thing that my hands mostly are accurate in communication which is my most heartfelt desire."[63] And in his novel, he relates that writing gave Anthony the hope that became a salve for his spirit.[64] While as himself, he describes the sense of purpose and even duty—essentially, a movement towards the future—that comes from writing: "It is our inner determination that keeps us feeling hopeful and enables us to turn suffering into an opportunity and a mission."[65] This sense of purpose—the capacity to project the self forward—is also evident in Higashida: "If we know there is even a single person who understands what it's like for us, that's solace enough to give us hope."[66] Further, the sense of purpose that writing enables is experienced as a force that comes from deep within: "It's my prayer that

I help the world to find a better way to work with nonverbal autistic people."[67] And for Higashida, this force is what gives meaning to his entire existence: "I used to wonder why non-speaking me had ever been born."[68] And Mukhopadhyay puts it succinctly: "Did I want to write? Of course, I did."[69]

Kedar's writing is insightful as we feel the necessary inclination to silence—dependence on regression—he continues to experience, despite being able to write: "I like being anonymous, but I am determined to say what has to be said."[70] And elsewhere we find the following: "I face my pharaohs—autism experts—to see if we can't find a way to liberate autistic people from the solitude they face."[71] Higashida concurs and, in a stunning summation, he conveys how thoughts (interior) make it to the exterior to be shared in interhuman communication, while also relating the affective tethers of words:

> Since I've become better able to communicate with others via my alphabet grid, I've been taken aback by how much my words can affect and even move people. Exchanges of thought are, to a large degree, reliant upon this thing called language. Thanks to it, human beings—and we alone—can truly enter and explore the feelings of others. What an extraordinary skill.[72]

Along with pleasure—which is experienced as a capacity to invest affect forward (in future objects) and a confirmation of life—writing results in an accompanying reduction in anxiety. As himself, Kedar describes his relief, "once I could express my thoughts and connect intellectually to others."[73] And via Anthony, Kedar describes learning to write as the critical change in his life that enlarged his world, made him happier and calmer, and motivated him to do things other than stimming.[74] Furthermore, reflecting on the benefits of writing in reducing anxiety, Kedar demonstrates remarkable self-awareness: "I realized something interesting. Gradually my symptoms have been getting less intense."[75] Sellin comes to the same conclusion: "I've only been without permanent anxiety this long since I started writing[,] before that there was no hope at all."[76]

Second, we reflect on the enduring tension caused by **fusion (dependence)**. A passive disposition implies a dependence on a fusional other—and vice-versa. The conditions are inseparable, in that both are traceable to the archaic triangulation in which the self is passive and dependent on an indissociable other. If individuation is incomplete (i.e., stalled or impeded) because of an over-reliance on regression as a defence, then an individual will necessarily need an other to pull him forward—to provide objects, to offer a direction to follow. This dependence is at the heart of the problem for the nonverbal autist because he will need the continued presence of another during a long apprenticeship.[77] As Sellin relates, "I am so sad because it doesn't work so well on my own."[78] And elsewhere he states, "I am so disappointed because everyone doubts whether I write all this by myself."[79] Sellin is unequivocal about his desire: "I want to write properly because it is the way to independence."[80] He elaborates: "I would like to write entirely alone."[81] Nonetheless, he is dependent on support—on "how important it is for me to have a person always close to me firmly linked to my humble self."[82]

Sellin's reference to his "humble self" reveals the considerable suffering that comes from this dependence. Rationally, considering the immeasurable value of the reparation of writing, one might think that any "other" would do just to get the writing done. And yet, it is not so. For as predicted, given the unconscious processes at work in the condition of fusion, the witness-in-similitude needs to be both intuitively trustworthy and unconsciously recognized as affectively similar. These determinants are not amenable to planning, and there is no conscious selection process that can guarantee a suitable candidate. Assuredly, then, not every helper will be able to scaffold individuation through writing, as Sellin explains: "Not everyone is right for it working with support…so that I get the feeling I can speak dependently but freely."[83] Only the learner in question can intuitively feel whether the other will suffice.

Kedar elaborates how, "It helps many autistic people to have someone touch or even support their arm when writing or communicating. This is due to our trouble initiating and getting our bodies to obey our minds."[84] And he admits that even today, after years of independent typing (with no one touching him or his device), he "still need[s] a person nearby to help me keep my focus or I return so easily to my internal world which makes no demands and provides a drug-like trance to boot."[85] Kedar is detecting how the presence of the other enables progression to reality—whereas regression and the withdrawal to dream-work exerts its own force against progression. Kedar even notices that when he is more anxious, that regressive spiral is even more powerful: "In the past my fingers sometimes insisted on some letters that they kept repeating. It is rare now. If I feel nervous it happens more. I get trapped in the letters. I need to get unstuck somehow [from]… a trapped spiral."[86] Sellin describes the continuous draw of regression—that inner refuge of securing dreams—against which he struggles, even as writing helps individuation progress:

> A going out of oneself[,] a crate from which I am rising that would be a dream such as everyone dreams[,] but I don't see any way out of this crate which is me[,] even this important writing isn't enough a way out[,] destroys my old security[,] I am afraid of it … somethings will grow from walls one day that will rejoice the eye … there is a germ of hope in everything.[87]

Further, like Sellin, Kedar narrates how, as predicted from the unconscious processes at work, not just any helper will do: "I know people wonder why I am selective with whom I use my letter board. It leads some to doubt because people think I should use my board with everyone … but the process of trusting is slow."[88] And the fundamental passivity of the condition is palpable: "Slight touch seems to help unlock the sort of paralysis I have described."[89] In sum, therefore, support remains necessary throughout an apprenticeship that may naturally last for many years—or, as Kedar puts it, "autistic people require so much support to function and to emerge from our silent prison."[90] The result is a catch-22: learning written communication requires the presence of a facilitator, but the facilitator's presence is deemed to invalidate the written communication. I believe it is fair to suggest at this point that the main issue is a problematic focus on what is visible by the onlooker, accompanied by a neglect of what is invisibly at work in the learner.

Mukhopadhyay considers the support of a trusted, similar-enough other that must be gradually released—and the extent to which incomplete individuation engenders a problem with the body: "This time it was easy for the boy to write as he could feel the presence of the hand, his own hand linked to his body, at the shoulder point where his mother was holding him."[91] So, as Mukhopadhyay says, "The boy could relate his thoughts to words and express them by pointing and writing only when somebody held his shoulder."[92] In sum, as he puts it, facilitation—the apprenticeship through the continued presence of a trusted, similar-enough other—makes him "feel that part of my body with which I was to perform that task."[93] He elaborates:

> I have a concrete proof that to start with any new activity it is important for the autistics like the boy to be held at that part of the body which does the work as the "relating" ability develops slowly through practice. Then it can be faded out as the person gets the habit of the particular work.[94]

Crucially, also as predicted, Mukhopadhyay gives audition (rather than vision) priority in the unconscious recognition of affective similarity and the assurance of trustworthiness in the other on whom he needs to depend throughout his apprenticeship to writing—i.e., the witness-in-similitude: "The problem was that he needed time to get used to the person—his touch and most important—his voice."[95]

Third, we contemplate the residual tensions impacting **individuation (awakening)**. Individuation is scaffolded by writing as it enables two "positions" of self in triangulation with one's own words (some of which necessarily carry unconscious affects). This circulates affect, restoring the unconscious security needed for individuation to proceed. The result is the liberation of affect and the securing of reality. I believe no one expresses this better than Higashida:

> Passing to and fro between the world of the story and my daily reality, the dreaming boy I once was coexists with the adult I am now. Time loses definition. Translating into words the thoughts and landscapes that appear in my head brings me profound fulfillment.[96]

Kedar elaborates on the pleasure that comes from the liberation of unconscious affect: "It's amazing to be liberated from silence. No one should have to face this hardship. Communication is what makes us fully alive."[97] He adds, "I think autism is like solitary confinement. Communication can't be accessed without help and the right kind of instruction."[98] And because individuation implies a gradual emergence from the refuge of regression—that passive dream-like state—it is naturally experienced as a feeling of awakening. Poignantly, Kedar relates that his character, Anthony, felt like a sleepwalker who was waking up at last.[99]

On the other hand, writing will not enable (access to) the capacity for speech. For it seems that the developmental window for speech as a conscious motor movement is only open for a limited time—and by the first year of schooling, that time has long passed. Kedar, even as a published author of two books, shares his regrets about this: "I want so badly to speak … It's awful to live in such silence."[100] And although writing is hugely beneficial to unconscious securitization by reanimating archaic triangulation, it's still an anomalous form of communication in the social—perhaps akin to how the Deaf are easily subject to exclusion because Sign is seldom used by the general population. So even while attending higher education and being active in the community, Kedar reports that, "It's lonely because no matter where I am, I am the only one who points or types."[101] Likewise, Sellin confirms that while "most of my help inside my crate has come to me from writing"[102]—and writing is a "fabulous help"[103] out of a "dreadful labyrinth"[104]—he is still subject to the problem of non-inclusion:

> If a miracle happened let's say this restless spirit became calmer articulated better so that everyone could understand what he was saying the ways speaking people easily understand each other[,] then all the same it's a fact it would be too difficult for me[,] but I haven't entirely given up that hope.[105]

In sum, Kedar relates the following, not without bitterness: "Though I still get sad, it's true, I'm not hopeless. Now I'm living in a flashcard-free world."[106] Sellin seems to share Kedar's opinion that, at least, "writing is my first step out of that other world."[107] Poignantly, Sellin also shares why independent writing—though it has such a long apprenticeship and slow output—still matters so much: "A mute person wants to articulate too[,] he has a right to language too[,] without language we are dead isolated outcast apparatus[,] an important work[,] bringing language to the mute."[108] And Sellin closes our discussion with this invaluable advice:

> I would also learn how to behave to people who actually cure lonely growing up people of autistic agitation to express a hope[,] its true there are no stupid autistics[,] there is no way out without hope[,] anyone can see that.[109]

In closing this chapter on exteriorization and witnessing, I believe that we can reasonably infer (i.e., theorize) that writing leverages enduring unconscious processes to enable self-triangulation. For writing restores the circulation of affect between invested phonemes and the self in echo. True, it is a late repair developmentally. But it is a formidable one that is constantly accessible, making the long apprenticeship worth the effort. Also true, it will not guarantee social inclusion—nor speech—and some barriers to complete integration will remain, more so the later that writing is learned. But writing significantly reduces anxiety, and this alone makes a highly significant and deeply humane contribution to an autist's quality of life. Even more crucially, writing returns a voice—agency—to the muted self.

Notes

1 Canadian Broadcasting Corporation.
2 As seems apt to call it in translation, as explained previously.
3 In Halmos 1994, 262.
4 In Guillerault 1997, 245.
5 Dolto's word is «reconnaissance,» whose phonemic play has already been suggested.
6 In Kouki 2005, 86.
7 In Manier & Kouki 2003, 186–187.
8 We have only to think of academic research (including works like the present one) to locate this dependence.
9 1932, 243.
10 «Le Héron» is in the public domain.
11 2012, 119.
12 1995, 92.
13 2007/2013, 120.
14 2005, 218.
15 1995, 88.
16 2012, 109.
17 2000, 67, 69 & 70–71; also 2005, 155.
18 2017, 237.
19 2007/2013, 120.
20 2017, 58.
21 Ibid, 100.
22 2000, 11.
23 In De Sauverzac 1988, 13.
24 Dolto's highly respected «Maison vertes» remain prominent as grassroots associations around the world, especially in Europe and Canada. I expand on the concept in my previous work on Dolto.
25 Dolto 1985b; also De Sauverzac 1988, 13.
26 French curiously divulges this relation homonymically, for «je suis» means both "I am" and "I follow"—with perfectly identical orthography and pronunciation.
27 2008, 118.
28 2005, 205.
29 Ibid, 220.
30 Dolto 1981, 189.
31 2015a, 68.
32 2012, 109.
33 Ibid, 121.
34 2005, 164.
35 2000, 87.
36 2005, 197.
37 2015a, 80.
38 2007/2013, 92.
39 2017, 264.
40 Ibid, 58.
41 2005, 211–212.
42 2007/2013, 104.
43 Ibid, 120.
44 2000, 67.
45 2005, 206.
46 2012, 119.

47 Ibid, 122.
48 2007/2013, 123.
49 Ibid, 124.
50 2017, 214.
51 Ibid, 98.
52 2012, 109.
53 2007/2013, 120.
54 2012, 102.
55 2017, 99–100.
56 1995, frontispiece.
57 Ibid, 57.
58 Ibid, 77.
59 Ibid, 56.
60 Ibid, 95.
61 2008, 216.
62 Ibid, 160–163. (His word "record" in Dolto's mother tongue and my own is «record»; this is homonymically two phonemes, «re/corps» [body again] as another enigmatic suggestion from words seems to helpfully feed thought.)
63 2012, 55.
64 2018, 171.
65 2012, 106.
66 2017, 89.
67 2012, 66.
68 2007/2013, 40.
69 2008, 159.
70 2012, 66.
71 Ibid, 115.
72 2017, 86.
73 2012, 57.
74 2018, 170.
75 2012, 155.
76 1995, 125.
77 Learning to speak also requires the continued presence of another. A child playing alone (and capable of speech) will invariably be discovered talking to stuffed animals, pets, shadows, toys, etc. For language is learned in exchanges with others (real or not) because the echoes of our invested phonemes securitize reality. As Dolto narrates, the child's acquisition of the mother tongue begins with the pre-conscious exposure to phonemes *in utero*, followed (from birth) by the language input of familiars and the wider sonar landscape. From here, the child receives support, including (hopefully) gentle corrections of mispronunciations—the perfection of phonemes. The child then imitates what he hears. Ostensibly, he receives pleasure from the approval his attempts elicit among caregivers, and from his newfound capacity to articulate choices. With regards to a second language, it is also common knowledge that there is a critical period, after which it is nonetheless learnable but not as perfectly or easily. Yet no one would accuse a bilingual child of five of not really speaking because his apprenticeship in that code is still being scaffolded. In fact, we readily accept that 10 years of support (on average) is required for the acquisition of speech in anyone's mother tongue—if we include the first years of primary education, where intrafamilial orality and idiolects are progressively corrected to conform to social norms. Furthermore, children learning to write (at home or school) have long apprenticeships until their work is readable and their spelling is standardized. Yet no one questions the merits of a four-year-old's journal as a demonstration of learning because the teacher (who is present

during "shared writing") typically transcribes the learner's thoughts in standard form below his invented spelling. Yet when nonverbal autists learn to scribe or type, the support of another is routinely taken as an invalidation of their learning and products. Educationally speaking, this seems illogical.

78 1995, 54.
79 Ibid, 69.
80 Ibid, 84.
81 Ibid, 136.
82 Ibid, 71.
83 Ibid, 95.
84 2012, 78.
85 Ibid, 98–99.
86 Ibid, 163.
87 1995, 25.
88 2012, 76.
89 Ibid, 78.
90 Ibid, 98–99.
91 2000, 32.
92 Ibid, 32.
93 Ibid, 74.
94 Ibid, 32.
95 Ibid, 30.
96 2017, 99–100.
97 2012, 66.
98 Ibid, 62.
99 2018, 216.
100 2012, 72.
101 Ibid, 91.
102 1995, 139.
103 Ibid, 144.
104 Ibid, 144.
105 Ibid, 60.
106 2012, 59.
107 1995, 225.
108 Ibid, 128.
109 Ibid, 59.

Summary for Part Two

Dolto theorizes that autism is a regression to the archaic, and nonverbal autists confirm critical aspects of the lived experience of regression. As Dolto's theorization predicts, a number of defining traits are observable: a passive disposition; the dominance of audition; abundant daydreaming; creative symbolization; vibrant thinking; a passion for words; precocious reading; difficulty with change; a love of nature; reliance on regression; and the most powerful indicator of all—overwhelming, persistent anxiety. We should also discover, as predicted, that once writing is enabled—despite its relatively long apprenticeship, the extended dependence on an other, and its admittedly slow output—this greatly reduces anxiety by facilitating the resumption of individuation: a sense of self as freedom and purpose. And while writing does not restore speech nor guarantee full social inclusion, it is a good-enough substitute for speaking in terms of its restorative unconscious work. For like speaking, writing enables an echo of our words to be made "present," offering securitization on the pattern of archaic triangulation. In fact, the evidence from the corpora of four nonverbal autists confirms these predictions decisively. In addition, their testimony attests to the truth that not being able to speak does not entail not being able to think.

A passive disposition signals a reliance on regression as a defence—and vice-versa. This implies a continued dependence on an other to provide objects. But individuation requires precisely the opposite. Individuation is the self-securing condition of mental and emotional dissociation from that other. It is the realization of affective self-sufficiency. When sufficient individuation is achieved, affect can be invested readily enough in new objects that one finds for oneself. Thus, individuation is experienced unconsciously as self-provision, the capacity for ensuring one's own survival. In every sense, then, individuation requires the ability to self-triangulate—that is, to continually restore (i.e., reanimate) the witness with whom objects are automatically secured through being dreamed as co-experienced.

Privileging Dolto's theorization on the role of language in circulating unconscious affect, we focus on phonemes as objects. In any triangulation, circulation is continuous from one "position" to another. So affect flows from the pre-self and indissociable other to random phonemes that become invested via their engagement in unconscious triangulation. Further, affect also returns to the pre-self from

DOI: 10.4324/9781032655123-13

the indissociable other (and the affect this other invests). Effectively, then, archaic triangulation enables the diffusion of affect by association in proliferations of triangulations that create rich associative networks for circulation. And crucially, along those same pathways (albeit at incalculable associative distances), archaic triangulation enables the pre-self to (re)experience unconscious affect as a proof of life.

Reading can deliver chance encounters with our pre-invested phonemes. Enigmatically, this means that a text is unconsciously an environment for the provision of objects. Mind you, this assumes reading freely, letting the passive reader follow his intuition along archaic traces, in a secure mental and emotional condition that allows him to take a chance on being unconsciously lured. Along the pattern of archaic triangulation, the benefit of finding pre-invested phonemes—and/or words richly associated with them—is the return of affect to the self. This is unconsciously self-securing. Small wonder, then, that someone in the throes of mortifying anxiety would be precociously hyperlexic. It might even be that an author in the mother tongue, with a sufficiently generous corpus, would serendipitously offer an abundance of one's own archaic phonemes—texts imbibed with archaic echoes, criss-crossed with archaic traces—a veritable water table of unconscious affects. In dream-work, this abundance of invested phonemes might even return a good-enough witness, making an author a means of unconscious securitization. And in dream-work, that securitizing witness might even be the storybook character who speaks those invested phonemes, or who delivers a good-enough "version" of the self to be deemed unconsciously similar. For this restitution is happening in dream-work after all—unconsciously—so a character that seems alive *is* alive, functionally speak. Besides, a character is also associated with the author, who is or was alive. And through all these means, texts can scaffold individuation.

By extension (i.e., by association), we can infer that nature affords similar opportunities for the restitution of archaic security—the means being just as enigmatic. For nature is, by definition, an all-providing environment offering an abundance of random living things. Any of these living things might deliver a good-enough other—a witness—for someone passively disposed to follow unconsciously, triggering forward displacements of affect through an enticement (i.e., lure) to engage new objects. So wild nature harbours an unlimited potential for restoring archaic security in reality and returning affect to the self. Small wonder too, then, that an anxiogenic, passive individual would find calming relief and unspeakable pleasures in natural surroundings.

Archaic triangulation continuously invests the phonemes of the mother tongue with affect during the critical first months of mental and emotional development—when what is "mental" and "emotional" is inseparable, as is always the case in the unconscious. This means that associative thinking is also affectively driven by associations to phonemes that are invested during the archaic stage. The affective legacy to one's mother tongue is formidable. Reciprocally, one can easily infer the considerable affective sequelae of migrating to a second language with few phonemic correlates.

But beyond reading and nature, the most permanent reparation of unconscious security comes from writing. As Dolto explains, our own words coincidentally include some of our affectively invested phonemes in an unconscious (latent) register inscribed in language. We cannot help it. Further, Dolto describes how the child first learning to speak repeats the mother's phonemes to evoke her dreamed presence. Effectively, he is ensuring his own unconscious security by that archaic resonance. Put another way, the child's own voice expedites his unconscious individuation. And what I have suggested is a leveraging of Dolto's unprecedented and highly usable theorization of the role of the phoneme in archaic triangulation to formulate the simple but indispensable notion of an echo.

In the archaic triangulation of any phoneme (by which it is invested with affect), there is functionally a play—an echo—between two archaic "positions" of the self: the pre-self and the witness blurred with it. In fact, this unconscious tandem between "I" and "(s)he/you" (and/or referring to oneself by name, as-if an other), leaves its traces in the developmental passage of every young child learning to speak, as can be easily observed in homes and classrooms worldwide. It also discloses its continued, permanent residence in the autist's texts as an enduring inscription of the archaic triangular situation. In short, in producing language, we inevitably triangulate invested phonemes between two "positions" of the self. This generates unconscious echoes that, along abundant associations, reanimate archaic triangulation. In short, this resonance taps trapped affect, recirculates it, returns affect to the self, and thereby delivers an unconscious proof of life.

We can further express the resonance of any echo in terms of two overlapping opportunities for unconscious "play." On the one hand, there is an echo between what is inside (a phoneme in associative thinking), and what is outside (a phoneme in a spoken or written text). Perhaps we could call this a spatial echo. On the other hand, there is also an echo between the self as speaker (or writer), and the (later) self as listener (or reader) at some later date. Perhaps we could call this a temporal echo. But whether the echo is spatial or temporal, as it were, echoes make manifest some latent content in reality—i.e., in space and time. And this is what enables the restitution of archaic triangulation that automatically delivers unconscious security. Additionally, in terms of the unconscious processes at play, writing self-secures reality just as well as speaking. It may be slower (i.e., less immediate) than speech, but it is a more durable record. Thus, writing provides a good-enough experience for stalled individuation to restart, providing an invaluable benefit in nonverbal autism. For the archaic triangular situation is a permanent installation beneath consciousness that remains as a lifelong unconscious resource.

I hope that readers will be compellingly affected and genuinely informed by the impactful material these nonverbal autistic authors provide, and by the sheer strength of their intellectual and creative contributions. In a style unique to each, these writers relate the lived experience of being trapped in silence in a refuge—regression—that ironically holds the indelible appeal of dream-work and security. Reading and word play offer consolations, though the precocious capacity to read is often undetected or disbelieved. And the ability to write independently—which is inherently subject to suspicion due to a lengthy apprenticeship dependent on the sustained presence of a trusted other—lessens anxiety while restoring a sense of personal freedom and improving quality of life.

In terms of a conclusion to Part Two, the nonverbal autist thinks creatively, reads competently, and needs nature more than most people. He also has the right to write. For the child who cannot travel on the superhighway to self-securing individuation that speech offers can nonetheless find an inviting trail in the woods. And given that autism *is* a regression to the archaic, how can interventions better address it? This is the question we will engage as we consider applications for practice in Part Three.

Part Three

Practice

Preamble for Part Three

As I am writing this book, the global COVID-19 pandemic seems to be waning, at least in my corner of the world—Toronto, Canada. On Friday, 13 March 2020, my Grade Sixes were having a pre-Spring Break party when news came to take a few school materials home as we would be out for an extra week or two. Everyone was in a festive mood about having a longer holiday, as we waved each other off. Little did we know that we would never be back in our classroom again. Come June, teachers were posted outside their respective schools, handing back pencil cases and indoor shoes in labelled bags to students showing up at intervals, everyone in masks on a hot, sunny day. We had "pivoted to online"—as we learned to say—and children I had seen on camera for four months seemed so much taller than I remembered. Forced onto remote platforms, teachers had identified enduring understandings and trimmed all else. Math ran on instructional videos, subtopics in science and social studies were skipped because they simply weren't do-able, and the arts became a means of entertainment and relaxation rather than being a proper subject. Like teachers everywhere, I spent months reinventing my practice because online school required so much preparation and students easily became unhooked, turning off their cameras and falling off the radar—with many families being naturally too strained to do much about it. By June, everyone was exhausted but at least it was over. Next year would be different.

But as it turned out, the next school year, 2020–2021, was not very different at all. Locally, teachers and students chose between "online" or "in-person" environments—and students went back and forth all year, creating complete mayhem for plans and assessments. While working in-person, teachers wore masks, face shields and gloves; and we were instructed to leave collected work untouched for three days. Education had become a vector for contamination. Alternately, while working online, teachers faced a struggle to keep kids present, virtually speaking, and turning in any work at all. By June 2021, we were back on the same sidewalks, handing out labelled bags to fewer kids, though, because most had learned by then to never leave anything at school. I saw about half of my Grade Sixes and they looked so much paler than on camera.

My seniority enabled me to transfer to a much smaller school the following year, as I deliberately sought less exposure to COVID-19. Sure enough, 2021–2022

DOI: 10.4324/9781032655123-15

continued to be disorienting and dangerous: masks, sanitizer, filters, protocols and endless checklists. Kids routinely missed 40–50 days of school due to illness and/or the family's obligation to isolate. There were no sports, clubs or field trips. Entire cohorts got sent home again and again, pivoting unpredictably from home to "bricks and mortar" until we were all dizzy and completely drained—students, families, teachers and administrators. Worst of all, student engagement—what teachers most care about—was impossibly hard to secure.

Retired and reflecting, I realize now how we had all turned to reading and writing through those deeply challenging years. I leave it to future historians to chronicle the inner workings of the epidemic in schools and its sequelae on so many levels. But I personally know of no teachers who did not drive their programmes with novels or some kind of shared reading. In turn, we gauged how our students were feeling and managing mostly by their writing: journals, projects, paragraphs, online chats, emails, etc. Throughout the devastating destabilization, reading and writing were the tethers that held us together. Literacy became the remains of education in impossible times.

In fact, the question of education in impossible times is something Dolto spent her whole life considering. How can a child who manifests stigmatized difficulties be socially supported? How can learning be restored in the child who seems not to be listening? How can a child who never (or no longer) speaks be supported in communicating? How might a child with debilitating anxiety be helped to deal with change? How can the child who seems passive and withdrawn be nurtured to regain a force for living? These are some of the queries about learning that Dolto spent decades of clinical work trying to address. Her interest in education had begun early in life. By the time she was only eight, she was telling people that she wanted to be a "doctor of education."[1] Family members would jokingly prod her about what that was. She would reply very seriously that she had no idea, but this is what she would become. In time, she would go on to be a medical doctor and psychoanalyst. Yet even then, she saw herself in an educational context, referring to her most influential clinical supervisor in the hospitals of Paris, the great Sophie Morgenstern, as her "principal teacher."[2]

From such beginnings, I believe that a very strong case can be made for how Dolto spent her entire working life being a teacher. When she was already in her 60s, she was hosting seminars on psychoanalytic work with children at l'École Freudienne de Paris,[3] and on children's art (in lieu of toys) in therapy at the Institut Océanographique.[4] Her seminars were attended by hundreds; for example, 400 were registered for her sessions at the Institut National des Sourds in 1981.[5] There were waiting lists for her training clinics, where attendees became "choral witnesses."[6] And she personally invested in educational initiatives—for instance, by supporting L'École Neuville (outside of Paris).[7] Lifelong, Dolto presented at countless conferences, including one in Canada as late as 1983[8]—when she was already 78 years old. And in 1988, at the age of 80, she was still training others during her sessions with infants from a local orphanage. She became known in her neighbourhood for her unsurpassed dedication to children, as she went about to her seminars and supervisions dragging the oxygen tanks needed for the pulmonary insufficiency that would take her life in August of that year.[9] Even as she lay in bed in her last weeks, she read manuscripts being sent to her[10]—an activity any teacher can recognize, for we routinely spend both ends of the day marking and reviewing student work. More than anything, Dolto manifested a teacher's attitude towards children, for we occupy our liminal moments wondering what to do about a certain child, issue or concept. And as Dolto put it, her life's goal was always "to question there where I feel questioned."[11]

In Part Three, with the benefit of years of further reflection and a specific focus on Dolto's belief that autism is a regression to the archaic, I revisit the directions for future work that I left open at the end of my previous project on Dolto.[12] The most pressing directive I articulated then, the need to presume competence in non-verbal autism, is the incentive for the present project in its entirety.[13] Beyond this overarching concern (or rather, because of it), I began to hear my earlier questions differently and to sense how the "phoneme in echo" might be a useful formulation. As a result, four of my prior considerations now seem more pressing. So these inform the chapters that follow, as I leverage Dolto's theorization of the phoneme to address some practical questions in the field of education.

But first, we begin with a necessary recap of the theoretical context thus far. The archaic stage of psychosexual maturation begins early in gestation and extends until birth, when the umbilical castration (i.e., birth) triggers the oral stage. During the archaic stage, the child begins an unconscious mental and emotional activity that will be unceasing as long as he lives: he dreams. Dreams, like all unconscious processes, are driven by the instinct of conservation. So by definition, this dream fulfils his wish to live—and its continuity it is a proof of life. Diverse objects enter the infant's dream-work, as they do for any of us.

The onset of our mental and emotional life has its origins in the archaic stage, then, alongside the dawn of our physiological life. And it is a physiological fact that audition develops somewhere around 24 weeks gestation (or earlier). Thus, audition is prominent and precocious in the infant—compared to vision, for example, which only becomes dominant postnatally as the infant progresses towards a greater share of consciousness. In contrast, *in utero*, in the unconscious beginnings of our mental and emotional life, audition dominates. Precocious audition—which is continuous and cannot be turned off—provides a preponderance of objects for the infant's dreams.

Not only that, but the infant is not ever alone, is he? He is completely fused with an indissociable (m)other without whom he cannot survive. And this indissociable other provides all his objects. Thus, this indissociable other is not experienced unconsciously as separate: rather, he confounds this similar other with himself, as-if he were her. So the pre-self begins in a dream where every object that arrives is co-experienced with an indissociable other. This is functionally a triangulation of pre-self, indissociable (similar) other, and an(y) object.

Crucially, archaic triangulation circulates affect as a flow of libidinal energy that characterizes unconscious life and drives psychosexual maturation. Affect circulates in triangulation beginning in the archaic stage—and we thus infer that archaic triangulation is the precursor of the Oedipal triangulation. As the infant receives everything from his indissociable other, affective circulation is experienced as a dream of provision—the continuous arrival of objects and affect. Put another way, unconscious affect circulates from the other through objects to the pre-self and keeps returning affect to the self. Thus, archaic triangulation is self-securing.

During growth in the archaic stage, unconscious affect naturally increases in quanta to enable the fueling of psychosexual maturation. And, in dream-work, objects that are associated with each other become pathways for the flow of affect, as triangulations form from other triangulations, and so on, in proliferations that ensure the continuous circulation of affect—its liberation. The continuous circulation of affect enables self-regulation. On the other hand, anytime the flow is impeded, there will be a surcharge as affect is blocked from liberation, generating the experience of anxiety. Therefore, the instinct of conservation (in the interest of survival) drives the system to seek pathways for the liberation of affect. Conversely, in the absence or limitation of sufficient means for liberating affect, affect is conserved by the instinct of conservation—resorbed into pre-existing pathways.

Since audition is so precociously dominant, and audition provides so many of the earliest objects, the phonemes of language become indispensable in creating associative networks for the circulation of unconscious affect. The phonemes of any language are syllable-type units that are audible in repetitions within the long indecipherable strings of voice to which the infant is exposed *in utero*. So phonemes are common objects in unconscious triangulations: pre-self, indissociable (similar) other, and phoneme. Phonemes that are repeated and/or highly invested by the mother are naturally more invested by the infant. Furthermore, phonemes that are associated with other pre-invested phonemes (i.e., auditorily, phonetically) are automatically invested as affect flows between them, perpetuating pathways for affective circulation through associations.

In the unconscious, what is mental and what is emotional is indissociable. For unconscious affect that is invested in phonemes (along pathways) seeds associative thinking. And as associations proliferate—and perception and proprioception develop—the infant's mental and emotional world expands exponentially. The most ubiquitous objects, phonemes, become perceptible more clearly and in greater numbers, enriching associative thinking, as affect is diffused (i.e., displaced) along pathways for its liberation. Thus, audition is unconsciously attuned to finding issues for affect since liberation enables self-regulation—and self-regulation is driven by the instinct of conservation. So the infant, while inherently passive, is phenomenally receptive.

Meanwhile, the indissociable other slowly starts to be dissociated unconsciously as the infant acquires a liminal experience of his own difference from this other. Developmentally, he still experiences himself in the continuous presence of a self-similar other, but his sense of otherness becomes more flexible. In particular, there is a growth in his nascent awareness, by repeated associations, of the other of the mother whose phonemes—thanks to the dominance of audition—are frequently encountered and invested. Unconsciously, he now experiences himself as blurred (in dream-work) with this other of the (m)other in taking in new objects. So the child's mental and emotional life becomes marked by a more generalizable formulation of archaic triangulation: pre-self, witness-in-similitude, and phoneme. The witness-in-similitude is the unconscious experience of a continuous, securing presence that vouchsafes for objects as paths for investment (i.e., the preservation of affect)—and who is unconsciously 'recognized' as being highly similar to the self affectively, being both present (in dream-work) and blurred with self.

The unconscious triangulation of pre-self, witness-in-similitude and phoneme that begins in the archaic is a permanent inscription far below consciousness. Needless to say, it legates a formidable heritage to the mother tongue and to associative thinking.[14] It is vital to note that this archaic history does not limit what we think, nor does it make us culturally bound to a fixed set of ideas based on our mother tongues. What it does, instead, is essentially "preload" affect in the phonemes we encounter during the archaic stage. And while these phonemes may reappear in phonetically similar languages, we can infer that we will best sustain affective circulation in the language of our archaically invested phonemes. To restate, the archaic stage does not constrain how or what we think based on our investment in certain phonemes. Rather, it predisposes our affective investments—that is, how (much) we feel in and through any given language.

Any phoneme with associations to archaic phonemes can be affectively invested; likewise, any other who is unconsciously recognized as a witness-in-similitude can be affectively invested. Note that since this is a process grounded in dream-work, the other may even be a non-human lifeform or a storybook character recognized as unconsciously affectively similar. And through the network of associations achieved by triangulation, the infant invests in new objects that are continuous with his archaic investments, thereby liberating affect: anxiety is decreased. Conversely, the incapacity to be unconsciously lured by new objects (and thus to liberate affect) precipitates the withdrawal (i.e., condensing) of affect along pre-existing pathways as the experience of regression: anxiety is increased. As a vital means for self-regulation, then, the transit of affect in language takes place in its unconscious (i.e., latent) register as we produce our own words—which accidentally, naturally include some of our invested phonemes—in speaking or writing; and we are unconsciously resonant to our invested phonemes when we haphazardly encounter them in listening or reading. Another vital inference is possible here: we can recover affect from our own phonemes, but only if consciousness is sidelined. This is, in fact, the work of the "talking cure."

It is worth emphasizing at this juncture that not all relations can sustain affective circulation. But ultimately, any relations that can sustain the continuous circulation of unconscious affect will necessarily involve (even at great associative distances) some circulatory tethers—affective pathways—to pre-invested phonemes and/or to a prior witness-in-similitude (ultimately reaching back to the indissociable other). Archaic triangulation is a dreamed relation installed deep beneath consciousness. And we are driven lifelong by the instinct of conservation not to squander affect.

So we invest unconscious affect only if, and when, returns of unconscious pleasure are guaranteed—that is, our chances for survival are enhanced. Otherwise, we automatically resorb it defensively, saving it from unquantifiable risks.

Since the circulation of unconscious affect is under the jurisdiction of primary processes, the critical restitution of the archaic triangular situation that we unconsciously seek (and need) in reality—namely, invested phonemes and the witness-in-similitude—are never findable consciously, nor in consciously manipulated (i.e., deliberately curated) spaces or texts.[15] As driven by unconscious processes that antedate consciousness developmentally—and that continue to exert their immeasurable strength far below consciousness—the accidental return of archaic investments in reality, being the experience of unconscious (re)securitization, will require free environments, chance opportunities, coincidences and serendipity. It is completely irrational and instinctive—thus it entirely eludes human planning.

Dolto explains the (re)finding of unconscious archaic security as "the articulation of a perception that has come from the exterior world to which he remains attached, that is, fragments of phantasms."[16] Put another way, it is an experience whereby "unconscious phantasies are externalized,"[17] as what is "perceive[d] of the interior … is articulated with what is perceived as coming from the exterior world."[18] Dolto stresses how important it is to our unconscious security in reality to refind (i.e., re-source in) our archaic investments, including that indissociable other needed to testify to our affective experiences. For, as infants, all of us are lured to reality—and build our sense of unconscious security in it—by being affectively woven with others. This proliferation of sufficient associations, through abundant objects for circulating unconscious affect, is what achieves self-regulation—increased pleasure and decreased anxiety. On the other hand, as Dolto elaborates, if no suitable objects come from the side of reality to continue our archaic dreams of security, we will keep our unconscious affect to ourselves, holding it in relatively small circulatory paths. This constriction of affect generates anxiety, as "nothing comes from the exterior to this individual to break the vicious cycle,"[19] as she puts it. At issue is that the flow of formidable reserves of affect is needed for all subsequent stages of psychosexual maturation. So the constriction of affect—its unavailability for forward displacements—limits the potential to invest in our futures, loves and work. It is therefore experienced unconsciously as a threat to survival.

Following Dolto, I am suggesting that archaic triangulation on invested phonemes is an unconscious echo. For a phoneme is effectively circulating between two "positions" in triangulation—self and witness—along the enduring archaic triangular pattern wherein the pre-self and witness-in-similitude co-experience objects. Thus, phonemes in echo restore the deep sense of security that is inherently associated with archaic triangulation. In fact, we can encounter echoes of our invested phonemes in reading—as words on the outside echo what is inside (i.e., our invested phonemes in associative thinking). This can also happen when we read the works of an other who we recognize unconsciously and affectively as a witness. And, enigmatically, this can happen when we read our own works with conscious distancing—refinding them after forgetting, for example. At issue is that the process of recovering unconscious security is ungovernable and inaccessible by conscious planning. Archaic triangulation also leaves a significant trace in our relations with nature as an all-providing environment of objects, including non-human lifeforms, any of which might serve as good-enough witnesses.

Birth—physical separation—neither entails nor compels unconscious separation. The pre-self will still feel fusional and passively dependent on the continuous presence of an other for his objects and security until his individuation can be achieved. Individuation—the self—requires affect to circulate freely onto new objects along associations that ultimately source their affect in archaic triangulations, without the reliance on regression. Individuation is the ability for unconscious self-securing. This is (very) difficult to achieve for an infant who is born somewhat or deeply regressed as a result of suffering or setbacks in normative progression during gestation that were (necessarily) unnoticed and unnarratable. Few objects of reality are likely to find associative links to deep objects of dream-work; few unconscious lures can be engaged; and regression will become even more entrenched. This delays the normative, gradual shift towards consciousness that relies on affective investments and that is necessary for intentional movement—including the motor act of speech. Physical growth proceeds nonetheless on its own agenda, but a developmental window for speaking may be missed and, thereby, foreclosed. Language comprehension will be developed and thinking will be vibrant—but the child will be functionally mute.

This is precisely the conclusion that Dolto compels, namely that autism is a regression to the archaic. So doing, Dolto provides the theoretical rationale for why (and how) nonverbal autists are mute but thinking. In turn, the evidence from four nonverbal autistic writers confirms Dolto's theorization decisively. For these authors attest that the lived experience of autism is dominated by a reliance on regression as a defence, with all the expected markers: passivity, attuned audition, daydreaming, symbolization, thinking, love of words, precocious reading, difficulty with newness, affinity for nature, and unrelenting anxiety.

Dolto demonstrates persuasively that thought is rooted in the archaic stage as a natural progression from dream-work. This is so because precocious, pre-conscious audition *in utero* invests unconscious affect in repeated phonemes of the mother tongue that proliferate in/as associative thinking for the continuous circulation of affect that ensures self-regulation and continued psychosexual maturation. Unconscious processes do not depend on conscious ones (e.g., the conscious motor act of speech). Instead, the reverse is true. For unconscious processes develop first, entirely independently—and they continue so long as the human organism lives. As a result, thinking begins long before any child is expected to speak his first word. So not being able to speak never means not being able to think. From this, I believe that we can now advance further proposals about the unconscious work of phonemes—their impact on language, literacy and learning—to make education an instrument for the preservation of affect and a reparation for the difficulty of living.

Chapter 7 analyses the unconscious affect invested in early phonemes—names, home languages and sonar landscapes. What are the implications for migration and

Indigenous children deprived of their mother tongues through forced assimilation? What happens to a child who no longer encounters his affectively invested phonemes, or can no longer use them? What is the affective cost of changing a child's name—or of bilingualism? What might losing associations to the witness entail? And what are the repercussions of invested phonemes for nonverbal autism?

Chapter 8 explores the persistence of archaic object relations as these relate to reading. How might reading return pre-invested phonemes, or reanimate archaic objects? How might reading offer a witness? Why is it important for the reader to choose what to read? How does reading produce self-securing echoes? How might reading reduce anxiety? How do unconscious echoes in reading support individuation? Why might someone reject reading? Why are books and libraries so important? And what are the repercussions of securing reading for nonverbal autism?

Chapter 9 investigates the role of writing in a kind of witnessing that secures triangulation. How does writing produce unconscious echoes? How can writing produce echoes in space—that is, between words in our thoughts (interior) and in texts (exterior)? How can writing produce echoes in time—that is, between when we put words down and we encounter them later? What is uniquely operational about note-taking as transcription? What is the unconscious work of writing that makes it so essential? And what are the repercussions of writing/transcribing for nonverbal autism?

Chapter 10 considers the archaic continuity that is securable from our experiences in nature. How might nature support an emergence from regression? How might a random lifeform in nature serve as a good-enough other to follow? How might a random lifeform serve as a good-enough witness? How can enabling self-provision in an all-providing environment scaffold individuation and reduce anxiety? What is the unconscious work of nature? Why is an access to wilderness not just pleasurable but indispensable? And what are the repercussions of exploring nature for nonverbal autism?

The questions arising out of Dolto's unprecedented project are deeply provocative for education. And while interventions inspired by Dolto are grounded in what we understand about nonverbal autism from a theoretical and evidentiary standpoint, they can benefit not only nonverbal autists but all children. At issue is that pre-conscious learning is happening in the human infant during the archaic stage under the influence of unconscious processes, particularly because of our affective investments in the phonemes of our mother's tongue to which we are precociously exposed. This earliest learning permanently impacts our ability to liberate unconscious affect: to be happy as a self, to minimize our anxiety, to learn (i.e., invest in new objects)—and to love our familiars, jobs and lives. And what is perhaps most curious about Dolto's theorization is that is it so hard to explain yet so easy to implement. For the prescriptions that issue from it incur almost no costs, are simple to learn, and are risk-free for learners and teachers. Unconscious processes require little accommodation, in other words, but they can secure formidable returns.

Notes

1 Dolto 1985a, 231–232; Dolto 1986b, 68–69; Dolto & Roudinesco 1986/1988, 17; Potin 2008, 112.
2 In Dolto & Winter 1986, 23; Nobécourt 2008b.
3 In Djéribi-Valentin 2005, 495.
4 Ibid, 523–524.
5 Ibid, 698.
6 Dolto 1977b, 28; Coronel & De Mezamat 1997b; Charial, Eliacheff & Valentin 1999, 50–53.
7 D'Ortoli & Amram 1990; D'Ortoli & Amram 2009a; D'Ortoli & Amram 2009b.
8 In Djéribi-Valentin 2005, 859.
9 Ibid, 602, 606, 639, 820, 855 & 890.
10 For example, C. Dolto 1989, 9.
11 Dolto 1984, 323.
12 Saint-Onge 2019, 219–220; its pre-publication drafts are dated 2016–2018.
13 Due to time and logistical constraints, my doctoral dissertation, from which my previous project on Dolto arose (2019), could only cover so much. Although the implications of Dolto's work for nonverbal autism were patently evident then, I received sage counsel to defer a deeper inquiry to a later date. I am truly thankful for this advice because the delay of years and the quiet space for thinking has, I believe, been fruitious.
14 Dolto's theorization does not support linguistic determinism. As should be evident, her exploration of the archaic stage addresses the unconscious, affective register of language and the emotional world—not cognition. Archaic experiences with phonemes do not prescribe or limit what we can think; what is at issue instead is the unconscious affective charge of words.
15 The grave implications for texts formulated by artificial intelligence (AI) are beyond the scope of this project.
16 Dolto 1984, 276.
17 Freud 1914b, 150–151.
18 Dolto 1982, 146–147.
19 In Kouki 2005, 88–89.

Chapter 7

Name—Awaiting Echoes

Preliminary Words

The 19th-century Canadian poet, Emily Pauline Johnson (1861–1913), was the child of a Mohawk chief (father) and an immigrant from Bristol, England (mother). Considered Canada's first performance artist, she appeared on a stamp issued in 1961; she was shortlisted for the recently issued $10 bill; and she is apparently on the candidates list for the next $5 bill. It seems Johnson lived on the Chiefswood reserve[1] throughout her childhood and was spared off-reserve (i.e., residential) schooling due to poor health, so she would have learned Kanyen'kéha at home—her father's (but not her mother's) tongue. Nonetheless, the 10-page introduction to her collected works written by an English critic does not even mention her Indigenous name, Tekahionwakeh: "double wampum"[2]—effectively, "double life." Johnson writes in a rather formal literary style about Indigenous people as if they were "other," often using familiar tropes. For example, a corn husker is described as "rich in tawny colouring of her race";[3] and she writes of the "war-cry of a long-forgotten brave."[4]

Throughout Johnson's corpus, there is no personal record of any favourite words in Kanyen'kéha—no traces of the names of any loved ones, toys, dolls, neighbours, pets, songs, trees, rivers, special places, etc. For though Johnson apparently understood Kanyen'kéha well, she wrote in a manner that was deliberately pleasing to her English audiences. And while her theatrical performances strove to showcase her Indigenous roots, her writing seems to have entirely lost Kanyen'kéha—and that part of Johnson rooted in it. As it happens, only one century after Johnson, Kanyen'kéha faces the risk of being entirely lost. It is a threatened language, with only a few thousand speakers left who are actively trying to save it by teaching it to a new generation. In fact, language death is a real danger that impacts Indigenous cultures worldwide. In 2022, for example, the last speaker of Yagan (an Indigenous Chilean language) died, and the language perished with her.[5] Enshrined is the enigmatic proposition that humans and their languages are mutually interdependent.

People speak of cultural memory disappearing when languages die because an intrinsic and irreplaceable aspect of human history seems embedded in words

DOI: 10.4324/9781032655123-16

and the stories they make uniquely tellable. In Canada, we are currently barely beginning to acknowledge the uncountable sequelae of a devastating social project of erasure launched in the prior century. It is widely known that more than 150,000 First Nations, Métis and Inuit children were forced to attend church-run, government-funded schools between the 1870s and 1990s. They suffered every form of abuse, including the prohibition against using their mother tongues (L1s) or seeing their families. Thousands died while in supposed "care."[6] In fact, the deliberate eradication of language was shamefully at the forefront of national policies. As Duncan Campbell Scott, the infamous superintendent of that system stated in 1920: "I want to get rid of the Indian problem."[7] Thus, 139 residential schools in Canada operated for 120 years[8]—four generations. As a result, not only were survivors stripped of their mother tongues but so were their children, grandchildren and great-grandchildren.

And while the obliteration of cultural memories is a highly significant loss that should never be minimized, Dolto draws our attention to an even more pernicious and pervasive consequence of mother tongue attrition: the loss of pathways for the circulation of unconscious affect. For the circulation of unconscious affect in language—its phonemes—is what liberates it, minimizing anxiety and helping us invest in new learning. This circulation of unconscious affect in language fuels networks of associations that nurture our earliest mental and emotional development—our associative thinking—while assuring our existential security. And when we haphazardly encounter echoes of our archaically invested phonemes in the social, we are unconsciously scaffolded in our progress towards conscious action in reality. As a result, the loss or suppression of a first language implicates potentially serious regressive impacts.

A. Inscription

I freely confess that my preferred genre of literature is language memoirs, wherein bilinguals reflect on their sense of self and their different emotional lives in each tongue. Eva Hoffman is credited with a work that defines the genre as she exquisitely narrates her own feeling of being "lost in translation"[9] between Polish (L1) and English (L2). A single example is illustrative:

> "River" in Polish was a vital sound, energized with the essence of riverhood, of my rivers, of my being immersed in rivers. "River" in English is cold—a word without an aura. It has no accumulated associations for me, and it does not give off the radiating haze of connotation. It does not evoke.[10]

Taking up Hoffman's astute observation, what happens if a word does not evoke? Or, if no words ever evoke? I believe Hoffman is touching on the power of words to animate and enliven us—to nourish our affective investments in our own lives. For invested words secure an affective experience of being immersed and of being bound to associations that are indelible to the self.

It is because phonemes are affectively invested in the archaic stage that language has the well-documented effects discerned across disciplines. For example, the Canadian researcher and educator, Sandra Kouritzin, has explored language attrition. One of her respondents lost then relearned Cree as an adult; he believes that he "never completely lost the language, it just 'went to sleep' for a little while."[11] Kouritzin adds that, "Many seemed to feel that the language was buried deep within themselves somewhere, if only they knew how to find it."[12] This introspection is stunningly accurate, for mother tongue phonemes are deeply webbed with unconscious affects below consciousness, and formative in networks of associative thinking beneath conscious thought. One of Kouritzin's other respondents, who lost Finnish, reports the following: "I no longer have the capability of understanding the stories I grew up with."[13] She is relating not only the loss of family and cultural lore, but the absence of stor(y)ing in words and names.

In addition, the internationally esteemed linguist, Aneta Pavlenko, relates that in her world-renowned studies of bilinguals, the "majority of respondents … perceive their L1 as most emotional and favor it as the language of emotional expression."[14] Pavlenko's explanation confirms both the affective and associative filiations:

> Languages into which speakers have been socialized in natural contexts, in particular at a young age … are perceived as embodied and emotional, which means that they are processed not only through cognitive channels but also through affective ones, triggering associations in autobiographic and emotional memory, bodily sensations, and physiological responses, examined through levels of autonomic arousal.[15]

There is further confirmation of the affective investment of phonemes from the clinic. In a rich and informative collection, RoseMarie Pérez-Foster describes how in therapy, "operationally, the second language served as a coping or defensive operation against the significant losses and anguish symbolized by the mother tongue."[16] This confirms that strong affects are embedded in the mother tongue, and that the second language provides a kind of defensive shield to functionally stabilize the self—an affective dampener, if you will. As Pérez-Foster et al. explain it, there is a "role of bilingualism in the reconstruction and working through of early memory in treatment, the development of transference."[17] For "language … becomes intimately yoked to the objects associated with the language learning, to the environmental ambience in which the language learning took place, and to the internal psycho-developmental state of the child at the time of acquisition."[18] Pérez-Foster concludes that, "Bilingualism can serve a highly dynamic and defensive function … [as] a formidable binder of anxiety that can effectively isolate and dissociate affect initially experienced in another language system."[19]

The poignant testimony of Susan Brison, an American scholar who was a victim of rape in France, corroborates this research: "Even after I regained my ability to speak, more or less reliably, in English, I was unable to speak, without debilitating difficulty, in French."[20] This defensive function leads to an essential inference:

speaking our most invested phonemes has a role in securing reality, so trauma that threatens our existential security and thereby leaves an unconscious trace (i.e., a record) can also become indelibly associated with certain phonemes. Thus, on the one hand, producing archaically invested phonemes (in speaking or writing)—or hearing them (in listening or reading)—securitizes reality by transiting unconscious affects. On the other hand, producing or hearing phonemes that are unconsciously associated with trauma is profoundly de-securitizing, leading to a degree of mutism in that language. For unconscious affect is inextricably bound with phonemes. Effectively, then, the situation for residential school survivors is such that not only was their L1 lost but the enforced L2 (i.e., in Canada, English or French) is replete with phonemes associated with personal, familial and cultural traumas. As a result, using (or encountering) these phonemes in daily communication cannot help but evoke unconscious associations that re-traumatize.

Dolto explored this defensive function of language—that we secure reality through the unconscious circulation of affect in the social by which we come upon echoes of our own invested phonemes. In fact, the young infant, passively disposed, is always awaiting echoes—they are his lures to reality. But if phonemes are deeply associated with trauma, the speaker (writer) using those phonemes will be constantly subject to encountering associations (from his own voice) that recall a threat to survival. We can infer that the instinct of conservation will drive the organism towards mutism in the interest of self-regulation (i.e., to reduce regressive events). Furthermore, also in the interest of self-regulation, any other proximal language may be adopted to enable at least some affective venting. Certainly, the new language will not easily circulate the unconscious affects associated with mother tongue phonemes. We can also infer, then, that the more different the salvific (new) language is from the traumatizing (prior) language, the fewer phonemic overlaps there will be. Put another way, the defensive aspect of the second language will be perfectly achieved, but at a high cost to affective circulation. Meanwhile, languages with multiple cognates (i.e., phonemic overlaps) will enable affect to circulate at least somewhat: the defensive function will be less perfectly achieved, but some affect will find its way to being liberated. In sum, a near-language will be ironically both more and less securing.

Dolto discovered this difficult tension in her clinic. For example, she stressed that it is important to never change a child's first name—as happens frequently during adoptions and migrations—because of a potentially "toxic effect"[21] on primary narcissism. Her word, "toxic," is intentionally powerful. For the infant has affect invested in his mother's voice and words; in the voice and words of the other-of-the-mother (usually but not necessarily the biological father); as well as in the auditory landscape of his family, community and neighbourhood. From birth, his name is invariably invested by family and may even have profound resonances to family history, invested persons and places, and so on. In early infancy, people will speak to and about this child, addressing him by name, playing homonymic games with it, nicknaming him, and embedding his name in familiar phrases repeated daily. Thus, the phonemes of his name alone will become the nexus of countless associations in the affect-driven proliferation of associative thinking—the ontogeny of thought. Yet, as Pavlenko observes, "Given the elusive nature of inner speech, it is not surprising that the research on bilingualism has, for the most part, steered clear of the phenomenon."[22] For her part, Dolto approaches the question head-on and offers critical supports.

In what is essentially a summation of the whole situation with the unconscious affective investment of phonemes, Dolto states that, "saying his name can wake up the subject."[23] So we can predict that the child whose name is changed will feel less "called." That is, he will feel less "lured" to reality due to not hearing a crucial word to which so much unconscious affect is associatively bound from birth. In turn, in not producing those critical phonemes daily (i.e., "I am…"; "My name is…"), he will lose an important means for "waking himself up" in the normative manner by which any speaking child begins to secure himself through the diffusion of his invested phonemes in his own auditory environment. In this way, the problem of the name represents the much larger problem that happens when invested phonemes fall off the sonar.

Dolto is clear that the mother tongue—of which the child's own name is central—has an indispensable value in carrying affect. Dolto stresses that, "the first name is the phoneme(s) accompanying the sensorium of the child … from birth to death."[24] So it is for the family name, in being a set of phonemes frequently heard in the family that may even have some geographical correlates in street, square or place names—or in a cultural history that is valued and shared. In sum, the mother tongue has a "historicizing function."[25] So what happens to a child who is not easily awakened? Necessarily, this would be a child inclined towards passivity and insecurity in reality—and tending towards fearfulness (anxiety) and mutism. This is indeed what the nonverbal autist testifies to. In sum, we predict that losing the mother tongue precipitates comparable effects along a spectrum—less gravity, but considerable similarity.

Yet at the same time as Dolto acknowledges the importance of the mother tongue to affective circulation (liberation), thanks to the unconscious investment in phonemes of the first language during the archaic stage, Dolto also upholds the defensive (i.e., impeding) function of a second language. For while encountering the unconsciously invested phonemes of the mother tongue that were experienced during the archaic stage is securitizing, encountering and/or using phonemes that have (since) become unconsciously associated with trauma is de-securitizing. Dolto recounts a case somewhat reminiscent of Brison's, wherein a French psychiatrist who was a victim of incest fled to English by moving to Australia.[26] The second language is a way to "run from yourself,"[27] Dolto believes, stressing that the salvific language merely needs to not conform to the mother's rhythm.[28] It is a kind of security in "camouflage,"[29] she offers. This use of language as a defence is even available to a deaf child, for in the literature of the Deaf, we can find this poignant account: "Imagining a more mature self, and embarrassed by past behaviors, he asked his mother to 'throw [old name] away. I'm [new name].'"[30] For the phoneme can transit affect in any languaged medium—through speaking, writing or Signing.

Freud gives a full description of the speech of the famous first patient of psychoanalysis, Bertha Pappenheim ("Anna O"), whose first language was German, but who was during the worst months of her illness "at her best and most free" in French and Italian.[31] As Pavlenko explains it, "More than a century ago, Freud and his disciples noticed that some of their patients favored the L2 for anxiety-producing topics and the use of 'obscene' words."[32] Pavlenko adds that, "language serves as one of the organizing principles in bilingual autobiographical memory, offering differential—or at least preferential—access to different life periods and events … [as a] *language of encoding affect*."[33] And her emphasis on language reception—audition—is a consequential one.

The defensive function of the second language is useful in the case of trauma, enabling affective quieting and associative distancing. But as Dolto stresses, it "risks breaking filiations."[34] So abandoning (or losing) the first language traps unconscious affect by disrupting the free flow through networks of associations. The result inclines the survivor towards less security (i.e., greater anxiety) and difficulty investing affect in love, work and reality. In fact, the incapacity to invest affect progressively is the hallmark of a regressive defence. And what we can conclude is that the oldest defence we have—regression—is working on the level of language, i.e., through language. I believe we can also infer that communicating in the salvific language becomes, ironically, a way of not fully communicating. For it is tantamount to a functional mutism of the true self, of the fully invested self, in an attenuation of affect. The second language defence comes at a considerable cost.

What Dolto's work lets us deduce is bold yet simple: the loss of access to one's invested phonemes in the social negatively impacts psychosexual maturation. In other words, the child just born already has an influential history with words that facilitates or impedes the quanta of affect at his disposal for encountering all future objects and transiting all further psychosexual stages. At stake is the unconscious circulation of affect in triangulations that return, by association, the securing presence of a witness that vouchsafes new affective investments. When the circulation of unconscious affect is continuous, reality is more easily secured; the individual "awakens" to invest in new objects (i.e., new relations and new learning); and he progresses well towards the conscious mastery of motor acts (including speech). Conversely, when affective circulation is impeded, reality is inherently de-securing; the individual defensively remains anchored to securing dream-work; passivity is installed; there is a preference for sameness (rather than new objects); and there is difficulty in progressing towards the full consciousness required for the intentional control of motor acts (including speech). I would like to argue that the evidence from nonverbal autistic authors confirms this profile in its entirety.

There is also strong confirmation for Dolto in the works of that highly influential educator, Maria Montessori.[35] Montessori describes the young child's passive receptivity as absorption: "The child … 'absorbs' language."[36] And she stresses how language comprehension happens long before speech (and independent of it): "There is a great disproportion between the powers of expression and the inner work the child is doing."[37] Following Freud,[38] Montessori muses on the daily evidence of unconscious processes: “Is not the kingdom of the subconscious to be found in sleep?”[39] Furthermore, she points out the overwhelming contribution of unconscious processes to the child’s development: “If we call our adult mentality conscious, then we must call the child’s unconscious … The child has an intelligence of the unconscious type, and that is what brings about his marvellous progress.”[40] Montessori concurs that unconscious processes are deeply implicated in “performing the mysterious inner work of his [the infant’s] auto-formation.”[41] And like Dolto, she locates their onset in *in utero*:

> If a mental life exists even in the newborn babe, this must be already there, otherwise it could not exist. In fact, it must also be present in the embryo … As we know, a child is sometimes born at seven months instead of at nine—and at seven months he is already complete enough to be able to live.[42]

In turn, Montessori emphasizes the critical unconscious role of language in development:

> The child does not “remember” sounds but incarnates them … this language comes to form part of his psychic life and of himself … There is in the child a special kind of sensitivity which leads him to absorb everything … to adapt himself to life. He does so in virtue of an unconscious power that exists only in childhood.[43]

In mentioning adaptation, Montessori acknowledges that the child is being formed from the start by the language he hears around him, insofar as human beings are an inherently communicative species. Her contention is not that unconscious processes are only active in childhood—for we recall her reference to sleep. Rather, her thesis is that the very young child—for whom consciousness is not yet reliably established—is singularly under the dominant influence of unconscious processes; and these processes are responsible for his adaptation, starting *in utero*, to his particular communicative environment. She expands on this pivotal point:

> The child receives from the nebula of language suitable stimuli and guidance for the formation in himself of his mother tongue, which is not inborn in him, but something he finds in his environment and absorbs … The child, it is clear, does not inherit a pre-established model for his language, but he inherits the power of constructing a language by an unconscious activity of absorption.[44]

This notion of unconsciously constructing the self in (through) language is a vital one that informs the onset of associative thinking—its flexibility and its dynamism. And in her own observations, Montessori detects the centrality of precocious audition in this early learning: “The hearing organs are connected to the mysterious seat of mental life where the child’s language is evolved in the depths of his unconscious mind.”[45] She adds that, “first to become fixed in the little one’s unconscious are the single sounds of language."[46] Her notion of single sounds seems to be a clear reference to audible chunks within spoken streams—i.e., phonemes. In addition, Montessori affirms the luring effect of phonemes: "He has a special sensitiveness for words; they attract his interest."[47] And she comes to the same overarching conclusion as Dolto—namely, that the infant "needs mental food almost more than physical food."[48]

B. Reverberations

What, then, is the consequence for the infant whose family has just immigrated to a country where his first language is not spoken? Suppose, then, that the mother tongue (L1) is still in circulation, but only in the home. Street and location names are entirely different than they used to be—so nothing echoes on daily walkabouts. The richly textured sonar landscape—familial, cultural and geographic—has effectively been silenced. Even in the best-case scenario, there will be a limited flow of phonemes within a small social sphere comprising a few proximal others. Beyond that, the L1 is nowhere to be found. At preschool, it is likely that no one will speak it. Perhaps the child will even be given a new nickname in these novel surroundings, something "easier" for locals to say. The child will naturally feel insecure—withdrawing and/or acting out—and professionals will put it down to his being "ESL."[49] In response, he will be given even more English (or other L2)—the new language as a misguided prescription. And, ostensibly to help the child, well-motivated staff will go out of their way to furnish labels in the language of school and community, to support his vocabulary growth. Meanwhile, however, his own invested phonemes will become ever-more distant and less reachable by association.

All the infant's networks of affectively-driven early associations—literally years of associative thinking, wherein mental and emotional life are fused—are built up around the invested phonemes of his mother tongue. Removing access to the L1 not only impedes affective circulation—and thus, the unconscious security needed to invest securely in new objects of learning—but it denies the affective influence of his formative first years of development. The forcible abandonment of the L1 severs (i.e., dries up) affective networks formed over the months of associative play with phonemes. In short, it silences an idiosyncratic archaic history of unconscious wealth that is intrinsic to the self. It thereby relegates quanta of affect to be trapped in circulatory pathways that are increasingly disassociated from the objects of reality, as affect effectively becomes unusable for future investments.

So if an individual reaches a certain age of responsibility and, following trauma, prefers to live, love and/or work in a second language (L2)—as a defence—then that trade is consciously made and its consequences can be judiciously assumed. But for the infant who experiences migration, for example, that trade is made on his behalf, without his consent. Yet up until then, his sense of self and security—and his thoughts—were intimately bound to the unconscious affect of his mother tongue's phonemes. The unconscious development of his mental and emotional life, contingent on those phonemes, was already advanced. As a result, the importance of sustaining the invested phonemes of his infancy cannot be overstated. Creative means will need to begin with the valuation of the L1 for its tremendous role in affective circulation, unconscious security and associative thinking. At home and school, and throughout the community, the language(s) of the infant's archaic stage—from which he is now distant due to his personal, familial or social circumstances—will need to be given generous and ubiquitous representation across contexts.

Note that it is entirely possible that words from a language other than the mother tongue may have been deeply invested *in utero*—for example, liturgical languages or the father's tongue (if different from the mother's). It is equally important to consider the names, words and voices of loved ones (including those left behind); the words of favourite books or sports (or even media programmes) that featured in the family's daily life; and even the language in circulation during conversations around themes that preoccupied the household in the prior location. Even street names that were frequently uttered on walks or transit rides may be relevant. At issue is the restitution of the sonar landscape—its most affectively invested and/or frequently repeated phonemes—in the new landscape, sprinkled amid the words of this new environment. Because not only does the infant's unconscious security depend on this continuity, but so do his associations in thought and his capacity to fully invest his fledgling self affectively in the new environment—and in new learning.

Assuredly, it is not ever possible to know which phonemes have been deeply invested and which have not. But I believe that an attempt at an anamnesis of affectively invested phonemes becomes worthwhile. In therapy, clinicians use anamneses to begin analysis—and Dolto was famous for the depth of detail in hers.[50] Yet any family or school can do the same easily enough, informally, focusing only on language. It is a matter of trying to discover the child's history with words beginning in gestation: the mother tongue, any other language of exposure *in utero*, the local geography (place names, streets, frequent stores, etc.) where the infant was carried and born—plus the names of family members and close friends, and the child's own true name, properly pronounced. The task of helping the regressed infant—including the deeply regressed nonverbal autist—and/or of preventing regression (however temporary) following a language shift would then involve trying to put invested phonemes into circulation subtly and naturally.

Critically, this is not about producing endless lists that sound artificial. Nor is it about coaxing the child to speak (in either the old or new tongue). Rather, securitization and scaffolding self-regulation involves facilitating a passive engagement with phonemes by providing access within a safe, non-coercive environment to words that are continuous with a young child's prior language investments—i.e., his archaic history. It requires his listening haphazardly (rather than systematically or intentionally), without any demand for language production. Unconscious securitization is a relatively simple project of audition that enlists the child's own capacity for an auto-recovery. The instinct of conservation does the work.

Phonemic play seems advisable as well, not only as an intervention for the regression provoked by first language loss but for sustaining archaic learning—i.e., for supporting the type of learning that is thriving in the archaic stage, wherein the phoneme is the critical conduit for affectively-driven associative networks. Ironically, teaching literacy based on phonemes (e.g., rat, bat, cat, sat, mat, etc.) has largely gone out of favour—though phonics is coincidentally poised for a resurgence in the revised language curriculum coming into force in the next school year in my current home province, Ontario.[51] In fact, the importance of phonemes in unconscious processes that begin *in utero* suggest the productivity of phonemic play—and the benefits of instructional practices that privilege phonemes—in nurturing the child's associative thinking and the healthy circulation of unconscious affect.

The unconsciously restorative potential of phonemic play implicates everything from nonsense words (e.g., Dr. Seuss) to poetry. Not coincidentally, Tito Mukhopadhyay—the most published of the four nonverbal authors studied—reports enjoying writing in new poetry styles, such as the ghazal[52] and villanelle.[53] He even titles one of his books, *I'm Not a Poet But I Write Poetry: Poems from My Autistic Mind.* I believe we are observing the securing of pleasure via a return of affect through the use of phonemes (in writing), experienced as (in) a de-muting of the self. On this view, the nonverbal autist's mutism appears once again to be on a continuum with the affective impedance provoked by language attrition.

For both nonverbal autism and language attrition reveal a de-secured self in the throes of anxiety who is muted in the capacity to circulate affect via invested phonemes. Thus I believe Dolto enables us to infer that both conditions are manifestations of regression, albeit to considerably different degrees of severity. And insofar as an individual suffering language attrition needs the environmental provision of archaically invested phonemes to coax investments in reality, the autist needs the same. Of course, this recommendation is entirely at cross-currents with the trend towards PECS[54] at home and school, and the widely held conviction that the autist—who struggles with eye contact and intentional motor control—appears to not be listening so that very few words are ever addressed directly to him. As Dolto has made abundantly clear, such a stance is grievously ill-advised. For not only is the autist constantly thinking but he is ardently listening—despite appearances. To stress, any child who is muted in/by language, with his unconscious affect trapped, needs more—not fewer—words.

The reparation of, with, and through language is entirely unconscious. Thus the process is not aided in the least by drawing conscious attention to it. Instead, the language needs to be put into circulation in the environment as a kind of auditory background. And another element of the infant's listening during the archaic is worth recalling here, too: the child is passively co-experiencing objects with a witness while in that all-providing environment. Along this pattern, the child will listen better when he is not the direct addressee but words are instead addressed to a group or another person. Ambient words that are available in a benevolent environment allow him to be a passive recipient, just like in the archaic stage. Phonemes cannot, therefore, be explicitly taught. Crucially, it is also worth noting that for some indeterminate time, there will be no measurable way to be sure if something is working or not. For unconscious processes are not amenable in the least to quantitative studies. Progress—gains in well-being, learning and communication—will be slow and subtle.

Unfortunately, the role of affectively invested phonemes is never discussed in education. Newcomers in JK[55] are immersed in second language classrooms, as families and staff comfort themselves that the children will learn the new language easily and adapt quickly—and they will. Meanwhile, young autists are integrated into schools as their teachers busy themselves creating signage to minimize the need for speech, counselled by outside specialists to keep language to the simplest instructions. But a rich affective and associative history is at risk. The mental and emotional development of every young child requires meaningful language, a harvest of invested phonemes—an alimentation of words to facilitate associations and affective circulation. Even the neurologist, Henry Charlton Bastian, who wrote the definitive work on echolalia in autism back in 1898, stated: "It is the auditory word-memory which is first revived in silent thought."[56] So the young child—immigrant or autist—needs his invested words in abundance. Thus, the reparation of education requires audition, whereas silencing phonemes affectively mutes the self.

In fact, this seems to be a particularly auspicious time to disseminate Dolto's theorization of the archaic stage and the unconscious work of language. For UNESCO declared 2022–2032 the International Decade of Indigenous Languages, launching "an unprecedented initiative to preserve, revitalize and promote global linguistic diversity and multilingualism as a unique heritage and treasure of humanity."[57] Its summative report gives the current count at "8,324 languages spoken or signed in the world."[58] Other researchers report that 3,045 languages (42 per cent) are endangered;[59] and that, on average, one language has become extinct every three months over the past 100 years.[60] UNESCO chronicles the devastating consequences:

> Language loss entails an impoverishment of humanity in countless ways. Each language—large or small—captures and organizes reality in a distinctive manner; to lose even one closes off potential discoveries about human cognition and the mind. The death of a language inevitably leads to the disappearance of various forms of intangible cultural heritage.[61]

We should not be surprised that language is described using environmental tropes—diversity, endangered, extinction—for as Dolto demonstrates, language is learned environmentally beginning *in utero*. And Dolto's elaboration of how archaically invested phonemes circulate affect, provide unconscious security, and seed associative thinking makes an invaluable contribution to all projects that support the preservation of languages.

In conclusion, beginning during gestation, the phonemes of our first language are invested with unconscious affect and seed associative thinking. Henceforth, we are unconsciously susceptible to our archaic echoes since these enable the free flow of affect and secure reality. The loss of such paths—deliberately or accidentally—carries formidable consequences for the availability of unconscious affect in daily life: our loves, work and learning. Children deprived of their mother tongues due to migration or forced assimilation suffer consequences that reduce the flow of available affect; provoke formidable anxiety; and hamper the developmental shift from passivity to activity. A child who no longer encounters his affectively invested phonemes or can no longer use them will need to be scaffolded to (re)establish his unconscious security, while building associative bridges between the L1 and L2.

Meanwhile, the affective costs of changing a young child's name—or early language migration—are significant, so the advantages need to be carefully weighed against the disadvantages. Finally, the loss of invested phonemes makes it harder to unconsciously experience associations to the securing witness, provoking the loss of a sense of self, of not feeling "real" (i.e., affectively connected) in one's own life. The repercussions for the nonverbal autist, who is deeply regressed from the start, are such that anxiety will be greatly reduced if the environment can supply (for passive consumption) rich vocabulary in the languages encountered beginning *in utero*, and the individual can enjoy an exposure to more rather than fewer words—preferably as an indirect addressee. For, from infancy, we humans are storied by our dreams on phonemes. We are always awaiting echoes.

Notes

1 Chiefswood Park (near Brantford, Ontario) is now a National Historic Site and a centre of Haudenosaunee culture.
2 A ceremonial beaded belt that serves as a living historical register; e.g., see Onondaga Nation 2022.
3 Johnson 1917/2022, 95.
4 Ibid, 20.
5 Cambero 2022.
6 As of the time of writing, the unmarked graves of 1,638 children have been found "by accident" throughout Canada, on the former sites of these schools; Indigenous nations seek much greater funding for ground-penetrating radar (GPR) to find and honour all the missing children.
7 Union of Ontario Indians 2013.
8 For more information, see e.g., Assembly of First Nations 2022.
9 Examples of full-length language memoirs include titles by Marjorie Agosín, Gloria Anzaldúa, Cathy Bao Bean, Patrick Chamoiseau, Evalina Chao, Isabelle de Courtivron, Sadiqa de Meijer, Ariel Dorfman, Padma Hejmadi, Eva Hoffman, Quiara Alegría Hudes, Nancy Huston, Alice Kaplan, Maxine Hong Kingston, Jhumpa Lahiri, Shirley G. Lim, Kyoko Mori, Richard Rodriguez, Luc Sante, Ilan Stavans, Olivier Todd and Jane Jeong Trenka (as well as mine: *Bilingual Being*).
10 1989, 106.
11 1999, 183.
12 Ibid, 83.
13 Ibid, 95.
14 2005, 141.
15 Ibid, 237.
16 2004, 252.

17 Pérez-Foster, Moskowitz & Javier 2004, 178.
18 Ibid, 260.
19 Ibid, 261.
20 2002, 114.
21 In Halmos 1994, 239–240; Dolto 1984, 46.
22 2014, 224.
23 Dolto 1984, 46 & 94.
24 Ibid, 46.
25 In Chaperot & Celacu 2010, 439.
26 In Djéribi-Valentin & Kouki 1998, 54.
27 Dolto in Potin 2008, 140.
28 Dolto 1987, 16.
29 In De Sauverzac 1988, 237; Dolto 1987, 33; Djéribi-Valentin 2005, 213.
30 Gulati 2003b, 38.
31 Breuer & Freud 1893a, 25.
32 2014, 283.
33 Ibid, 194 (emphasis hers).
34 In Caldaguès 1982, 99.
35 Note that I have no affiliation with any Montessori school or programme.
36 1949/2010, 100.
37 Ibid, 103.
38 Ibid, 76.
39 Ibid, 70.
40 Ibid, 22.
41 Montessori 1914.
42 Montessori 1949/2010, 61.
43 Ibid, 56–57.
44 Ibid, 73.
45 Ibid, 105.
46 Ibid, 79.
47 Ibid, 158.
48 Ibid, 182.
49 I.e., a learner of English as a Second Language (a common designation in educational systems).
50 For example, in De Sauverzac 1985, 60–62; Djéribi-Valentin & Kouki 1998, 180–183.
51 Government of Ontario 2023.
52 2012, 20.
53 Ibid, 41.
54 Picture Exchange Communication System.
55 Junior Kindergarten—i.e., the usual point of entry, in Canada, at age three or four (depending on birthdays).
56 1898.
57 UNESCO 2022.
58 Ibid.
59 Eberhard, Simons & Fennig 2022.
60 Nuwer 2014.
61 UNESCO 2011, 6.

Chapter 8

Library—(Re)Finding Echoes

Preliminary Words

Bertha Pappenheim was a feminist and community activist who strove to curtail the «traite des blanches» [white slave trade].[1] She opened and managed orphanages, schools and shelters, and her legacy to the field of social work is widely acknowledged. Yet in 1880–1882, intensely disturbed after her father died, Pappenheim became the first patient of psychoanalysis: "Anna O." As Anna O., Pappenheim is rightly credited for the nickname she gave the new field—the "talking cure";[2] and its therapeutic process—"chimney sweeping."[3] Following her treatment, she published edifying stories for children under the pseudonym, Paul Berthold—melancholic life lessons related by unsold objects in a junk shop. An omniscient narrator relates how, in the dark of night when the little store is closed, all sorts of objects that might seem lifeless and unimportant begin to whisper, relating their peculiar histories, each with a heavy share of grief. Overhearing the objects as they talk, the narrator concludes that there is so much sorrow everywhere that his own is but an insignificant portion of the overwhelming misery in the world.[4]

Possibly, some sadness has been inadvertently layered (through word choice) by her respected translator (Renate Latimer), in transporting these unusual tales from German to English. But Pappenheim herself seems frank that misery grounds her tales, and she dedicated her life to alleviating the suffering of others. In her narratives, she speaks through a thimble, coffee grinder, streetlamp, and so on. But any reader of the original, *In der Trödelbude*, would be privy to a deeper level of interpretation on the German phonemes of the names of those objects (and her title) in relation to Pappenheim's history. This game of words is rampant in any text because we always seed our works with our unconsciously invested phonemes—we cannot help doing so.

Dolto thus helps us realize that every corpus—and every theory—cannot help but be autobiographic.[5] And any invested object (including a character) is necessarily a later edition—a secondary revision—of the author's invested phonemes. We infer this because of the direction of the developmental process: first, affect is unconsciously invested in phonemes; second, phonemes are associated to objects of reality and confer affect to them. So while we may feel consciously drawn to

DOI: 10.4324/9781032655123-17

a character or setting, Dolto reveals that beneath any overt connections, readers have powerful unconscious filiations—in being lured or not—through echoes of their idiosyncratic archaic phonemes. And if archaic echoes are strong or numerous enough, an unconscious slippage happens—a blur of identity (identification) between self and author (or character)—that restores archaic triangulation and makes a book (or corpus) an environment of provision. Reading is archaic-syntonic.

Pappenheim lived the remainder of her relatively long life (1859–1936) as the Anna O. of literature, dying only three years before Freud passed, aware that her struggles (including her institutionalization) were a matter of public record. Yet by reading the extensive memoirs of her ancestor, Glückel Von Hameln—a prominent 18th-century businesswoman—Pappenheim found strength and direction for her future. So it was that after recovering from an illness so acute that, at its peak, she could only speak in English nursery rhymes,[6] Pappenheim had herself painted as Glückel.[7]

Through her migration of names—Bertha Pappenheim, Anna O., Paul Berthold, Glückel—I believe we are being alerted to a progression of the self through writing. For the reader who meets Pappenheim is invited to follow her paths forwards and backwards—to read about hysteria, her children's tales, the white slave trade, social work, and even Von Hameln. Thus, Pappenheim's texts become an invitation to divergent fields of thought associated with her, and with each other. With Pappenheim, therefore, I suggest that we are encountering the notion of a chain of custody, so to speak, in reading: our capacity to follow an author, or object, by association. In other words, we grow our fields of thought—our investments in new objects—based on a witness vouchsafing directions for new investments. We may read whoever an invested author reads, as typically found in marginalia—footnotes and indices. In fact, we are simply detecting a derivation—a later edition—of the archaic triangular situation: self, witness and phoneme. For an author can serve as a witness in whom we place our trust, as one triangulation proliferates from another, and so on. We also detect how the assurance of security—truth and trust—underpins triangulation. As a result, finding a new author to love along such filiations is a promise of joy—a harvest to feed our daydreams.

Interestingly, in the 19th-century archives of autism, the physician Martin W. Barr noted that an echolalic child "learned the alphabet and to repeat with facility Mother Goose rhymes."[8] So we have Bertha Pappenheim (temporarily regressed) speaking only in nursery rhymes—and an autist (fixatedly regressed) speaking predominantly in nursery rhymes. Uncannily, both records were etched in 1882. And insofar as Mother Goose rhymes (unlike songs) are typically learned from shared texts, reading is a possible source of words for their particular echolalia. On this view, echolalia may be an attempt to communicate by repeating the words of a loved one—precisely what any infant does when learning to speak. Once again, then, the nonverbal autist seems to be on a continuum with the non-autist. Pappenheim is right: there is an echo of Cinderella in the need to sweep away ashes of the past congesting affective paths so life can move forward. But perhaps there is also an echo of Snow White and Sleeping Beauty: you can sleep a long time, years even, until the right object comes along to wake (i.e., lure) you back to reality. On this view, reading is an intervention for the problem of regression—and the prince is a phoneme.

A. Inscription

During the peak of the COVID-19 pandemic of 2020–2022, I observed numerous times how line-ups at local second-hand outlets were longer than those at the grocery stores. Having lost their social moorings—schedules, employment and gatherings—people felt themselves falling through the cracks of their own lives.[9] So intuitively, it seems, they were drawn to junk shops, searching for meaning, for some affirmation of security. Row upon row of people examined or picked up random things—I was among them—seeking through chance environmental encounters with objects to refind on the outside what felt lost on the inside. Freud shares a related example from his own life wherein, walking on holiday in an unfamiliar town, he reads, "every shop sign that resembles the word in any way as 'Antiquities' … betray[ing] the questing spirit of the collector."[10] He is narrating how echoes carry an element of daydreaming, of wishful thinking and pleasure—and that such echoes can happen at the word level. Freud also reminds us that finding archaic echoes liberates affect, as "pre-cathected word-images provide a passage for discharge."[11] Reciprocally, it is possible to encounter phonemes that are unconsciously associated with trauma—phonemes that do not lure (exteriorize) and thus do not enable affective liberation—but trigger anxiety instead. I believe that Freud is highlighting this phenomenon when he describes "an intense wish to reject what we have read."[12] And in his use of the term "intense," we confirm that self-regulation conveys a powerful experience of pleasure.

Reading offers fodder for our daydreams. And because unconscious processes drive the development of capacities that are both mental (i.e., associative thinking) and emotional (i.e., affective self-regulation), the words we encounter while reading not only liberate affect—securing us and reducing anxiety—but they also enter our thoughts and seed our associative thinking. Furthermore, any environment for the abundant provision of words, of which some will inevitably be invested phonemes (or have associations to them) will evoke the dreamed presence of the witness. This will make a book—even more so, a corpus—inherently securing. And since this process is unconscious, the stuff of dream-work, a character (even a non-human one the author creates) can be a witness.

It is well-documented, for example, that children naturally have imaginary companions that acquire a great importance in their lives. For example, the educator and researcher, Marjorie Taylor, states: "Many children have several imaginary friends at a time, and some acquire new ones as others disappear … many preschool children pretend to be an animal or another person on a regular basis."[13] Further, the imaginary companion serves as a trusting witness: "Most invisible entities in children's fantasy lives embody the desirable characteristics of a loving friend."[14] This is arguably the entire basis for children's books, as bears, dogs and myriad others deliver their invaluable life lessons.

As we are learning, a witness is indispensable at the boundary between dreams and reality. Adults may experience this when they wake from a dream or recover from states of altered consciousness (e.g., after medication or trauma)—they feel the need to immediately check with a trusted witness about what really occurred. But all humans live in this liminal space for their first years of life. Put another way, we won't always believe in talking rabbits or invisible mice—but for a time, we must. And in dream-work, a witness from a text is as good as a real one.

When we take on (in) the objects (including phonemes) of a witness, we are (as we were in the archaic) both *with* and *as-if* this very similar other—thus, we are unconsciously secured. This is the crucial process of identification that is so necessary to individuation—to freedom from regressive (fusional) dependence. It is just another example of the stunning explanatory power of archaic triangulation—that begins as self, witness and phoneme—that it can account for this common human experience. In time, along unconscious associations, triangulations will proliferate to enable changing witnesses through progressions of the self. Not just our ideas will change but our feelings, too, because the unconscious processes involved—namely, affective circulation and associative thinking—conflate mental and emotional activity. And that is why (and how) a book is a such a great way to help change your mind—literally.

Universally, parents and educators are familiar with children taking on the words or objects of invested characters in daily life—dressing as so-and-so for weeks; repeating a set expression *ad infinitum* (blurring the distinction with echolalia); or carrying around a story-related prop all day long. The witness found in reading can even seem to appear (arrive) in reality—or at least to be witnessing our reality—when we come upon associated objects as coincidental events, or we fortuitously find associated objects on the street, in a park, or even in a junk shop. The environment outside us begins to echo the environment inside us.

There is a clear suggestion here, it seems to me, for carers of significantly regressed children (i.e., nonverbal autists) to enhance the permeability between the environments of books and reality. We can also infer an important contribution to prevention. Perhaps it is possible for the family, in reality, to travel to the landscape of a story, to meet live versions of characters, or to find costume accessories, for example. Most vital of all, however, a respect for the child's archaically informed passivity must prevail: the child needs to be invited to opportunities that are facilitated with a minimum of conscious attention drawn. In other words, this is not about saying, "Look, there's the donkey from your story!" Rather, it is about safely being near the donkey, for example, while caregivers talk about other things, filling the auditory space with their own random phonemes—and thus, letting the child enjoy the potential for self-securing.

In truth, kindergarten is a wonderful place for observations. A wood chip on the playground looks just like a jewel from the book read to the class that morning; classroom toys find roles in story plots; children act out a favourite character's words and deeds; they take on text-inspired names for the day or week, and so on. Anyone familiar with young children knows how such accidental objects—echoes of stories—are a great source of pleasure. For they carry an unconscious conveyance: the witness is here so the world is secure. It is a proof of life. In truth, the world abounds with cultures that honour finding external evidence of internal symbols. As Taylor stresses, "There is not one objective truth about the boundary between fantasy and reality. Essentially the same belief can be judged as a delusion or a non-delusion depending on the culture of the believer."[15] Further, Taylor notes that "Some children, typically at about 9 or 10 years of age, create 'paracosms'—entire societies or worlds for the imaginary people to inhabit."[16] For the capacity to re-experience the witness through the objects of reality nurtures forward investments of affect by securitizing reality. The environment is made porous.

To stress, refinding our stories in reality lures our further engagements in it, as the unconscious (re)experience of the witness enables new learning. For, just like in the archaic, new objects—particularly phonemes—are inscribed with affect by virtue of being co-experienced (i.e., associated) with the witness, enabling new paths for investment. As such, finding archaic echoes confers on reality the security of the archaic environment. So doing, archaic echoes sustain individuation, which is exactly what a regressed individual needs—including, but not only, young children and nonverbal autists. No wonder it feels so tragic to reach the end of a favourite series, or to discover that we have read everything an author ever wrote—or to want to reread favourite stories, to relive them, as it were. For a book is an offer of objects within an all-providing environment laced with traces of affect and replete with unconscious associations. Reading is self-securing.

We now recall what is most crucial about archaic triangulation with respect to the phoneme: it is a relation of self and witness co-experiencing a phoneme in a kind of echo—and by this triangulation, affect circulates and returns to the self. The witness fuels triangulations upon triangulations—in a wild diffusion of associations and proliferations of circulatory pathways that keep reinvesting the self. Thus, archaic triangulation is a precursor and a model for the ubiquitous human phenomenon that certain echoes of experience—i.e., echoes of the self on an invested object—return unconscious affect. For example, revisiting a childhood landscape is highly evocative—the self then and now, triangulated on a place (wherein objects, including words, are invested). So is touching a special object from childhood, such as a blanket or toy—the self then and now, triangulated on the object. Note that an echo implies both positionality and return—a (re)encounter with an invested object from another direction. And the reassurance—i.e., the return of affect to the self—happens via a revisited path. Perhaps, then, we are detecting a relation to the widely acknowledged and observable preference of nonverbal autists for going somewhere on the same set path every time and returning along an equally fixed path—as if new paths were phobic, or as if existential anxiety were at stake. Perhaps it is.

Dolto shares her own experience of learning to read with her beloved governess using an orientalist collection of short fiction, *Les Babouches de Baba-Hassein*.[17] For months, people thought she was reading because she could sound out "syllables that meant nothing" until one day, her governess told her to listen to herself reading.[18]

As Dolto describes it, the sense she obtained from hearing her own voice seemed miraculous, as words became "activated, enchained."[19] Here, then, is the securing role of hearing one's invested phonemes in the environment—and the lingering influence of the unconscious work secured via that childhood text will be formative. For in 1943, the first of Dolto's three children, then an infant, appears in a tunic and turban, the photo caption reading, "Asian prince taking a walk incognito."[20] And in 1956, Dolto will visit Egypt—the setting of *Babouches*—sending home a postcard from Ptolemy's Door that perfectly evokes that deeply invested text.[21]

Dolto's other autobiographical insights about reading are equally informative. She recalls reading a weekly magazine delivered to her grandparents' home, «La Semaine de Suzette,»[22] calling it, "an enormous thing that helped me live in reality."[23] For it served as testimony, she explains, that outside her family, there existed other humans who cared about the same things she did.[24] Her example also points to the fact that the witness is nowhere in sight but presumed "present" due to creating this work. In Dolto's narrative, I believe we also can detect something of her own difficult childhood—her need to find in reading what was not findable at home. Dolto's elaboration of the archaic stage allows us to predict that since finding passages for discharging affect is crucial to self-regulation, the incapacity to do so is anxiogenic. And we have already confirmed that nonverbal autists read precociously to enable affective self-regulation. Now, with Dolto, we come upon a simple formulation for affective continuity: we are driven to find archaic echoes, wherever and whenever, as a solution for regression.

Montessori herself has a considerable body of work on regression. Foremost is her observation that the inherently passive child will be lured by only some—but not all—of the objects in his environment, and driven by unconscious processes from the start: "They are more attracted to some things than to others. Thus, they do not take in the whole of their environment. They have a guide within themselves … The guide within them exists from the first."[25] Montessori also notes critical periods for objects to "arrive" to enable normative progression: "If the child is prevented from enjoying these experiences at the very time when nature has planned for him to do so, the special sensitivity which draws him to them will vanish, with a disturbing effect on his development."[26] If objects do not unconsciously lure within such developmental windows—i.e., if objects do not manifest in his environment, or if the child is so regressed that his objects lack associations to the lures—regression results, as Montessori explains: "I hold that many regressive tendencies are due to a lack of the vital urge which guides the child to make his social adaptation."[27] This is exactly what we theorize about nonverbal autism. Montessori concludes that a regressive position provokes anxiety: "But suppose we have another type of child, who does not feel this irresistible attraction for his environment. In this type, his love for it has been thwarted and replaced by fear."[28] So if regression is seriously anxiogenic, and phonemes are the best lures, why not promote reading?

Reading is conducive to self-regulation because it facilitates new pathways for the circulation of unconscious affect. From this, we draw two inferences with momentous consequences for schooling. First, reading a text that one has chosen (or written) is potentially self-securing in facilitating the dissemination of invested phonemes, since these appear haphazardly in works that lure us. Conversely, reading a text that one has not intuitively chosen (e.g., that a teacher or parent has selected) is potentially de-securing since it is not as likely to contain invested phonemes, thus it is unlikely to lure or secure us; it might even include phonemes unconsciously associated with trauma in ways no one may know. Therefore, being compelled to read can be phobic. And all these effects of reading—securing or de-securing—are magnified if one is "forced" to read aloud, since doing so not only activates internal echoes but also populates the external environment.

In effect, then, external echoes that are securing enhance language production, while those that are de-securing precipitate regression. Enigmatically, to remain unconsciously secure, the reader must be guided by instinct—a call to read (or not). Certainly, informative texts can be read for research and conscious acquisitions. But reading for self-regulation is something different: it leaves the text choice to the reader's intuition. For if we can find our archaic echoes, the unconscious experience of the witness returns and regression slowly gives way to progression. As it turns out, then, the solution for the temporarily regressed is the same in kind as that for the profoundly regressed—nonverbal autists. At issue is the capacity for self-securing defined as a need to establish on the outside (reality) a reliable access to the witness securing us on the inside. Of course, the notion of unconscious influences in reading seems unreasonable and illogical. But as the nonverbal autistic writer, Birger Sellin, shares: "You can learn nonsense from us and … a nautical view of life which is by no means ontologically simple."[29] Precisely.

B. Reverberations

There is cause to worry, then, when community libraries are repurposed; when school libraries are stripped of books and turned into "tech hubs"; when artificial intelligence writes novels and replies to our messages; and when the metaverse impinges on the human universe. Dolto's elaboration of the unconscious role of phonemes in human development makes it abundantly clear that we are awakened and secured in reality as a function of finding our archaic echoes in the social. Humans wake each other up, so to speak: we enable interhuman affects to transit between us (right from gestation), by which we self-regulate and thus survive in a co-constructed reality. Since self-regulation is in the balance, human beings are instinctively resonant to the presence of another real human being, whether that person is alive or not at present. It is our defining *modus operandi* as a communicative species. And because the unconscious is moot for time and space, then old books, papers, dictionaries, letters, diaries and even maps are all worthy documents to read for the restitution of affective circulation. In fact, these marginalized materials—the very things libraries may discard (perhaps due to mould or dust mites) or remove from circulation (i.e., limiting access or locking up)—are incredibly potent as reparative instruments because they have been invested by others and thereby convey a sense of another to follow. Thus, I believe Dolto shows us why our relationship with reading is another proof of unconscious processes—one that is as obvious as dreaming. For reading circulates unconscious affects via the transference in texts.

In this context, another beneficial practice worth highlighting is that of "Social Stories."[30] We have already encountered the conflation of pronouns that is common in autism. In fact, this trait was observed over one hundred years ago, when Barr wrote of an autistic patient "invariably speaking of himself in the third person."[31] What Dolto crucially shows is that fusion—a passive, regressive position of unconscious affective dependence on another—is a normal stage of mental and emotional development in which autists simply linger. Thus, when a child speaks (or writes) in the third person, I believe that we can assume a continued state of fusion—i.e., that individuation is incomplete. It is curious but true: grammar delivers a diagnosis. In working with autists, the highly regarded American educator, Carol Gray, innovated the genre—now used productively in educational settings worldwide—more than 20 years ago.

The concept of Social Stories is brilliant and fully theorizable along the model of archaic triangulation. For limited phonemes invested by the child are put into circulation in a text and repeated within the language environment of the story: "include reference to Audience interests, perhaps using a favorite character to demonstrate Story content";[32] and story creators are encouraged to "add custom photos and/or images that the student recognizes and can relate to."[33] The story is an experience of self in the third person, wherein this other (that is self) serves as a witness: "Social Stories are documents that are worthy of the trust of their Audience."[34] And the reduction of anxiety (the most debilitating symptom) in confronting new learning is patent: "The improvement of behavior that is frequently credited to a Social Story is the result of improved understanding of events and expectations."[35] In short, the child is scaffolded for success in reality and supported in the long and much-delayed challenge of individuation.

Given Dolto's theorization, we can easily derive further inferences about reading. Reading in one's first language (L1) will be more likely to offer invested phonemes—and the return of the unconscious experience of the witness—than reading in a second language (L2). By the same logic, someone traumatized in their L1 will find books in the L2 less anxiogenic. And as the unconscious work of reading implicates a relation in dream-work within the self—rather than a conscious relation with others—anyone reliant on regression as a defence (i.e., an infant, autistic individual or trauma survivor) will benefit from their books never being disrupted by others. Their texts should be left to lie wherever they are, to whatever page they are open, with no attention whatsoever drawn to them. In effect, this is an environmental provision of words (book), where words reciprocally mark the environment (living space). The process is passive and private.

This is obviously a completely different matter than sharing books with children, which is always a worthy goal—especially if the child selects the reading(s). But the unconscious work of reading is something else, something other. It occurs beyond the purview of consciousness through dream-work on words. Thus, the regressed reader needs to come upon books or authors by accident or circumstance—discovering a title or text by happenstance, perhaps overheard in the conversations of others, or found in a junk shop. The text becomes a path to follow—and in turn, it may suggest the work to read next. For self-regulation is governed by the instinct of conservation, driving humans to intuitively refind their pre-invested phonemes. Thus, we infer that all children read silently long before they are acknowledged to be readers.[36] For even as we progress into the future, we unconsciously seek the past—to (re)find our archaic history. Freud invoked this matter by simply saying that humans universally retain "the desire to go to sleep where one has slept in childhood."[37] We are driven to seek the echoes of our archaic dreams.

In conclusion, our archaic relations with invested phonemes persist lifelong and impact reading at the level of the word and witness. Reading that is self-selected offers the best chance of encountering pre-invested phonemes to reanimate archaic affects. Through this unconscious process, reading can return the experience of the witness that delivers existential security. In turn, re-experiencing the witness confers affect on new relations and objects along a filiation of trust. The unconscious experience of the witness also invests (by associations) new objects for learning, diffusing affect. As such, it supports individuation in that the self becomes capable of self-securing objects.

It is crucial for readers to choose their texts because affective security is contingent on re-experiencing invested phonemes along associations—whereas an environment that fails to lure or presents phonemes associated with trauma is anxiogenic. And however irrational a reading refusal might seem to be, it is entirely justified in terms of the unconscious processes crucial to self-regulation. The plain reason is that phonemes that lure us (and/or that we ourselves write)—and that we feel instinctively "called" to read—enable the liberation of affect that reduces anxiety. In addition, reading such texts aloud produces self-securing echoes in the environment. The repercussions for nonverbal autism are evident: presume that precocious reading occurs—and facilitate the passive play between textual and real environments. Thus, the abundant access to books in community and school libraries is more than a matter of literacy. For the formidable potential to refind archaic echoes makes reading unconsciously reparative.

Notes

1 Pappenheim 1924/1986.
2 Breuer & Freud 1893a.
3 Jones 1953/1982, 224.
4 1888/2008, 34–35.
5 I do not read German but I read French. In my previous project on Dolto, I take up this transference of the autobiographical in any text (or theory) with numerous examples from Dolto's life—including an entire chapter dedicated to the play of the phoneme /do/ in her corpus.
6 Breuer & Freud 1893a, 39.
7 Guttmann 2001, 191–192; the portrait of Pappenheim as von Hameln is readily findable online.

8 1898, 27.
9 There was a reported 25 per cent increase in anxiety due to COVID-19 (United Nations 2020 and World Health Organization 2020).
10 1901b, 110.
11 1895, 365–366.
12 1916a, 71.
13 1999, 5.
14 Ibid, 18.
15 Ibid, 144.
16 Ibid, 136.
17 Balesta 1894/1902.
18 In Potin 2008, 116.
19 Ibid, 114.
20 Ibid, 178.
21 In Djéribi-Valentin 2005, 267.
22 Published 1905–1960; e,g., see BD Anciennes.com.
23 Dolto 1986b, 67.
24 Ibid, 68.
25 1949/2010, 91.
26 Ibid, 87.
27 Ibid, 74.
28 Ibid, 77.
29 1995, 181.
30 I have no connection to Gray or any organization promoting Social Stories.
31 Barr 1898, 27.
32 Gray 2010, xx.
33 Ibid.
34 Ibid, xxxiii.
35 Ibid, xxxi.
36 Barring complete blindness.
37 1907/1962, 156 [Meeting of 27 March 1907].

Chapter 9

Transcription—Producing Echoes

Preliminary Words

Charles Darwin's son, Francis, edited an unassuming text of barely 80 pages that holds claim to being his father's authoritative autobiography. Darwin's[1] recollections were apparently set down during his leisure time—"for nearly an hour on most afternoons"[2] from 28 May to 3 August 1876—and written for his children, "without any thought that they would ever be published."[3] Francis assures the reader that he left the words as he found them except "to make a few corrections of obvious verbal slips."[4] Francis does not explain, however, why every entry is within the stated time frame except for a single inscription five years later, 1 May 1881. In this stunning afterthought of a passage, Darwin mentions every book he has written, thanks "Frank" for helping with his publications, and spends most of the lengthy entry reflecting on his writing style:

> There seems to be a sort of fatality in my mind leading me to put at first my statement or proposition in a wrong or awkward form … I used to think about my sentences before writing them down; but for several years I have found that it saves time to scribble in a vile hand whole pages as quickly as I possibly can … then correct deliberately. Sentences thus scribbled down are often better ones than I could have written deliberately.[5]

Darwin also describes how he plans a book from "the rudest outline in two or three pages, and then a larger one in several pages, a few words or one word standing for a whole discussion or series of facts."[6] And he bemoans how, "My mind seems to have become a kind of machine for grinding general laws out of large collections of facts,"[7] while "so poor in one sense is my memory, that I have never been able to remember for more than a few days a single date."[8] Darwin also narrates how he condenses his reading into notes:

> I have bought many books, and at their ends, I make an index of all the facts that concern my work; or, if the book is not my own, write out a separate abstract, and of such abstracts I have a large drawer full. Before beginning on any subject

DOI: 10.4324/9781032655123-18

I look to all the short indexes and make a general and classified index, and by taking the one or more portfolios I have all the information collected during my life ready for use.[9]

Discovering this priceless text is an infusion of pleasure. Googling, I learn that 1 May 1881 was a Sunday and, haphazardly, the wedding of Ivan Pavlov, Nobel laureate and father of behaviourism. In the context of autism, the coincidence is astounding. For on that day, Darwin—who died before the first Nobel prize was awarded but would surely have been a worthy recipient—puts to pen what is arguably a profound antithesis to behaviourism in a postscript intended to remain private. In it, Darwin seems to candidly acknowledge the crucial share of unconscious processes in his writing—and in his theories, so widely recognized for holding such explanatory power.

Foremost is the fact that the text is an intimate one, so he feels free to speak. Also pertinent is that the distal entry comes after five years of leaving his autobiographical reflections untouched. This is the hallmark of the *après-coup* of dream-work—that thoughts make their way slowly as returns come unpredictably, sometimes (much) later, after a deep, unconscious reworking. This phenomenon is familiar in psychoanalysis and often witnessed in therapy. Further, Darwin's outlines are a testament to the potency of associative thinking as single words represent entire chapters, he tells us. And his note-taking vouches for the work of condensation, as he reads huge volumes of material, producing indices, and indices of indices, until the organization of his thoughts is associative—a collection of words in relation to one another. Surprisingly, Darwin also divulges that his memory is poor—i.e., that he has a predilection for consciously forgetting. So his indices are his *aide-mémoires*: external records of his internal thinking, which he later reads as he prepares to write.

By producing these condensations, Darwin inadvertently enables the formation of an echo of his most invested words between his thoughts and his notes. From his notes—these outer reserves of inner condensations—he will then wildly diffuse his invested words in a free stream of writing, displacing them in myriad sentences without overthinking—as he divulges. It is only after this initial free displacement without deliberate intention—almost like the expression of dream-work—that Darwin returns to his writing and, with the gain of self-observation, clarifies the expression of his ideas. We should not forget that slips of the pen (akin to slips of the tongue) were present too—Francis tells us so—as evidence of unconscious "slippage" between intention and production. What Darwin arrives at in this manner—i.e., from enabling, even prioritizing, an unconsciously-informed methodology—is decisively better, he says. And his unprecedented theories are memorials to the fecundity of the unconscious influences in his process.

We should not be surprised to see the two main mechanisms of dream-work—displacement and condensation—being so active in free writing, as Darwin exemplifies in this rare volume. For as Freud explained it, "creative writing … is a continuation and substitution … for the play of childhood."[10] But dream-work is not only play, it is formative work. In the Darwin family's lovely little book, mental and emotional worlds entwine, as a text written for the love of his children also traces his foundational ideas and contributions.

In fact, Freud explained over a century ago—within a decade of Darwin's musings—that any word is associative in nature: "A word, then, is a complicated concept built up from various impressions, i.e., it corresponds to an intricate process of associations."[11] Freud's work on unconscious processes disturbed the general public (as it often does now), at least as much as Darwin threatened the status quo. Ample proof is that Freud was nominated for the Nobel prize 33 times—32 times in physiology and medicine, and once in literature—but never won.[12] And as Freud explained, "writing … by which the intensity of self-observation may be increased varies considerably according to the subject-matter."[13] Freud is implicitly suggesting that all writing is autobiographical and that it enables self-observation: a second view on one's own thoughts. Since then, through her work on phonemes, I believe that Dolto elaborated the mechanism for what Freud described. For the unconscious inscription of our most invested phonemes makes every text we write (or speak) incidentally autobiographical as we displace and disseminate affect, liberating it. Furthermore, in reflecting on the outside (i.e., the external environment) the words circulating on the inside (i.e., the internal environment, our thinking), writing produces natural echoes that are securitizing.

A. Inscription

Funnily enough, Freud underwent formative training in physiology and medicine at l'Hôpital Pitié-Salpêtrière, in Paris, where he attended lectures on hysteria by Jean-Martin Charcot and translated them into German.[14] At the "Pitié" today, there is still a trace of Charcot, Freud and the prominence of unconscious processes in the ongoing work of the sleep disorders clinic. The well-respected researcher who currently heads that facility, Isabelle Arnulf,[15] reports some highly pertinent observations impacting dream-work and writing. First, she notes a reparative process among her patients: they write out their nightmares, later reread those transcriptions, change the ending, and read the new scenario before falling asleep; by this technique, recurring nightmares disappear within two weeks.[16] Through rereading, she narrates, "comfortably installed, in broad daylight, to minimize emotions and physical manifestations of fear … associated with the narrative,"[17] new associations are formed in connection with a secure environment. To this, we can now add that associations are also formed by writing itself, as phonemes are immersed in new grammatical contexts.

We should not forget that homonymic play is also a source of associations that blur affect and thought. Dolto was famous for the emphasis she gave homonyms, as exemplified in the long-format publication of her therapy with Dominique.[18] Here, it seems particularly apt to reference an autistic patient of the great psychotherapist, Frances Tustin: "Peter, like other autistic children, had the notion that words which sound alike must be connected in some way."[19] If ever she had been asked, Dolto would surely have insisted that Peter was right.

For we will come upon some anomalies of logic when we begin to explore the unconscious work of phonemes, and things that do not seem to make sense at all are nonetheless true. For example, in therapy with her famous patient, Dominique, Dolto interprets homonymic plays: how the word for a mother's «lait» [milk] is a homonym of the antonym, «laid» [ugly], of his patronym «bel» [beautiful]; how his nursery, which he called «la salle» [the room], is a homonym of «la sale» [the dirty one]—representing his new baby sister; how his sister's name, Sylvie—phonemically «s'il vit» [if he lives] was experienced as foreboding about an uncle who died; how Dominique wants to be a «voleur de mer» [pirate], a homonym of «voleur de mère» [thief of the mother], disclosing his jealousy towards his sibling; and his recovery being due to learning that a man can be a «maire» [mayor]—a homonym of «mère» [mother].[20] Another teen patient, Tony, who is truant, speaks of acute pain in his «genoux» [knees]; but homonymically, this is «je – nous» [I – we/us]—which Dolto takes up as a game of «mots» [words] and its perfect homonym, «maux» [pains].[21] Her patient, Katia, only four, states that she wants a medal on a «ficelle» [thread], and Dolto takes up the homonym, «fils-elle» [son – she], to start the analysis.[22] And her work with nine-year-old, Robert, who talks about falling out the «fenêtre» [window], centres on the paradox vested in its homonyms: «feu – naître» [fire – being born] versus «feu – n'être» [fire – not being].[23]

Dolto's approach admittedly seems so radical and so bizarre. Yet she had phenomenal success—the historical record is unequivocal about this. So something about phonemic plays is highly significant in analysis and reparation. We recall that audition is the most crucial sense *in utero*, offering objects and facilitating continuity to reality—and that homonyms are heard as a single (i.e., the same) phoneme. Dolto says the infant has "intuitive hearing."[24] For it isn't until reality arrives that homonyms can be distinguished by association to objects or relations—that the "knee" and "I – us" can be correctly discerned. Phonemic play conveys thoughts and affect because mental and emotional life are interwoven in the unconscious investment of phonemes. Thus, any witness who is receptive to latent content—i.e., open to unconscious conveyances—can learn a lot about another in the transference. This is arguably the whole basis for psychoanalytic therapy.

Dolto assumes that archaically invested phonemes issue suggestions during the early months and years of the child's coming to consciousness. So the child "lives" invested phonemes—rooting truth in them. And we should not forget that homonymic play is also a source of pleasure—it remains so even when children are old enough to become irrepressible punners. Through her detailed anamneses and extensive note-taking, Dolto is alert to the child's phonemes in her listening—it is the focus of her practice. And by taking up (i.e., speaking) the child's invested phonemes in her sessions, she becomes a witness in triangulation, enabling his individuation. Thus, Dolto becomes a resonator, as she puts it, to awaken the child's "own analyst."[25] She is pointedly clear: this is an auto-recovery.

What Dolto also reveals is that in writing extensive notes of her sessions and rereading them later, she came to better understand her patients and she could experience their affective situations more clearly. Dolto was considered by some of her critics to have "too much intuition and not enough method,"[26] yet her clinical approach precisely aims to privilege intuition—i.e., archaic, unconscious processes pertaining to the phoneme. Through acute listening, Dolto is privy to some strange confusions in the child's mind that have arisen from homonymic plays and suggestions on phonemes—dream-work on audition—as what is «malentendu» [misheard] creates a (perfectly homonymic) «malentendu» [misunderstanding]. In turn, hearing those invested phonemes in circulation enables the child's individuation to proceed.

Crucially, homonymic play is an auditory pleasure only. When we transcribe, we will need to decide, for instance, between "die" and "dye," or "fir" and "fur" (or their equivalents given the phonemes of any language). Meanwhile, for example, the infant named *Di*ana or *Fer*nando is invited to some wild, unconscious plays as homonyms bounce auditorily while issuing wild suggestions. This is also why phonemes are easily subject to slips of the pen—like Francis Darwin found in his father's reflections. For as a legacy of the archaic stage, phonemes are subject to unconscious plays. Thus, when we write and commit to a spelling—the sentence as a sentence, so to speak—we become more conscious of these plays and suggestions emanating from the archaic environment where dream-work commences its productivity.

Note-taking—transcribing—is a given of the psychoanalytic method that, as it turns out, is central to it. For archaic triangulation—the phoneme in echo between self and witness—has spectacular explanatory power. The therapist jots a patient's most invested words and/or most repeated words—that is the nature of note-taking. As Darwin explains, the process is a form of indexing—of compressing long strings of audition (from reading or hearing) into condensed units of words. Strings are stripped of non-essentials (prepositions, articles, etc.) as heavily weighted words—nouns, adjectives and verbs—become dominant. Words that repeat may get underlined or bolded, conveying their affective load. And over repeated sessions—i.e., through successive listening or rereading—some words begin assuming greater importance, taking on the role of headers that open entire fields of associations.

In sum, in notes, one word comes to stand for a long set of facts and reflections—an entire story. Note-taking concentrates affect and ideas onto fewer phonemes—and condensation is a principal means of dream-work. As such, transcribing—i.e., condensing words collected over multiple repetitions and encounters from what someone says or writes—creates a very special situation for the conveyance of unconscious material: a resource of condensed and invested phonemes, with associations to each other, circulating in a language bath (i.e., in a full body of notes). The phonemes another has invested are not only repeated and charged with affect but also include (necessarily, accidentally) the phonemes that have seeded that individual's associative thinking. And that is why Dolto could better grasp her patients' emotional situations upon rereading her case notes—and why being a "script-girl," as she put it, has such huge theoretical value. This is also why Dolto was both intuitive and successful in treating Dominique, Tony, Katia, Robert and countless other child (and older) patients over the decades.

In effect, writing serves two vital functions: communication and individuation. The notion of writing for communication is one everyone is familiar with. And for the nonverbal autist, learning to write fundamentally offers the same kind of empowerment as Signing does for the Deaf. It is necessary for personal agency—and after all, "attaining language fluency is more important than which language the child becomes fluent in."[27] It also puts words into circulation—dispersing them in the environment, thereby continuing the dream-work (i.e., diffusion) that securitizes new objects (i.e., reality). So why not let the nonverbal autistic child become fluent in writing for communication?

Writing for individuation, however, carries additional possibilities because it enables triangulation. This happens as words on the inside—silent thoughts—appear in echo on the outside, reanimating through this echo in space the circulation of affect that delivers the unconscious experience of the securing witness. It also helps words in circulation in our thoughts appear for our own witnessing days, months or years later—as an echo in time—and, once again, this delivers the unconscious experience of the securing witness. So, again, why not help the nonverbal autistic child achieve individuation?

What we learn from prolific note-takers like Darwin, Freud and Dolto—and from the value of note-taking to therapeutic work, including the fact that homonymic plays offer their suggestions to thought—is that transcribing enables a particularly potent form of triangulation, returning both affect and thoughts due to the unconscious weave of the mental and the emotional. We also confirm that research is a special relationship with formidable unconscious concomitants. For in being invested in a relationship of close listening (or reading), we invite the transference—especially if we freely allow ourselves to be available, like in the archaic, rather than imposing conscious controls or over-planning the process. Through transcribing, the transference that is securable blurs affect and content, influencing our thoughts and feelings. Transcribing also feeds our dreams because it taps archaic processes steeped in dream-work. So transcription helps us migrate our thoughts and receive new insights—often, as is the case for dream journals, upon waking. And as it is with dreams, the more we engage in transcription, and the more we feed our dreams, the more there is to write, and so on. Thus, on the word, the continuity of affective circulation is restored in the play between reality and dreams.

The "environment" of note-taking is archaic-syntonic: it evokes the presence–absence of someone whose key words (read or heard) we absorbed. We note their most invested, most frequent phonemes, and we become invested in these phonemes through this witnessing—precisely in the manner that objects in the archaic gain affect by association to the indissociable other who provides them. We do not write everything the person says—we concentrate their points. And as we do, we feel something for those words and ideas. Mental and emotional activity are synchronous because in the act of condensing words, we are engaging in a process conducive to dream-work and associative thinking. Through this, it is as-if the words themselves echo—resonating the affective investments of the absent witness and of ourselves. So within a language bath of words, pages of notes, some phonemes become more important, precisely in the same way that affect influences the formation of pathways for associative thinking from invested phonemes. The notion of the language bath—a fluid auditory environment of words—is determinative. For phonemes in the archaic are always perceived within a soundscape—not alone, but in streams of language serving a kind of echo-location.

Thus, the free flow of language in the environment is imperative for giving phonemes their distinction, in terms of being more invested and more repeated relative to the wider auditory input. In any event, it is well within the explanatory power of archaic triangulation to account for how transcribing (aka note-taking) revives affective circulation and stimulates thought. But beyond this is the truly therapeutic, reparative power of transcription: archaic triangulation is a continuous flow of objects that nourish dream-work and serve as food for thought. So transcription becomes a form of self-feeding. Phonemes enter into triangulation, restoring affective security by opening new pathways that also grow associative networks simultaneously—since what is mental and emotional converges.

As such, the enigmatic "presence" of the absent witness—the speaker or writer from whom we took notes—satisfies the archaic condition of the witness. And as a result, new objects (in reality) are secured by association to the witness, and the persistent condition of fusional dependence—passivity due to sustained regression—is loosened, thereby enabling progression. The individual becomes self-luring, so to speak. Once this mechanism of self-recovery is triggered, it proceeds in earnest because it supports self-regulation. For unconscious processes, in being driven by the instinct of conservation, naturally leverage any opportunity that benefits long-term survival. Only a little salts the soup.

What is at stake in triangulation is the capacity to circulate affect because an invested phoneme is co-experienced in dream-work as an echo between the self and the witness who is felt to be affectively similar and indissociably present, whose presence returns archaic security. In fact, Tustin herself noted with Peter that, "Throughout his treatment, I would need to be constantly on the alert for this overlapping or fusion of the two of us … as an 'undercurrent' in our interaction."[28] Tustin also touches on the blur of inside and outside that is at stake during the process of individuation: "They [autists] feel part of the outside world and feel it is part of them without feeling separate from it."[29] For her part, Dolto is theorizing that this blur of inside and outside is an essential developmental process that enables our progression from a natural primary dependence on regression (unconscious defence) to the development of the ego (conscious defence). It is only that in the nonverbal autist, progression has stalled or slowed significantly, and it is the continued dependence on regression as a defence that simultaneously compels and reveals the fusional state. Understanding this allows us to infer a reparation: facilitate the triangulation of phonemes on the "outside" to scaffold individuation. And in modestly describing her stunning work as simply "a witnessing put into words,[30] Dolto introduces herself to her patients as their transcriber—telling Dominique, for example, that she is merely "the one who writes what you say."[31]

Arnulf conveys an abundance of valuable results in her studies, including the fact that recollections increase over time when patients are asked to keep a dream journal.[32] So something about writing our invested phonemes—putting them into echo in triangulations (self, witness and phoneme)—nurtures further dream-work. I believe we are detecting the proliferation of associative thinking in/as dream-work, and how dream-work makes use of phonemes. As if in a direct confirmation of this prediction, Arnulf discovers that when accounts are written in a dream journal, they are more condensed than when dictated orally.[33] I suggest that what this reveals is that affect on phonemes is condensed by transcribing, whereas speaking is a later capacity that diffuses phonemes into auditory space. I believe we can infer, then, a two-step process: phonemes are triangulated in dream-work, circulating affect and proliferating associative thinking; and only secondarily do we speak our phonemes thanks to later developmental processes involved in the physical maturation of the motor apparatus for speech. The logical conclusion is a momentous one for nonverbal autism: while speaking requires thinking, the reverse is not true.

B. Reverberations

In fact, we previously considered this division of labour between thinking and speaking. In nonverbal autism, the first step has been achieved so that associative thinking is vibrant, developing wildly—not despite dream-work but because of it. On the other hand, regression has impacted the far later development of conscious motor control (including speech). As such, writing facilitates triangulation—putting phonemes in echo—while bypassing speech. As a case in point, in educational programmes for Deaf children in Italy, "The written language is taught as a foreign language through the medium of the fluent sign the child already knows."[34] Speaking is simply sidelined. And returning to Arnulf once more, 49 per cent of "deaf-mutes" (her term) dreamed they could hear and 43 per cent could speak in their dreams. Conversely, those who speak and hear without impediment dreamed of being deaf or mute.[35] This is further evidence that external speech (as a motor movement) is entirely distinct from internal speech—thought—that derivative dream-work.

In fact, speaking itself is so late developmentally that, from research on the Deaf, we learn that, "Linguists speculate that sign acquisition precedes spoken language acquisition because it is easier for infants to articulate the hands than their vocal tracts."[36] And as a prominent Deaf writer generously admits, "I am prone to slips of the fingers while typing that are quite often meaningful."[37] There is a wonderful record of dream-work from the same field, as "Laura [Bridgman] fingerspelled in her dreams and in daydreaming."[38] Further, from Montessori herself, we have a strong argument for teaching writing early:

> The child's explosion into writing is closely connected with his special sensitivity for language … the age of five and a half or six, this sensitivity has ceased to exist; so it is clear that writing can be learned with joy and enthusiasm only before that age.[39]

Writing out one's own thoughts—putting down on the "outside" what is on the "inside" is the pre-eminent echo. It is, like speaking, a means of filling the environment with words, some of which cannot help but carry the archaic echoes of our invested phonemes. Thus, in writing and rereading, we gain the capacity for self-observation that Freud detected in creative writing, and that Dolto so eloquently theorized. At stake is a triangulation of self, witness and phoneme, in that the self writes and later serves as a witness. The witness is yourself—but a different version in time and space (environment). Exactly how (much) later will impact the capacity for self-observation. For what we predict is very simple: the less the share of consciousness, the greater the impact of unbridled unconscious processes.

Therefore, letting some time go by—or perhaps even rereading the transcription in a different environment (evoking different associations), or in a varied format—will enable the return in echo of an invested phoneme linked to a whole set of pathways in associative thinking. Letting even more time go by generates a more powerful echo as a strong return of affect and a new way of thinking about an object. Thus, we reach a surprising but compelling conclusion: unlike the assumption that rationality dominates critical thinking, the capacity to consider divergent views, and to turn over ideas in bold and original ways, inherently relies on unconscious, associative thinking. What we can also observe is that critical thinking is effectively a return to (of) our invested phonemes (i.e., condensations) in associative thinking—from another direction. Thus it is archaic triangulation—the phoneme in echo—that grounds innovation. We also note the ironic gains of regression: it is debilitating in reality but proliferates an associative wealth. Thus, we can infer with confidence that the nonverbal autist thinks more—not less.

The implications for self-publishing are substantial because transcribing and later rereading—especially after forgetting—is a potent means for returning affect to the self. So doing, it also liberates affect, encourages affective investments in new objects, and stimulates associative thinking. Of course, learning to write will require an apprenticeship. A facilitator will need to be nearby to reread, offer spellings, guide the hand in using tools, and/or issue encouragement. As with any educable skill, the time required for independence will depend on the age at which the skill is introduced, the learner's full profile, the frequency of sessions, and the quality of the support offered.

In this light, it seems curious indeed that nonverbal autists struggle to be facilitated in acquiring writing[40]—and that when they do receive support, their texts are considered invalid. In fact, one of the most authoritative and well-respected researchers on autism, Lorna Wing,[41] stressed this need for support almost 50 years ago:

> A very useful approach with autistic children is to teach the steps needed to accomplish practical skills by guiding the child's limbs through the necessary movements … Initial resistance or complete passivity may be met, but, if the teacher perseveres, the child eventually begins to perform. He may continue to demand the touch of the adult hand and refuse to do anything by himself, but this can be overcome by reducing the amount of contact very slowly until finally there is no touching at all.[42]

As any regressed individual is necessarily fusional (i.e., incompletely individuated), as we have elaborated it with Dolto, the nonverbal autist's dependence on another will naturally be indispensable—perhaps for years—until individuation is achieved. And it is writing that will gradually enable his individuation.

I believe there is an excellent articulation of writing practices in education already afoot in Reggio Emilia programmes.[43] For example, it is considered central to be "listening to the words of children and then offering them back to the group to restimulate and extend their discussion and joint activity."[44] Student speech is "enlarged [as] written quotes as parts of displays,"[45] and the "rereading of the experience"[46] is considered to be pivotal. Part of the design entails "encouraging children to make symbolic representations of their ideas."[47] Thereby, teachers become "transcribers and documentors,"[48] "writing down what the children say, then reading back their comments."[49] To stress, documentation is fundamental, "providing a verbal and visual trace of the children's experiences and work."[50] Furthermore, this "documentation stays on display in the classrooms for years."[51] So schools become securing environments to revisit, which is especially helpful if a child has been fragilized into a temporary regression. For the space is full of a child's phonemes—recalling the archaic experience of a language bath while securitizing reality by association with the phonemes present in that space-time. And in a process we now understand to be clearly leveraging unconscious archaic triangulation, the children's invested descriptions are used to plan new learning through what is termed *progettazione*—a form of "'projecting ahead' … [as] 'reconnaissance,'"[52] and a "basis for planning next steps."[53]

At first, adults are the documentors in these and other programmes, recording the phonemes children utter about (or while) completing work—in an evocation of anecdotal note-taking during parallel play. But children should soon learn to be their own documentors since this step is momentous to the beneficial unconscious processes at stake. Writing should be started as early as possible, for example by helping students to sign their art or label other products (e.g., photographs)—if only with marks; and enabling opportunities for them to transcribe words they love from texts they love—even, whenever possible, *on* texts they love. Crucially, writing should not wait for reading but precede it. Of course, writing implements of all kinds will be valuable resources for these projects of private pleasure that require others to facilitate without co-opting. At issue is that the fuelling of dreamwork that enables affective circulation and proliferates associative thinking is governed not by the conscious capacities of carers but by the unconscious capacities of learners.

Thus, when children write on things (including pre-written surfaces), create endless lists, intensely copy (and recopy) words in acts of writing that seem pointless to others, or even cut up their own written words (as if to keep one letter or phoneme over another)—as commonly occurs with all young children—these works should never be discarded without permission from the child. It is likewise if they colour over and/or trace words repeatedly, for even simply changing the format (e.g., the font or colour of words) might fulfil the minimum conditions for creating simple echoes—not terribly powerful, perhaps, but a worthy first step. And as transcriptions do private work within the self, they should never be inspected, displayed or judged without consent. In addition, if the creative writer insists on keeping scraps and bits, space should be found. Eventually, the child can be expected to disinvest these materials and allow them to be discarded—but not yet.

In fact, this need to put our fleeting thoughts outside ourselves—to note what seems to matter most in a moment of time-space—is not only the business of childhood. Thanks to archaic triangulation, human thought is designed, beginning *in utero*, to thrive on echoes—our ability to experience our invested words at even some small distance (of time or space). For in the archaic, this separation-individuation with a witness (i.e., the absence-presence of a similar other) generates unconscious affect and associative thinking. So we think better and develop convictions, like Darwin did, from having the words we collect in life available for our return. Thus, a child's transcriptions should be respected as educational texts—no less valuable to growing thought than Darwin's portfolios were to him.

It is commonly said—and indisputably true—that everyone has a right to a fluent first language. Therefore, writing is a successful intervention for autism because it supplies the archaic conditions for individuation—for securely exiting a regressive position—thanks to the triangulation of invested phonemes in an environment of words delivering the unconscious experience of the securing witness. Transcription, as a specific writing practice, is predicted to be particularly beneficial: writing out notes (i.e., favourite words and phrases) from (or even on) a beloved author's text(s); and freely enjoying rewriting notes, reorganizing and shifting words around, indexing and condensing. It is writing as playing. One of the nonverbal autistic authors studied, Naoki Higashida, advances a bold challenge: "I want to ask you what we can do so that we can survive for the future."[54] I believe Dolto answers this question: nonverbal autists need to write.

In conclusion, writing is not just a means of communication but a crucial scaffold for individuation in reality (time and space). This is because writing produces unconscious echoes of invested phonemes. It is naturally conducive to archaic triangulation, enabling the phoneme to be experienced from two "positions" of the self in time (as writer and later reader); and/or from two "positions" of the self in space (as thoughts on the inside are findable on the outside). Further, transcribing (i.e., note-taking)—writing out the most invested words of a trusted other—produces powerful echoes as the phoneme plays between the self and witness, restor(y)ing triangulation along the archaic model.

Transcribing is especially susceptible to archaic echoes because it condenses a stream of language to its most invested phonemes. Thus, transcription returns affect to the self while stimulating associative thinking. This makes writing an essential educational activity and gives it a place of privilege far ahead of learning to read in terms of its reparative potential. The repercussions for autism are such that writing should be facilitated as the best means of restoring progression (individuation) to address a profound regression, even though the presence of another human being will be necessary—admittedly for years—until individuation (self-securing) is achieved. In sum, we can write our way out of regression by producing self-securing echoes of our unconscious dream-work, to guide our journey to reality.

Notes

1 Except where otherwise stated, "Darwin" refers to Charles.
2 Darwin 1881/2015, preface.
3 Ibid.
4 F. Darwin in ibid, preface.
5 Darwin 1881/2015 (dated 1 May 1881), n.p., third page of the 10-page entry.
6 Ibid.
7 Ibid, sixth page.
8 Ibid, sixth page.
9 Ibid, third and fourth pages.
10 1908a, 152.
11 1891/2011, 77.
12 Nobel Prize Outreach 2022.
13 Freud 1900a, 103.
14 Freud 1925[1924], 21.
15 Translations of Arnulf are my own.
16 Arnulf 2014, 151.
17 Ibid.
18 As mentioned already, I discuss the homonymic play in Dolto's corpus (in both her autobiographical and case materials) in greater detail in my previous work on Dolto.
19 Tustin 1981, 228.
20 Dolto 1971.
21 Dolto 1984, 363.
22 In Caldaguès 1982, 51.
23 In De Sauverzac 1988, 88–90.
24 In Halmos 1994, 339.
25 Dolto 1985/1989, 134; Dolto & Winter 1986, 61 & 143; Guillerault 1997, 77; Djéribi-Valentin 2005, 219.
26 Roudinesco 1986, 496; see e.g., Littner 1974.
27 Gulati 2003c, 37.
28 1981, 198.
29 Ibid, 177.
30 In Dolto & Winter 1986, 31.
31 Dolto 1971, 110.
32 2014, 17.
33 Ibid.
34 Gulati 2003c, 53.
35 2014, 40.
36 Gulati 2003c, 41.
37 Gulati 2003a, 361.
38 Lane 1984, 291 (Bridgman is considered to be the first Deaf-Blind student formally educated in the US).
39 1949/2010, 157.
40 I have no direct affiliation with programmes or schools for Facilitated Communication.
41 Wing actually wrote the foreword for two of Mukhopadhyay's fine books—*Beyond the Silence* (2000) and *The Mind Tree* (2003)—in her capacity as Consultant Psychiatrist.
42 1976, 201.
43 I have no affiliation with any Reggio Emilia school or programme.
44 Edwards 1996, 169.
45 Rankin 1996, 196.
46 Ibid, 208.

47 Fraser & Gestwicki 2000, 11.
48 Ibid, 51.
49 Edwards 1996, 154.
50 Ibid, 11.
51 Fraser & Gestwicki 2000, 156.
52 Wien 2008, 11.
53 Katz 1996, 27.
54 In Wurzburg & Biklen 2011.

Chapter 10

Forest—Following Echoes

Preliminary Words

I went looking for a classic fable from Aesop to include in this momentous final chapter—one I might recall from over 60 years ago. I first came upon "The Olive-Tree and the Fig-Tree,"[1] a lovely story featuring my two favourite foods. In it, the olive tree is smug about how she never loses her leaves and thereby looks beautiful year-round. But come winter, a snowfall causes her to bend and break, whereas the bare fig tree is unharmed. Some versions, translated from Greek or prior renditions, add terrifying elements to the storm; some even deliver the moral that boasting about your wealth invites disaster. But children are easily frightened, and they are not independently wealthy. Besides, any child would be far more likely to identify with the fig in the first place, since it looks less perfected (developed) yet survives. So is it not possible, instead, to consider the valuable lesson of this fable to be that one's ability to adapt to the seasons of life is what best ensures survival—or that appearances are not everything?

I soon found another that I remembered almost as fondly, "The Oak and the Reeds."[2] In it, a huge oak tree is thrashed by the wind until it is uprooted and falls into a stream, landing in some reeds. Broken, the oak asks the reeds how it is possible (given that they are so much weaker than he is) for them to not be flattened by the powerful wind. They answer that rather than trying to stand fast against the force, as he attempted to do, they simply bend. A frequently suggested moral for this fable is the common idiom, stoop to conquer.[3] But I respectfully disagree. For the child is already stooping due to his age-related social standing; he rarely conquers adults (even with the greatest effort); and it is frankly cruel to encourage a child to belittle himself. Is it not possible, instead, to consider that the valuable lesson here is that those who believe themselves to be mighty will eventually fall through forces beyond their control—and that things will turn out well in the end?

I believe it is fair to ask how it is possible for popular interpretations in wide circulation to be so often wrong about how these fables are likely to be received by a child—and which part of the story the child might need to hold onto in the search for meaning and edification. Unlike some of Aesop's interpreters and translators across the centuries, Dolto perfectly understood the child's predicament—his

DOI: 10.4324/9781032655123-19

inherent weakness due to his situation of dependence—for which she innovated her famous «poupée fleur»[4] [flower-doll] as a therapeutic instrument. She successfully used it in her treatment of autistic children and others who manifested grave communicative and/or relational difficulties:

> It is a foolish being if we compare it to an animal and a human, but it is a being that seems complete … the child judges it to be thinking and feeling like him when he is inferiorized by a situation that is stronger than his will, a situation of dependence by nature … Perhaps the absence of nutritional questions makes its originality … [as] a creature freed from its familial relations of dependence.[5]

What we find in this remarkable quote is that the child takes the flower-doll as a witness—as well as the intrinsic relation between the witness (who is, by definition, "in similitude") and the process of identification. What Dolto is elaborating, in fact, is that the human child is coming into the world from a natural position of inferiority relative to those around him, one that is intrinsic to the extended conditions of reliance on others in which he begins.

We cannot know whether animals experience a similar sense of weakness issuing from their relations to their carers. But humans apparently have the longest period of infant dependency of any lifeform on Earth (relative to the length of our lives), one that lasts many years. And during those years, beginning *in utero*, the child begins to develop his mental and emotional life—and to form himself as a being who, while dependent, is destined to achieve individuation. Therefore, throughout his long period of dependence, the child develops an awareness of his own limits and of the extent to which he needs others who, if all goes well, will support him. And through experiences in nature, the child can observe two trees on a winter's day, or after a storm—one that seems perfectly formed and one that seems less so—and quietly learn, all by himself, that the one that seems inferior for a time may turn out to be stronger in the end; or that being the biggest lifeform in any environment guarantees nothing in the end.

It is not a far leap from the flower-doll to a tree being a good-enough witness. It has the same defining attributes, only on a larger scale. On this view, it becomes possible to consider that the animals that populate Aesop's fables—foxes, dogs, crows, lions, donkeys, and so on—are later editions, developmentally speaking, on the long and winding continuum of individuation from unconscious passivity to conscious activity. For they have mouths—they find their food and they talk—and they move about. But the reparation nature provides also includes witnesses like trees and vegetation whose greatest virtue—as Dolto demonstrated with the flower-doll—is that they are low on the scale of intentional capacities. As a result, they conform to the child's unconscious experience of himself, thereby sufficiently satisfying the unconscious reconnaissance of similarity that triggers triangulation. And in triangulation, the affective investments of the witness become the child's own, like in the archaic. It is a condition of dependency, to be sure, but one that nonetheless enables the resumption of affective diffusion onto new objects.

A. Inscription

We have already described how invested phonemes in sufficient quanta trigger the unconscious experience of a witness. Here, crucially, triangulation is reversed: a good-enough witness triggers an engagement with new objects that are invested simply because they are invested by the witness. In this sense, we detect how the lifeform delivers a kind of self-observation—an echo of "positions" of the self in the encounter with objects—which is so necessary for critical thinking and developing individuation. For reification, our presentification in reality, is a process of having our co-experienced objects become affectively invested—and reciprocally, of having our common objects of affective investment be witnessed. The recuperation taps dream-work, so the recovery is a powerful one offering the best chance of liberating affect onto new objects that nourish associative thinking and enable progressions towards individuation. And insofar as progression is the antithesis of regression, the reparation of nature is instrumental for nonverbal autism.

Throughout her professional life, Dolto expounded the crucial role of the similar-enough other, the witness, in identification. As she explains it, health requires progressions of identification: successive "bereavements" of fetal sonority,[6] of identification with one's mother,[7] of childhood and even of the preceding hour[8]—i.e., to "separate from the oneself of yesterday to seek the oneself of tomorrow."[9] As such, the witness must be trustworthy, along the model of the indissociable other that ensures survival in the archaic. Perhaps it is a tree for now, and later a mouse or bird—who knows. But the closer the identification is to an age-appropriate witness, the more serviceable it will be in reality.

Critically, a good-enough similar other will necessarily impart invested affect—conveying that following it will secure a proof of life, survival. Even a kindly pet might do—as Dolto finds in young Robert, who is identified with his gardener's dog.[10] So what Dolto analyses in her clinic is identifications.[11] As she elaborates it, children need "proof of existence," and thus they employ each other for identification.[12] This is, in fact, another principle guiding her «Maison vertes»—giving infants this chance, with special concern for the eldest (or only), as needed especially in societies where large, extended families living near one another are in decline.

Through this unconscious mechanism, our identifications will change over the course of our development, in progressive iterations of the self. But, driven by the instinct of conservation, we will always seek to locate witnesses that are unconsciously securing in the interest of optimal self-regulation—that is, reduced anxiety through affective liberation. And an existing witness will not be abandoned until a suitable replacement is found—i.e., until sufficient affect can be displaced by association. Until then, the child remains naturally fixated on an existing set of securing objects, in what Leo Kanner described in the context of autism—not very kindly at all—as an "obsessive desire for the preservation of sameness."[13] And what Dolto helps us grasp is that the autistic child—like every child but to a greater degree—needs to find echoes of his perseverative objects in new objects to migrate his investments.

The problem is that regression as a defence is so effective in its conveyance of security that the longer the fixation, the harder abandoning it becomes. And because triangulation is an unconscious process, no one can deliberately locate or provide a witness through any conscious selection using intention, deduction or rationalization. Besides, it is not possible for anyone to know—including the person in question—what attribute of the witness makes it affectively similar unconsciously. Instead, the child needs to find the suitable similar-enough other for himself. It is unconsciously intuited. Thus space and time must be left open for play—for inviting an unconscious reconnaissance. This is why Dolto privileges the natural environment as offering opportunities for dream-work, for unconscious restoration, in that the child can find—like the flower-doll—a witness for himself.

Dolto invented the flower-doll in 1946, through her own intuition that this was precisely what was needed to help her five-year old patient, Bernadette. And it was. For the flower-doll proved to be instrumental in the full recovery of this young person who, when Dolto first met her, believed herself to be a wolf-child.[14] Dolto admits, a decade into her practice at this point, that she "had never seen such a grave case."[15] Yet even this early in her career, Dolto was alert to the identifications children make to natural lifeforms and how these reveal, by the similitude of the witness, the child's archaic relations. So disposed, she discloses her therapeutic approach: "Each time a child gives me a drawing, I take it as language; I ask, 'And if we said who it is?' Or else, 'And if you told me where you would be, if you were in the drawing?'"[16]

She narrates how, repeatedly, her young patients showed her flowers saying, "'It's me,' [while] there are in fact children who declare that a piece of furniture is them or another person, a house, a tree, a rock."[17] Dolto observed in clinic that daisies were often invoked.[18] She analysed these identifications as she simultaneously considered the words (i.e., phonemes) used to name the witness and describe the scene. She was searching—while being open to unconscious transferences through her unobtrusive, attentive listening (while note-taking)—for every possible archaic echo in "this phenomenon of identification, which is so important when it happens to the benefit of a detached flower that flies in the wind."[19] The individual's desire for freedom is so patent. And as with all things Dolto, she reflected productively by combining affect—her experiences in the transference with this patient—with thinking associatively about why the individual favoured this particular witness: "Flowers are the only creatures in which our senses perceive life (birth, blossoming, death), and to which they do not attribute voluntary motility, nor sonar emissions … all the while giving proof of their vitality by their existence, their colour, their perfume."[20]

We pause to take in the breadth of Dolto's stunning observation: at issue is a witness that is suitable to serve for the purpose of unconscious affective similarity simply because it is alive and passive—and because it neither moves nor talks. It cannot initiate action and it absorbs objects from its environment. In sum, this similar-enough witness is regressed. And it turns out that finding a regressed witness (for the regressed self) is sufficient to secure reality—to begin displacing some of the affect that has become fixated to such an extent as to prevent progression. Dolto considers the case for autism:

> The trauma that renders a child autistic can be a separation from his mother in space and in time … he does not yet know that he exists without her presence … That is why the child falls, as we say, into autism … the subject being unable to continue his progression … He is awaiting the return of the mother of prior times. A trauma is something against which the child abuts that makes him stay in place in a past that is no longer even a past … without associated desires, without landmarks.[21]

The witness is unconsciously experienced as lost—for whatever reason, perhaps even *in utero*, perhaps only for a moment of unpreventable suffering for the mother and/or child. To stress, the mother may not actually be lost, but she is nonetheless experienced unconsciously as being lost. The child regresses to securing dream-work and awaits the return of the witness. If the regression is deep enough, or long-lasting, it will be harder to lure affective investments to reality—i.e., to find associations to those dream objects in reality. This is the emotional situation of the child with autism. As we can infer it now, the autistic child has insufficient landmarks in reality, thus a limited (reduced) capacity to triangulate new objects; this slows (or even stalls) the transfer of affect to new objects that is needed to scaffold consciousness through the assurance of continued unconscious affective security. In other words, this is a child who needs a witness but is moored so deeply in an archaic terrain that finding suitable (associated) objects is challenging. Only a deeply regressed witness will suffice—and such is most easily findable in nature.

In truth, by the process of living, every human being cannot help but disperse affect onto ever-expanding fields of objects until it is spread pretty thin. It is as if daylight disperses our forces, making us neglect—literally, overlook—what used to matter most, what is most invested at the core of the self. So we need to let ourselves (day)dream to recall it. The case for each one of us becomes, then, an extremely minor example—same in kind, but not in quanta—of the distress that causes any infant to regress if he feels that continuity is lost with the one on whom his life depends—his witness—and he is compelled to wait, unable to progress until the witness returns. It is as if we could forget who we truly are—our deepest goals, our most invested archaic objects, what makes us truly ourselves, unlike any other human being—if these natural, random reminders did not arrive. A witness serves as a good-enough other to follow in the most idiosyncratic ways, unique to each one of us. Any of its movements, pathways, directional observations or objects—or associations to all these—might serve the unconscious reconnaissance of similarity. Thus, nature offers an uncountable, unnarratable abundance of possibilities.

But the witness is not the only archaic return securable from nature. The other is to be found in some vital regressive concordances—in silence, anonymity, and the continuous rhythms of organic life. As Dolto explains it, "I accord much importance to the thought of neutral «lieux»" [sites][22]—"these sites of nature … [and]

happy solitude[,] sites of beauty, of serenity, of softness, of impalpable matern-ing,"[23] where "an echo of archaic peace of being resonates."[24] This notion of neutral ground also touches on anonymity as safety, as Dolto narrates:

> We slumber with delight in reparative sleep ... in a recuperative solitude of his [mankind's] being in the world ... in a dive into his reassumed anonymity ... in forces that, on the margins of his unconscious, reanimate archaic faith through a living that ignores itself as an individuated creature.[25]

Anonymity is literally the condition of not having a name, of being alive prior to being called, before any individuation. It is a return to the restorative dream-work of the archaic—to a time when passivity was enough, as ambient sounds from the all-providing environment facilitated the arrival of objects for absorption. And the earliest experiences *in utero* are of a watery hush—much the same way that our nightly dreams require a muting of daily reality. It is what Dolto has called an "organizing silence"[26]—and it is one that enables a secure passive withdrawal.

The situation with autism, as articulated by Dolto, is that of a fixation on regression as a defence, as provoked by an unknown trauma—of unspecified duration and likely undetected—for the mother or child (or both) during the earliest developmental stages.[27] Archaic restoration through triangulation takes the child back to the neutral ground of a passive existence where there are no demands; the environment provides random experiences that serve unconscious securitization; and daydreaming, with its wild associative plays, is invited.

That is why Dolto recommends that patients be enabled in peacefully living out a stage that normally has been surpassed by then.[28] In other words, nature facilitates a state of passive receptivity, hence an acute alertness to the smallest signals of life—just as in the archaic. A propitious environment teaming with movement—unlike fabricated outdoor spaces—leads to an expectation of objects arriving that, in turn, encourages greater receptivity. So it is not enough to be outdoors—the space must be wild and authentically organic, beyond the conscious control of any human. It is a process of slow awakening that is self-reinforcing because, in facilitating self-regulation, it serves the instinct of conservation. Thus, nature nurtures our survival instinct.

Wild nature is a being-with what lives around us but without us. It is an all-providing environment that privileges the essential of life—movement—in relative mutism. The individual is alone, yet not, in a silence highly conducive to day-dreaming, as nature offers an abundance of unexpected forms. Plays of light make some things look like others, as shapes overlap each other in layers—like progressions—and fledgling forms sprout up through the decay in liminal spaces between what is coming and going. Forms that are not quite perfect anymore (e.g., drying, yellowing, rotting or falling), or not quite perfect yet (e.g., tiny shoots, buds and neonates), abound and thrive on grounds charged with possibilities. Nature offers living proof that there are different ways to survive, as an impressionistic world makes an impression on all our senses. In such open, vibrant spaces, there are no limits to what associations might be evoked, enabling an energetic stirring of unconscious circulation. For the offering of nature is both consciously unfathomable and unconsciously formidable. And even the most fleeting sign of life is enough to follow.

B. Reverberations

The archaic echoes securable from nature are those at the core of triangulation, through which everything pulses, as life begins for the human infant. As such, nature offers the deepest echo and the most archaic-syntonic repair. Even a semblance of a wind is sufficient, as Dolto has already explained—for, as Freud himself has already stated, "the indispensable attribute of all instincts ... [is] their capacity for initiating movement."[29] Unconsciously—in the overriding interest for self-regulation, under the instinct of conservation—we are always in search of the lost rhythm[30] that was (and remains) our primary source of unconscious security. Dolto narrates abundantly across the decades how a binary rhythm symbolizes the most basic sign of vegetative life.[31] For in rhythmic exchanges[32] inaugurated in the archaic stage—in rhythms of displacement[33]—one sound follows the other, and life begins in/as an echo.

Nature also seems to provide abundant examples on the "outside" of what we experience unconsciously on the "inside"—beginning in the archaic. For pathways—even blueways—that stretch in all directions and intersect randomly, changing with the seasons, seem to manifest associative paths to follow. Nature also offers multitudes of objects in associations with each other, in intricate relations within an inherently associative world—biodiversity—that can serve as an affirmation that we too are living in movement in this world. Perhaps, also, the trees and rocks that serve as markers along paths on the exterior terrain echo the interior "terrain," wherein phonemes serve as nodes along the affect-driven, associative paths connecting our thoughts. It is hard to know what to make of this odd proliferation of concordances between natural landscapes and the nature of associative thinking. But it is not impossible that it affords a measure of self-knowledge and/or helps delineate inside from outside—the boundaries of self—thus supporting individuation.

Resourcing in this archaic dream-work, we recover affective resources because triangulation returns affect to the self. It is an archaic reparation about which many of us have an intuition—the urge to sit on a beach looking at waves, walking quietly on a leafy path, staring at wild animals as long as they will let us, smelling our gardens, touching trees, and so on. It is an ancient call—an echo in itself—founded on archaic triangulation. Thus, the offer of a movement to follow that is obtainable from nature is an unconscious reparation that disrupts our fixity, liberating affect and reducing anxiety. So when a mole or egret seems to be looking at something, or heads somewhere down a path—on the ground or in the sky—this movement is enough of something to follow. The subtle stirring can loosen trapped affect, nurturing a bit of displacement. Herein, we are speaking of the most archaic echoes findable by a human being: the notion that from another lifeform whose life we follow—investing in what it invests in—we can commence our life, our self. And we should not neglect the capacity smell has for evoking similitude, insofar as smell is more archaic than vision. For it is a recuperative process that relies on the lifelong ability humans have for employing regression as a natural defence—a falling back to move ahead again.

In her own musings on regression, Montessori acknowledges the implications of the young child's special relation with a securing silence. For she describes, "lessons of silence [that] end with a general calling of the children's names ... the call is made in a whisper, that is, without vocal sound."[34] She adds that, "in the silent contemplation of nature, it may happen that a normal child will hear the call of her mysterious voice ... or perhaps he will feel that lure of nature."[35] The relation to the child's archaic history seems so stunning that perhaps we can fairly suggest that Montessori was also highly intuitive. For the child's relation with silence, as vocal sounds are muted by the watery envelopes *in utero*, will end with his naming—birth. And Montessori is clear that nature is the most auspicious place for re-experiencing archaic securitization: "The peace [is] offered to their subconscious minds by the simple places where they had lived as children."[36] Through experiences in nature, the child, "absorbs the life going on about him and becomes one with it."[37] This passive absorption from the environment reanimates the infant's mode of engagement with objects of the archaic stage. Montessori points to the unconscious processes at stake: "The child has a different relation to his environment from ours ... the child absorbs it ... they form part of his soul ... this [is a] vital kind of memory, which he does not consciously remember."[38]

I believe that Reggio Emilia programmes also demonstrate an approach to nature that evokes archaic triangulation: "We all tend to notice the environment and 'read' its messages or meanings on the basis of our own ideas."[39] Thus, in these programmes, "The environment is ... considered as 'the third educator'"[40]—"a third teacher."[41] This even extends to bringing objects of the environment into the classroom, enabling continuity with engineered spaces of learning, i.e., our shared reality: "Another principle in creating an environment that acts as a third teacher, [i.e.,] bringing the outdoors in."[42] This emphasis on continuity with the archaic is also evidenced in the approach to the child: "They [teachers] must learn to teach nothing to children except what children can learn by themselves."[43] Here again is an emphasis on self-recovery—on respecting that the child's natural unconscious programme, so to speak, is capable of proceeding without the conscious manipulation of adult teachers and/or carers.

In sum, education is about the facilitation of natural methodologies that privilege the innate affective, associative, archaic wealth of every child—rather than any indoctrination into specific, synthetic methodologies that privilege conscious, rational thought. Embedding the environment in education is a matter of preserving natural human resources. And whether the environment is considered as second or third seems moot because in archaic dream-work, relations in triangulation are blurry anyhow and confounded with the self. But it is useful shorthand to consider the role of the environment in education as/in triangulation. By this, we can correctly predict that the environment will be influential in securing affective circulation and fostering associative thinking. For "space does indeed speak,"[44]as this practice upholds, simply because the environment is the child's teacher from the start.

I believe that another relatively new practice in education that also deserves our attention—Forest Schools.[45] One of the objectives that is surely valid in its own right is that "forest school boosts the children's physical fitness and general wellbeing."[46] Also meritorious is that children educated in this way may grow up to care more about the environment. But what seems most significant about this practice, from the point of view of human health, is the, "original philosophy of forest schools, which is based on experiencing freedom by connecting with nature."[47] Of note, as well, "The outdoor environment appears to be an effective stimulus for children's interest and enquiry because it is flexible, natural and contains many varied, fixed and loose elements."[48] The stress on objects that are varied, fixed and loose is an important one, for this is the offer of nature—landscapes subject to huge, unpredictable variations, along with unexpected finds that can return unconscious pleasure and security.

One of the nonverbal autistic authors whose texts we examined, Kedar, shares this anecdote from his walks in the natural spaces around his home:

> The path is muddy from rain a week ago in the shady spots, and the sunny spots show dried horse hoof prints, mountain bike tire prints, and the sure proof that dogs have gone by, not to mention deer and owls too … On the path I feel calm.[49]

He is inadvertently invoking the notion of a path to follow, as the ground leaves its proofs of life. For the Earth itself is a surface already lived upon which, in continuity, we can follow a path that invites us. There is a joy in finding a new path—and in returning to an old path. The following day—or even mere moments later—we will find the path changed somehow by the wind and the other lifeforms that inhabit it, so that a space seems to manifest echoes from one time to another. As such, a wild, natural environment is a place of possibilities that nurtures a perpetual state of hope. We are lured by that hope so that even a memory of creatures who once walked the same trails, or arrived against the same landscape, is good-enough as a consolation for living.

Nature promises continuous movement sufficient to assuage our anxiety by liberating affect, as we daydream and secure triangulations following the echoes of other lifeforms. As Montessori put it, "How does he [the child] achieve this independence? He does it by means of a continuous activity … everything in the living world is active."[50] And in this process, she adds, the child remains anchored in the archaic: "Children feel a special interest for those things already rendered familiar to them (by absorption) in the earlier period."[51] Thus nature lures by appealing to even the youngest child's already-long history.

The return to nature also symbolizes a return to an archaic place of provision where an unexpected object could arrive anytime to engage our senses—suggesting random thoughts and their associations to follow. Nature is also the closest we can get to a regression in broad daylight—a withdrawal to mutism where passivity is good-enough movement, as we trade our interhuman communicative dependence for organic peace. Nature offers silent proofs of the continuity of life, a promise of survival. And as it does, the triangulation that is securable returns affect to the self. Yet the tragic truth is that environmental initiatives are few and far between in most schools, and "outdoor ed" is ironically often considered a luxury draining instructional time and financial resources.

Yet every child—the most regressed, nonverbal autist more than anyone—needs to be facilitated in accessing wild nature. The access needs to be a free one that is not consciously planned by a carer or teacher—except from the point of view of the child's physical safety and of preserving natural spaces for posterity. The experience should be as silent as possible and to the greatest extent (prioritizing safety) the child should be allowed to choose where he walks and what he touches. His experiences should not be openly questioned, interpreted aloud, or interrupted by those around him. The mandate is for facilitation rather than structuration. So it privileges the safe and silent company of others who, while ensuring the child's physical security, understand and respect that the auto-repair—internal affective security—is a highly individual process managed by unconscious resources, not conscious control.

In conclusion, nature is an all-providing environment, like the archaic, where anything can be found—unplanned and unintentionally. As such, it is highly conducive to dream-work as a source of securing pleasure. The two reparative returns that nature provides are in offering witnesses, and in manifesting the continuity of organic life. First, finding a witness and investing in its objects by association enables a resumption of triangulation in reality as the witness scaffolds individuation. Second, the demonstration of organic life that is open to all senses—including smell—represents the pathways, rhythmic exchanges and continuous movements that herald our existence as fledgling humans. As such, these outer echoes of inner life are unconsciously affirming, serving up a proof of life, while providing a retreat to anonymity and security in passivity. The repercussions for nonverbal autism are that this recovery taps archaic triangulation at its roots: by offering random witnesses that seem passive; by investing affect since the witness does; and by privileging silence and the most fundamental echoes of organic life. In brief, the invaluable unconscious work of nature is an intuitive access to a powerful passive reparation. So access to the natural world is not just pleasurable but indispensable. Via archaic echoes in nature, we instinctively follow life to have life.

Notes

1 Aesop n.d./2007, 40.
2 Ibid, 24.
3 For example, see Aesop n.d./1884, 7–8.
4 I discuss the flower-doll in greater detail in my previous work on Dolto.
5 In Faure-Poirée & Djéribi-Valentin 1999, 39.
6 In Caldaguès 1982, 147; De Sauverzac 1988, 11.

7 Dolto 1981, 215; Guillerault 1997, 210.
8 In Lévy 2002, 42.
9 Ibid, 46.
10 In De Sauverzac 1993, 170.
11 Dolto 1977a, 124 & 128; Djéribi-Valentin 2005, 208.
12 Dolto 1985c, 190; Dolto 1987, 31; De Sauverzac 1988, 13; Djéribi-Valentin 2005, 762; Kouki 2005, 41; Hamelin and Rabaté 2011.
13 1949, 416.
14 Dolto 1981, 142–145.
15 In Faure-Poirée & Djéribi-Valentin 1999, 25.
16 Ibid, 22.
17 Ibid.
18 Dolto 1981, 139; Potin 2008, 56.
19 In Faure-Poirée & Djéribi-Valentin 1999, 41, 24.
20 Ibid, 41.
21 In De Sauverzac 1988, 71.
22 Dolto 1988, 64.
23 In Kouki 2005, 79.
24 Ibid, 80.
25 Ibid, 78–79.
26 In Caldaguès 1982, 163.
27 A disturbance in the archaic stage has been the focus of the present work, but it is reasonable to suggest that the disturbance provoking the infant's unconscious experience of the indissociable witness who is felt to be lost may also occur during the earliest (entirely passive) part of the oral stage. A strict delineation (or rigid timeline) is necessarily precluded since premature births, in particular, can temporally shift the umbilical castration rather substantially.
28 In Marette 1940, 17; Dolto 1981, 149; Roudinesco 1986, 497.
29 1909a, 140–141.
30 Dolto 1981, 24; Caldaguès 1982, 148; Dolto 1986a, 213; Dolto 1987/1998, 62.
31 Dolto 1977/1984, 212; Dolto 1984, 90; De Sauverzac 1985, 157 & 241; Dolto 1986a, 48; De Sauverzac 1987, 70; Halmos 1994, 94–95, 257 & 350; Lévy 2002, 105.
32 Dolto 1981, 251; De Sauverzac 1988, 144.
33 In Halmos & C. Dolto 1994, 274; Djéribi-Valentin & Kouki 1998, 61.
34 1914.
35 1913/2017, 33.
36 1949/2010, 58.
37 Ibid, 92.
38 Ibid, 56–57.
39 Gandini 1996, 136.
40 Ibid, 148.
41 Fraser & Gestwicki 2000, 11.
42 Ibid, 118.
43 Malaguzzi 1996, 66.
44 Fraser & Gestwicki 2000, 100.
45 I have no affiliation with any Forest School or programme.
46 Lee 2022.
47 Ibid.
48 Waters 2013.
49 2011e.
50 1949/2010, 82–83.
51 Ibid, 157.

Summary for Part Three

Dolto was a dedicated educator, and her project is highly instructive in radical new ways. As evidenced by her remarkable theorization of the archaic stage, and of autism as a regression to the archaic, *early language acquisition is dominated by unconscious processes*. This developmental fact means that phonemes have a crucial role in circulating unconscious affect to secure individuation, and in seeding associative thinking. Thus, Dolto's discoveries issue very provocative questions for education. And ironically, while it is extremely challenging to explain Dolto's material—which is known for being "difficult for its density"[1]—the practical applications are absurdly simple to implement, cost little, and pose no risks to learners or their carers/teachers. It would not take much, then, for educational programmes of all kinds to accommodate unconscious processes—and every child's archaic history with words—whereas the returns to human health, happiness, and the potential for learning are truly immense.

First, the phonemes of our first language are invested with affect and inform associative thinking. Lifelong, we remain unconsciously susceptible, awaiting these archaic echoes that enable affective circulation and secure reality. The nonverbal autist thus requires a continuous (passive) access to more language, not less. And the implications for teaching all children seem evident. Use the child's true name and refrain from nicknaming. Respect his first language and facilitate bridges between the first and new language(s), such as by co-creating bilingual dictionaries and sourcing dual-language texts. Prevent language attrition. Nurture phonemic play through rhyming games and poetry—and showcase homonyms. Remain critically aware that a second language results in communicative gains (and emotional distancing, if such is needed)—but also in affective dampening. So the exchange implicit in language learning must be carefully weighed when working with allophones and diasporic communities. When supporting young newcomers (i.e., migrants), be sensitive to their emotional world, in that their unconscious security and associative thinking is tethered to the mother tongue.

Second, reading helps us to (re)find echoes of our pre-invested phonemes, recirculating archaic affects and returning (in triangulation) the unconscious experience of the witness that vouchsafes new objects for learning. The nonverbal autist benefits from precocious reading and extended, facilitated play between texts and world.

DOI: 10.4324/9781032655123-20

And the implications for teaching all children also seem clear. Advocate for school and community libraries. Make available books that nurture phonemic play, including series with controlled vocabulary (i.e., that repeat phonemes). Privilege printed books and label the environment. Prioritize silent reading. Source texts associated with loved books and follow authors. Keep favourites long after they no longer draw attention, including texts pertinent to family history. Let children choose what they read and refrain (unless invited) from asking about a story, judging a book or author, reorganizing bookshelves, or consciously influencing reading choices. Leave books to lie where they are. And without drawing undue conscious attention to them, accept games in which readers adopt their objects (including words) from texts.

Third, writing scaffolds individuation by reanimating archaic triangulation through relational echoes of phonemes in time or space. Transcribing (note-taking) condenses the invested words of a witness to produce a powerful, unconscious, self-securing restoration. So learning to write independently is the indispensable long-term intervention for nonverbal autism. And the implications for teaching all children seem patent. Introduce writing early—before reading is expected or confirmed. Support the graphomotor skills required to use implements, and consider teaching cursive because of its natural continuity.[2] Include keyboarding practice and offer different surfaces (e.g., bark, used materials, paper types, etc.). Defend publishing. Accept writing as a daily activity, even if the child cannot read what he writes. Create small books and encourage note-taking from books; and, as much as it is feasible, allow writing on favourite books. Develop opportunities for journaling—even for the child who can only scribe a crayon mark—by drawing daily activities or providing photographs of learning experiences. Support writing in all ways, with a gradual release of responsibility to secure independence. Review, publish or post the child's writing only with permission.

Fourth, nature is highly conducive to dream-work, offering witnesses to follow while manifesting the securing continuity of organic life as echoes of the archaic environment—its associative pathways and rhythmic exchanges. Privileging silence and a regressive position, natural spaces are unconsciously reparative for nonverbal autists. And the implications for teaching all children seem obvious. Find wild outdoor spaces and protect them for posterity. Save old trees. Support map-making for areas to visit (or walking paths) and collect atlases. Often bring children into contact with wild nature—beaches, forests and fields (rather than parkettes or manicured gardens)—and return to special places. Resist over-planning beyond getting there and staying safe. When children are engaged, refrain from over-talking or interfering with their experiences. Value silence. Avoid focusing on what a child seems drawn to unless invited. Between outings, bring the outdoors in while showing respect for lifeforms (e.g., supplying nutrients and ensuring a timely release). Keep in mind that the environment, indoors or outdoors, teaches the child.

In sum, accommodating unconscious processes in teaching and learning requires acknowledging that passive education is a formidable human capacity. It also necessitates being mindful that regression is every child's only reliable defence for many years, until the decisive establishment of the ego (dependent on consciousness). Our passive receptivity begins in infancy and endures beneath consciousness, impacting the circulation of unconscious affect on which our security in (conscious) reality paradoxically depends—as well as the proliferation of associative thinking. As such, education has a critical role in facilitating the learner's affective investments in new objects and lessening anxiety—as well as in nurturing associative pathways for creative thought. Thus, educational programs that assume the dynamic vitality and the enduring influence of unconscious processes can make significant contributions to preventing regression and enabling progression-individuation. In short, education is deeply implicated in the obligation to, and the benefit of, sustaining the unconscious circulation of affect.

After all, consciousness is a far later development in humans, one that commences many months after unconscious activity is well-established, beginning *in utero*. Furthermore, consciousness requires unconscious scaffolding to develop—that is, the capacity to move affective investments along associative pathways to self-secure new objects without a regressive dependence. In sum, unconscious activity not only precedes but steers the far later capacity for conscious activity (including speech as a motor movement). In this context, Montessori returns to the discussion one last time: "Unconscious psychological development has taken place in him [the child], and when he initiates his first movements, this begins to become conscious … he is working out, and making conscious, something that his unconscious mind has earlier absorbed."[3] As Montessori explains—of particular relevance to language learning and nonverbal autism—"an unconscious activity prepares speech, succeeded by a conscious process which slowly awakens and takes from the unconscious what it can offer."[4] For, as she says, "conscious will is a power which develops with use and activity … its development is a slow process."[5] Long before consciousness, then, there is learning.

In conclusion, every infant is unconsciously active before becoming consciously active, and every human being remains under the influence of powerful unconscious processes for as long as we live. These processes, driven by the instinct of conservation, work for our self-regulation—our survival. Thus, they are inherently reparative. This foundational attribute of our species, elaborated so compellingly by Dolto, holds tremendous explanatory power in confirming that the nonverbal autist is regressed—and though he cannot speak, he can assuredly think. It seems to be nothing less than the "arrogance of consciousness,"[6] to quote Freud, to believe otherwise.

Notes

1 Halmos 2000, 34.
2 Interestingly, in the same curriculum document that will return phonics to Ontario classrooms beginning in September 2023, cursive writing is also making a comeback in language programming (see Government of Ontario 2023).
3 1949/2010, 25.
4 Ibid, 104.
5 Ibid, 231.
6 1909b, 39.

Conclusion

Without question, Dolto's project is spectacularly successful. There is a Rue Françoise-Dolto in the prestigious «13e arrondissement» of Paris, and her artifacts are in the Archives Nationales de France. Colleges, schools, gardens and parks are named after her. In 1999, for the 10th anniversary of her death, a UNESCO conference was held to honour her work; and in 2018, a stamp commemorated the 110th anniversary of her birth.[1] Not only that, but starting in 1962—and continuing to this day—Dolto (posthumously) authors Santa's responses to children.[2] Dolto's letter has been revised only twice in 60 years[3] and continues to be delivered yearly as a free service of the state.[4] As of 2016, it was received by nearly two million French-speaking children in over 140 countries.[5] Further, as I write this, the largest online retailer offers 340 books by Dolto to their North American shoppers, while their French arm offers 825. And a prominent search engine turns up 1,230,000 hits for "Françoise Dolto." Yet, paradoxically, a strange silence inhabits Dolto's work at the boundary of geography and language.

When Dolto was a precocious five-year-old, she asked her family whether she was "born too early in a century too old"[6]—and this question seems to perfectly capture where her project stands at the start of a new century. For the crux of her work was disseminated when the 20th century was already old, yet her work narrates what is incredibly early—the archaic stage. Working backwards from Freud, so to speak—from the oral stage to what is prior, the archaic—Dolto strove for a half-century to deliver on a promise she made half a century ago: "I have come for this, to witness for you the unconscious."[7] For she truly is an eminent witness for the enduring unconscious processes responsible for human resilience and our earliest learning, as driven by the instinct of conservation. Archaic triangulation on phonemes, as Dolto explains, inscribes the unconscious aspect of language learning to which the present work seeks to contribute. However, explaining Dolto's boldly original thinking (and its clinical grounding) requires a deep dive into the archaic to trace the infant's mental and emotional trajectory from gestation. And as Freud put it, "It is not always easy to tell the truth, especially when one has to be concise."[8] Nonetheless, I hope I have achieved sufficient clarity in relating Dolto's material and its staggering implications.

DOI: 10.4324/9781032655123-21

The three chapters in Part One: Analysis articulate Dolto's thinking about the infant's presentification (i.e., becoming conscious in reality) from an unconscious state commencing early in gestation. The instinct of conservation has a formative and enduring role in human life, and the unconscious circulation of affect central to survival relies on an archaic triangular relation of self, witness, and object. Due to the dominance of audition *in utero*—that all-providing environment sustained by dream-work—the most ubiquitous archaic objects are phonemes. Phonemes serve our lifelong need for affective self-regulation and inform the ontogeny of associative thinking. Unconscious processes (blurring what is mental and emotional) develop first, and progression will require securing unconscious continuity through associations. Regression serves as an unconscious defence when objects for investing unconscious affect are experienced as absent. Regression impedes progression-individuation, provoking anxiety. The unconscious origin of early language learning legates a phenomenal role to phonemes lifelong (i.e., even at great associative distances) by restoring archaic triangulation. Triangulation provides unconscious security by returning the experience of the witness (similar to the self and intrinsic to survival) that echoes the archaic stage. The fact that words are the best means of transferring unconscious affect greatly impacts language and literacy education—and it is foundational to theorizing why (and how) nonverbal autism is a regression to the archaic.

The three chapters in Part Two: Evidence provide vital testimony from four nonverbal autistic authors. Commonalities evoked in their works reveal sophisticated creative thinking despite the absence of speech. Additional traits include a passive disposition (i.e., incomplete individuation); a perseverative reliance on regression as a defence; and formidable anxiety. These authors demonstrate convincingly that the inability to speak does not entail an inability to think. Considering autism anew, then, we presume competence. Moreover, we seek to address anxiety through a better understanding of the unconscious, archaic mechanisms that are in play. So while intentional speech will not be restored, communication can be. At issue is that affective circulation is restorable given a passive access to phonemes—reading—that reanimates unconscious triangulation as an archaic relation of self, witness and object. Additionally, writing emerges as the most determinative intervention for restoring pathways to progression that—while necessitating the presence of another for some time, perhaps many years—offer the best means of scaffolding individuation. Writing facilitates the return of the witness as a self-securing echo, while nature emerges as an archaic-syntonic environment that also enables unconscious reparation. Thereby, the insights shared by four nonverbal autists compellingly confirm Dolto's formulation that autism is a regression to the archaic.

The four chapters in Part Three: Practice unravel the ramifications of the infant's journey as the circulation of unconscious affect that commences in the archaic remains indispensable to his self-preservation. The phonemes of the mother tongue—being the most prevalent objects of archaic dream-work—root thought, transit affect and source security. This archaic terrain and means of the infant's earliest learning—entirely under the influence of unconscious processes—imprints a permanent legacy in mental and emotional life. Progression-individuation depends on the environment providing objects that are unconsciously continuous (i.e., associated) with prior objects of affective investment. Barring this, regression continues to be the child's most reliable defence. Interventions should acknowledge the vitality of passive education, and the value of the phonemes of the child's mother tongue in affective circulation (i.e., reduced anxiety) and associative thinking. Understanding the archaic role of phonemes and how they inform the child's engagements with language and literacy also helps us better comprehend nonverbal autism. In turn, nonverbal autists affirm that archaic echoes securable in phonemes, reading, writing and nature can guide a universal design for learning to benefit all children. Thus, education has a responsibility for supporting the continuous circulation of unconscious affect, serving as reparation and/or prevention.

In conclusion, the archaic stage is a theoretical construct of global significance. Dolto discovers the unconscious roots of the phonemes of the mother tongue; the affect-driven ontogeny of associative thinking; the role of language in affective circulation (self-regulation) and unconscious securitization; and the enduring influence of archaic triangulation—self, witness and phoneme—that is determinative in individuation and recoverable through literacy. In sum, Dolto shows that language plays a staggering role on the developmental bridge between being unconscious and becoming conscious—during human pre-conscious learning. And what her project prescribes is a complete reorientation towards what I believe we can rightly call the *infant's learning style*, simply because so much learning is going on passively, long before consciousness, that impacts a child's potential.

Dolto's work also poses serious ethical questions for teaching and learning because the continuous circulation of affect is necessary for self-regulation (including managing anxiety)—hence the need for education to recognize the unconscious processes dominating the young child's engagements with the environment, including the language of instruction. Further, as I have attempted to demonstrate, Dolto's opening onto the archaic stage also prompts an urgent rethinking of autism. In fact, the depth and breadth of the infant's learning in the archaic stage should provoke nothing less than an epistemic shift in child development. Considering his own breakthroughs, Darwin once wrote to a colleague, "I cannot persuade myself that a theory which explains several large classes of facts can be wholly wrong."[9] I believe the same can be said about Dolto's theorization of the archaic and the phoneme. It is *that* consequential.

Dolto was well-known for her benevolence, as Élisabeth Roudinesco once noted: "Françoise liked doing good."[10] And my sincere wish is that I have done right by Dolto in representing her remarkable offering to human knowledge. It has taken me seven years of further research and reflection (from when I received my PhD in 2016), and six months of writing for 10 to 12 hours daily, with breaks to paddle. As winter came and I was forced off the Humber, I began hiking high along its banks, with a new vantage points and plaques to read. Thus, I learned that the river's true name is an Anishinaabe word, *Kabechenong*. I also found out that the place where I usually put in my kayak was the former site of a Haudenosaunee Confederacy village, *Teiaiagon*; and that my typical trajectory along the Humber was part of the Toronto Carrying-Place Trail, one of the oldest transportation (portage) routes in Canada, used for at least 5,000 years. So this beloved river is emblematic of the problematic encounter between Indigenous peoples and their colonizers—French Canadians, my ancestors. The reverberations are deafening.[11]

Government translations state that *Kabechenong* means a "gathering place to tie up." But I have discovered through further research that it is apparently better rendered as, "Leave the canoes and go back."[12] That seems much more fitting. For where we have landed after our explorations with Dolto—that unprecedented cartographer of infant development—is not a place to tie up but a place of continuous transits between water and land. And Dolto's message about the archaic is indeed that we should go back, way back, to acknowledge the enduring influence of our long, winding passage through foundational mutism. For the unconscious teaches us that an affective current is always coursing through the history we name the "self," and echoes of the archaic are perpetually resonating.

By following Dolto as she follows Freud, we learn that language acquisition is first and foremost a matter of self-preservation in our species. Affect that cannot be deployed in the service of survival is simply resorbed—conserved for our long-term health. Dolto makes clear that the first relationship every human child has with language is one of listening, not speaking. And any notion of a "language acquisition device" is not coherent without acknowledging the unconscious processes inscribing phonemes during our earliest learning. In fact, we each begin life attuned to an auditory environment that grows associatively and that is unique in its offerings of nourishment—our own syllable soups.

As I put the final touches on this manuscript in preparation for publication, I have been paddling again for about three months—ever since the ice melted, the boat launches reopened, and the geese began coming back to the river. I was about to get out of my kayak on a chilly April morning when a flock of 30 or 40 returned suddenly from their wintering grounds. They came in for a landing in a wild, rambunctious flurry, passing so close over my head that I felt feathers brush my ears and heard the air beating in their wings. They settled quickly on the river behind me, calling out loudly as if to celebrate their happy homecoming and the cooling water. Within weeks, I would be navigating around downy goslings swimming in single file, paddling with their webbed feet.

It is midsummer again now, and mature turtles are sunning themselves freely in the open—I counted 26 on a single low-hanging branch they shared with some peaceable ducks. And on dozens of water-lily leaves rest remarkable juvenile turtles with shells no bigger than 25-cent coins. There are fewer herons and cormorants this year, but more egrets and swans. There are also two Cooper's hawks on a high perch that seem to tolerate but question me; countless blue-green dragonflies hovering above my bow; young silvery pike jumping over my paddle; a tawny white-tailed fawn and mum nibbling on wild grape leaves; and red-wing blackbirds aggressively driving intruders, including me, away from their nests in the thriving reeds.

One of the giant maples that, from great distances in the fall, announced a turn in the river in bright reds and oranges, fell over during a winter storm and now lies sideways—its six-metre span of roots resting perpendicular to the ground, halfway up the ravine, while its topmost leaves brush the water. Another change is that the river is considerably higher this summer than last, so I can paddle further north now, about 100 metres beyond Mute Bridge, before encountering an unpredictable gush of water over uneven rocks, where the downriver current completely negates my best efforts. I feel as if I am moving forward, but abundant landmarks testify that I am actually idling. As always, getting closer to the source remains a risky undertaking.

Meandering one morning onto a much calmer stretch, almost exactly one year to the day when I began writing, I encountered an entirely unexpected phenomenon. The sun had just come up and the surface was absolutely still, without a whisper of a wave. But some 20 metres ahead of me, the water was bubbling vigorously, as if animated by a concealed spring or an enormous fish. It took me more than a minute to grasp what I was observing, for the first time ever—a group of six to eight river otters enjoying breakfast together, diving in and out, jumping over one another, occasionally revealing their sleek muzzles as they swam effortlessly beside my boat and kept right on playing.

Yet "quarter turtles" and "otter froth" are not the only river words added to my vocabulary this season. As the days become warmer, there are "stable flies"—fast-flying, persistent brutes carrying secondary pathogens from their favourite local ungulates, deer. Three quick bites reduced the mobility of my right hand for four days and gave me a left foot I could barely walk on for a week. I have enjoyed 65 summers in the Canadian woods so far, but I never encountered these creatures before. I can now joke about being "part deer," but the painful truth is that I was much happier never knowing their name—when I was occluded from that particular reality and able to simply daydream on the Humber.

We do not usually think of dream-work as doing actual work, but it does. And what Dolto reveals is that this dream-work is happening at the level of the constituents of words, phonemes, commencing during the personal prehistory of each one of us—when words have no firm definition but a formidable destiny. As it turns out, then, autism is perhaps the most distinctly human problem of all. For a valued member of the species that self-defines as communicative is prevented from full communication. Unconscious reserves are rich and healthy—and pre-conscious development has successfully proliferated thought—but the autist is challenged in executing conscious motor acts (including speech) right at the threshold of reality.

In his fine introduction to Freud's opus on dreams, James Strachey (his best translator) stresses that Freud identified dreams as "wish-fulfilling … [and] the regressive functioning of the mind … [involving] motor paralysis"[13]—a distinct mode of mental functioning under the primary processes.[14] Loyally Freudian while thoroughly original, Dolto simply considered, during decades of clinical experience with children, what this might mean for the infant *in utero*—whose mental and emotional life is governed by the primary processes, and whose main source of dream objects is language in all its rhythms and repetitions. So doing, I believe Dolto offers posterity one of the most understandable and viable applications of the Freudian legacy. In every sense, then, Dolto is also a superlative translator of Freud.

Ultimately, with Dolto, we discover that every fetus dreams in random streams of pre-conscious audition. And the infant needs to (re)encounter echoes of pre-invested liquid objects, phonemes, to successfully transition to reality—to an environment that is continuous with the unconscious archaic terrain heralding survival. Weaving threads from a watery world wherein every *infans* is non-speaking—as words arrive wildly, and whenever, upon an idiosyncratic sonar landscape—the affective security of coming to being, braided with others and open to offers, begins to form. Moving with the natural course (or moored for a time), such is the earliest journey of every member of the human species—of beings born(e) of, in, with and by language—whose love and learning always rely on an archaic river.

Notes

1 Bougault 2018.
2 *Notre Famille* 2015; *Le Point* 2012 & 2014.
3 In Djéribi-Valentin 2005, 712–713.
4 Chérer 2008, 34.
5 De Noétique 2017.
6 F. Dolto 1989, 46.
7 Dolto (in 1974) in Halmos 1994, 328.
8 1909b, 29.
9 1859.
10 In Dolto & Roudinesco 1986/1988, 39.
11 As this manuscript entered the production phase, in September 2023, I observed that the long-standing settler narrative (focused on European explorers), inscribed on a huge rock along the western edge of the river valley, had finally been replaced by new signage asserting the Humber's staggering historical value for Indigenous peoples for millennia.
12 Cote [Miskogayaashk] 2022.
13 1900, xv.
14 Ibid.

Bibliography

Aesop. (n.d./1884). "The Oak and the Reed." In R. Worthington (Ed.), *Aesop's Fables* [620–563 BC]. New York, NY: Frank F. Lovell & Company.

Aesop. (n.d./2007). "The Olive-Tree and the Fig-Tree." In *Aesop's Fables* (V. Jones, Trans. & A. Rackham, Illus.). Columbus, OH: Kahley House Publishing.

Arnulf, I. (2014). *Une fenêtre sur les rêves: Neurologie et pathologie du sommeil*. Paris: Odile Jacob.

Assembly of First Nations. (2022). "Residential Institutions." Ottawa. Retrieved from www.afn.ca/residential-institutions/

Authier-Roux, F. (Ed.). (2000). «Frédérique Authier-Roux: Entretien avec Juan-David Nasio.» In F. Authier-Roux, *Madame Dolto*. Paris: Erès, 15–29.

Balesta, H. (1894/1902). *Les babouches de Baba-Hassein* (J. Geoffroy, Illus.). Paris: C. Delagrave.

Bargh, J.A. (2014). "The Historical Origins of Priming as the Preparation of Behavioral Responses: Unconscious Carryover and Contextual Influences of Real-World Importance." In D. C. Molden (Ed.), *Understanding Priming Effects in Social Psychology*. New York, NY: The Guilford Press, 218–233.

Barr, M.W. (1898). "Echolalia: Some Notes on Echolalia, With the Report of an Extraordinary Case." *The Journal of Nervous and Mental Disease*, *25*(1): 20–31. Retrieved from https://ia600207.us.archive.org/9/items/b22407959/b22407959.pdf

Bastian, H.C. (1898). *A Treatise on Aphasia and Other Speech Defects*. London: H.K. Lewis.

BD Anciennes.com. (n.d.) «La Semaine de Suzette.» Retrieved from www.bd-anciennes.com/quelques-bonnes-raisons-de-sinteresser-a-la-semaine-de-suzette/

Bott Spillius, E., Milton, J., Garvey, P., Couve, C. & Steiner, D. (Eds.). (2011). *The New Dictionary of Kleinian Thought*. London: Routledge.

Bougault, S. (2018, 6 octobre). "Collection historique de timbre-poste français: Françoise Dolto: 1908–1988." [Postage stamp]. Retrieved from www.wikitimbres.fr/timbres/11361/2018-francoise-dolto-1908-1988

Breuer, J. & Freud, S. (1893a). "Case Histories, Case 1: Fräulein Anna O." *SE 2*, 21–47.

Breuer, J. & Freud, S. (1893b). "On the Psychical Mechanism of Hysterical Phenomena: Preliminary Communication." *SE 2*, 3–17.

Brison, S.J. (2002). *Aftermath: Violence and the Remaking of a Self*. Princeton, NJ: Princeton University Press.

Britzman, D.P. (2011). *Freud and Education*. London: Routledge.

Caldaguès, L. (Ed.). (1982). *Françoise Dolto: Séminaire de la psychanalyse d'enfants, Tome 1*. Paris: Éditions du Seuil.

Cambero, F. (2022, 18 February). "A Chilean Indigenous Language Vanishes as Last Native Speaker Dies." Reuters. Retrieved from www.reuters.com/world/americas/chilean-indigenous-language-vanishes-last-native-speaker-dies-2022-02-17/#:~:text=Cristina%20 Calderon%20died%20on%20Wednesday,language%20with%20translations%20to%20 Spanish

Chaperot, C. & Celacu, V. (2010). «La pensée et le langage par le corps dans la schizophrénie.» *L'évolution psychiatrique*, *75*: 435–444.

Charial, L., Eliacheff, C. & Valentin, J.-F. (1999). «De la transmission: Voir, écouter, sentir.» In Association Archives et Documentation Françoise Dolto & C. Dolto (Eds.), *Françoise Dolto aujourd'hui présente: Actes du colloque de l'Unesco, 14–17 janvier, 1999*. Paris: Gallimard, 48–62.

Chérer, S. (2008). *Ma Dolto*. Paris: Éditions Stock.

Cohen, L.H. (1995). *Train Go Sorry: Inside a Deaf World*. New York, NY: Random Books.

Coronel, E. & De Mezamat, A. (Producers). (1997a). *Françoise Dolto Film 2: Parler vrai* [Film]. France: Abacaris & Gallimard.

Coronel, E. & De Mezamat, A. (Producers). (1997b). *Françoise Dolto Film 4: Complément, Maud Mannoni, évocations* [Film]. France: Abacaris & Gallimard.

Cote, P. [Nodjmowin Miskogayaashk]. (2022). "Old Mill Subway Station Mural-Part 1." City of Toronto: ARTWORX. Retrieved from www.artworxto.ca/on-demand/old-mill-subway-station-rail-bridge-mural-part-1

Darwin, C. (1859, 13 November). "Letter to Leonard Jenyns." University of Cambridge: Darwin Correspondence Project. Retrieved from https://www.darwinproject.ac.uk/letter/DCP-LETT-2528.xml

Darwin, F. (Ed.). (1881/2015). *The Autobiography of Charles Darwin*. Middletown, DE: n.p.

DeGangi, G. (2000). *Pediatric Disorders of Regulation in Affect and Behavior: A Therapist's Guide to Assessment and Treatment*. Cambridge, MA: Academic Press.

De Mezamat, A. (2008). *Françoise Dolto parle de l'origine* [Television broadcast]. France: France 5/Abacaris Films.

De Noétique, PLK (2017, 17 novembre). «La réponse du Père Noël par Françoise Dolto.» Retrieved from www.plkdenoetique.com/reponse-pere-noel-par-fran-oise-dolto/

De Sauverzac, J.-F. (Ed.). (1985). *Françoise Dolto: Séminaire de la psychanalyse d'enfants, Tome 2*. Paris: Éditions du Seuil.

De Sauverzac, J.-F. (Ed.). (1987). *Françoise Dolto: Dialogues québécois*. Paris: Éditions du Seuil. (Original work published 1983)

De Sauverzac, J.-F. (Ed.). (1988). *Françoise Dolto: Séminaire de la psychanalyse d'enfants, Tome 3*. Paris: Éditions du Seuil.

De Sauverzac, J.-F. (1993). *Françoise Dolto: Itinéraire d'une psychanalyste*. Paris: Aubier.

Djéribi-Valentin, M. (Ed.). (2001). *Françoise Dolto: Père et fille, une correspondance (1914–1938)*. Paris: Mercure de France.

Djéribi-Valentin, M. (Ed.). (2005). *Françoise Dolto: Une vie de correspondances (1938–1988)*. Paris: Gallimard.

Djéribi-Valentin, M. (Ed.). (2008). *Françoise Dolto: Mère et fille, une correspondance (1931–1962)*. Paris: Mercure de France.

Djéribi-Valentin, M. & Kouki, É. (Eds.). (1996). *Françoise Dolto Essais: Sexualité féminine: La libido génitale et son destin féminin*. Paris: Gallimard. (Original work published 1960–1985)

Djéribi-Valentin, M. & Kouki, É. (Eds.). (1998). *Françoise Dolto, Articles et conférences 5, Le féminin*. Paris: Gallimard. (Original work published 1959–1988)

Doidge, N. (2015). *The Brain's Way of Healing: Stories of Remarkable Recoveries and Discoveries*. New York, NY: Penguin Books.
Dolto, C. (1989). «Préface.» In S. Ramstein, *Un pédiatre raconte: Histoires de bien grandir*. Paris: Hatier.
Dolto, F. (1940/1965). *Psychanalyse et pédiatrie: Les grandes notions de la psychanalyse, seize observations d'enfants*. (3e éd.). Paris: Éditions du Seuil.
Dolto, F. (1940/1971). *Psychanalyse et pédiatrie: Les grandes notions de la psychanalyse, seize observations d'enfants* (4e éd.). Paris: Éditions du Seuil.
Dolto, F. (1940/2013). *Psychoanalysis and Paediatrics: Key Psychoanalytic Concepts with Sixteen Clinical Observations of Children* (F. Hivernel & F. Sinclair, Trans.). London: Karnac.
Dolto, F. (1949). «La poupée-fleur: À propos des états narcissiques de l'enfant.» In C. Faure-Poirée & M. Djéribi-Valentin (Eds.) (1999). *Jeu de poupées*. Paris: Mercure de France, 19–42.
Dolto, F. (1956). «Introduction au dessin d'enfants.» *La vie médicale: Arts et psychopathologie, Numéro Spécial*, Noël 1956, 27–39.
Dolto, F. (1965). «Préface.» In M. Mannoni, *Le premier rendez-vous avec le psychanalyste*. Genève: Éditions Gonthier S.A., 5–49.
Dolto, F. (1971). *Le cas Dominique*. Paris: Éditions du Seuil.
Dolto, F. (1977a). *Lorsque l'enfant parait, Tome 1*. Paris: Éditions du Seuil.
Dolto, F. (1977b). «Préface.» In A. Muel, *L'Éveil de l'esprit*. Paris: Aubier Montaigne, 8–54.
Dolto, F. (1977/1984). «Heures et jours qui suivent l'accouchement.» In E. Herbinet (Ed.), *Naître et ensuite?* Paris: Stock, 187–266.
Dolto, F. (1978). *Lorsque l'enfant parait, Tome 2*. Paris: France Loisirs.
Dolto, F. (1979). *Lorsque l'enfant parait, Tome 3*. Paris: Éditions du Seuil.
Dolto, F. (1981). *Le jeu du désir: Essais cliniques*. Paris: Éditions du Seuil. (Original work published 1946–1978)
Dolto, F. (1982). «La boutique verte: histoire d'un lieu de rencontres et d'échanges entre adultes et enfants.» In M. Brown de Calstoun et al. (Eds.), *Enfants en souffrance*. Paris: Stock Laurence Pernoud, 137–156.
Dolto, F. (1983). «Françoise Dolto parle (*Dialogues québécois*.)» [Video]. Retrieved from www.youtube.com/watch?v=q_-DXyKF5RU
Dolto, F. (1984). *L'image inconsciente du corps*. Paris: Éditions du Seuil.
Dolto, F. (1984/2023). *The Unconscious Body Image* (S. Bailly, Trans.). London: Routledge.
Dolto, F. (1985a). *La Cause des enfants*. Paris: Robert Laffont.
Dolto, F. (1985b). «La maison verte.» Conférence au Centre de Recherches Psychanalytiques, octobre 1985. *Esquisses Psychanalytiques, No. 5, Actualités*. Retrieved from www.alaaddin.it/SITO%20DOLTO/Sito%20allegati/La%20maison%20verte%201985%20fr.pdf
Dolto, F. (1985c). "The Mirror's Child" (C. Vaughn, Trans.). In S. Benvenuto & A. Molino (Eds.), *In Freud's Tracks: Conversations from the Journal of European Psychoanalysis*. Lanham, MD: Jason Aronson, 185–200.
Dolto, F. (1985d). *Solitude*. Paris: Vertiges du Nord/Carrère.
Dolto, F. (1985/1989). «Conférence de Françoise Dolto au colloque organisé par le Centre Médico-Psycho-Pégagogique de Vigneux-sur-Seine.» In F. Dolto & C. Dolto-Tolitch. *Paroles pour adolescents ou le complexe du homard*. Paris: Hatier, 123–137.
Dolto, F. (1986a). *La difficulté de vivre*. Paris: Vertiges du Nord/Carrère.
Dolto, F. (1986b). *Enfances*. Paris: Éditions du Seuil.
Dolto, F. (1987). *Tout est langage*. Paris: Vertiges du Nord/Carrère.

Dolto, F. (1987/1998). «L'enfant dans la ville.» In *Françoise Dolto: L'enfant dans la ville*. Paris: Mercure de France, 9–52.

Dolto, F. (1988). *Quand les parents se séparent*. Paris: Éditions du Seuil.

Dolto, F. (1989). *Autoportrait d'une psychanalyste: 1934–1988: Entretiens avec Alain et Colette Manier*. Paris: Éditions du Seuil.

Dolto, F. & Nasio, J.-D. (1987). *L'enfant du miroir*. Paris: Rivages/Psychanalyse.

Dolto, F. & Roudinesco, E. (1986/1988). «Des jalons pour une histoire: Entretien.» In J. Aubrey et al. (Eds.), *Quelques pas sur le chemin de Françoise Dolto*. Paris: Seuil, 11–42.

Dolto, F. & Winter, J.-P. (1986). *Les images, les mots, le corps*. Paris: Gallimard.

Dolto-Marette, F. (1947). «Hypothèse nouvelle concernant les réactions dites de jalousie à la naissance d'un puîné.» *Psyché 9–10*, juillet–août 1947, 788–798.

Dolto-Marette, F. (1949). «Rapport de la 12ème Conférence des Psychanalystes de langue française (Paris, 4 et 5 juin 1949)» [Discussion]. *Revue française de psychanalyse*, XIII(4): 545–553. Retrieved from https://gallica.bnf.fr/ark:/12148/bpt6k54444473/f99.item.zoom

D'Ortoli, F. & Amram, M. (1990). *L'École avec F. Dolto: Le rôle du désir dans l'éducation*. Paris: Hatier.

D'Ortoli, F. & Amram, M. (2009a). *L'année de Vienne* [Film]. France: Fremeaux & Associés.

D'Ortoli, F. & Amram, M. (2009b). *Françoise Dolto & La Neuville* [Film]. France: Fremeaux & Associés.

Doyen, S., Klein, O., Simons, D.J., & Cleeremans, A. (2014). "On the Other side of the Mirror: Priming in Cognitive and Social Psychology." In D.C. Molden (Ed.), *Understanding Priming Effects in Social Psychology*. New York, NY: The Guilford Press, 14–34.

Durif-Varembont, J.-P., Bertrand-Oschwald, E., Boulanger, J., Fuchs, M. & Monasse, J. (1999). «Le transfert sur et dans le lieu.» In Association Archives et Documentation Françoise Dolto & C. Dolto (Eds.), *Françoise Dolto aujourd'hui présente: Actes du colloque de l'Unesco, 14–17 janvier 1999*. Paris: Gallimard, 295–310.

Eberhard, D.M., Simons, G.F. & Fennig, C.D. (Eds.). (2022). *Ethnologue: Languages of the World*.Twenty-fifth edition. Dallas, TX: SIL International. Retrieved from www.ethnologue.com/guides/how-many-languages-endangered

Edwards, C. (1996). "Partner, Nurturer, and Guide: The Roles of the Reggio Teacher in Action." In C. Edwards, L. Gandini & G. Forman, *The Hundred Languages of Children: The Reggio Emilia Approach to Early Childhood Education*. Norwood, NJ: Ablex Publishing Co., 151–169.

Edwards, C., Gandini, L. & Forman, G. (1996). "Introduction." In C. Edwards, L. Gandini & G. Forman, *The Hundred Languages of Children: The Reggio Emilia Approach to Early Childhood Education*. Norwood, NJ: Ablex Publishing Co., 3–18.

Eisenberg, R.B. (1976). *Auditory Competence in Early Life: The Roots of Communicative Behavior*. Baltimore, MD: University Park Press.

Fagard, J. (2013). "Early Development of Hand Preference and Language Lateralization: Are They Linked, and If So, How?" *Developmental Psychobiology*, *55*(6): 596–607.

Faure-Poirée, C. & Djéribi-Valentin, M. (Eds.). (1999). *Jeu de poupées*. Paris: Mercure de France. (Original work published 1949 and 1964)

Fraser, S. & Gestwicki, C. (2000). *Authentic Childhood: Exploring Reggio Emilia in the Classroom*. Albany, NY: Delmar.

Freud, S. (1888). "Hysteria." *SE 1*, 37–59.

Freud, S. (1891/2011). *On Aphasia: A Critical Study*. New York, NY: Literary Licensing.

Freud, S. (1893a). "Case 2: Fräu Emmy von N." *SE 2*, 48–105.

Freud, S. (1893b). "Case 5: Fräu Elisabeth von R." *SE 2*, 135–181.

Freud, S. (1893c). "Preface & Charcot (Obituary)." *SE 3*, 5–23.

Freud, S. (1893d). "On the Psychical Mechanism of Hysterical Phenomena: A Lecture." *SE 3*, 25–39.

Freud, S. (1893e). "The Psychotherapy of Hysteria." *SE 2*, 254–312

Freud, S. (1895). "Project for a Scientific Psychology." *SE 1*, 281–397.

Freud, S. (1896a). "The Aetiology of Hysteria." *SE 3*, 187–221.

Freud, S. (1896b). "Draft H: Paranoia." *SE 1*, 206–212.

Freud, S. (1896c). "Draft K: The Neuroses of Defence (A Christmas Fairy Tale)." *SE 1*, 220–229.

Freud, S. (1896d). "Heredity and the Aetiology of the Neuroses." *SE 3*, 141–156.

Freud, S. (1896e). "Letter 46, 30 May 1896." *SE 1*, 229–232.

Freud, S. (1896/1954). "Letter 52, to Wilhelm Fliess, 6 December 1896." In M. Bonaparte, A. Freud & E. Kris (Eds.). *The Origins of Psycho-Analysis: Letters to Wilhelm Fliess, Drafts and Notes: 1887–1902 by Sigmund Freud* (M. Mosbacher & J. Strachey, Trans.). New York, NY: Basic Books, 173–181.

Freud, S. (1900a). "The Interpretation of Dreams (First Part)." *SE 4*, ix–338.

Freud, S. (1900b). "The Interpretation of Dreams (Second Part)." *SE 5*, 339–627.

Freud, S. (1901a). "On Dreams." *SE 5*, 629–685.

Freud, S. (1901b). "The Psychopathology of Everyday Life." *SE 6*, vii–310.

Freud, S. (1905). "Three Essays on the Theory of Sexuality." *SE 7*, 123–245.

Freud, S. (1907/1962). [Freud's Remarks at Scientific Meetings in 1907]. In H. Nunberg & E. Federn (Eds.). *Minutes of the Vienna Psychoanalytic Society, Vol. I: 1906–1908.* (M. Nunberg, Trans.) New York, NY: International Universities Press, Inc, 81–275.

Freud, S. (1908a). "Creative Writers and Day-Dreaming." *SE 9*, 141–153.

Freud, S. (1908b). "Some General Remarks on Hysterical Attacks." *SE 9*, 227–234.

Freud, S. (1909a). "Analysis of a Phobia in a Five-Year-Old Boy ('Little Hans')." *SE 10*, 1–149.

Freud, S. (1909b). "Five Lectures on Psycho-analysis (The Clark University Lectures)." *SE 11*, 1–55.

Freud, S. (1910). "Leonardo da Vinci and a Memory of His Childhood." *SE 11*, 57–137.

Freud, S. (1912). "The Dynamics of Transference." *SE 12*, 97–108.

Freud, S. (1913). "The Claims of Psychoanalysis to cientific inlterest." *SE 13*, 163–190.

Freud, S. (1914a). "On Narcissism." *SE 14*, 67–102.

Freud, S. (1914b). "Remembering, Repeating and Working-through." *SE 12*, 145–156.

Freud, S. (1915a). "The Unconscious." *SE 14*, 159–215.

Freud, S. (1915b). "Thoughts for the Times on War and Death." *SE* 14, 273–302.

Freud, S. (1916a). "Introductory Lectures on Psycho-analysis: Part I, Parapraxes." *SE 15*, 1–79.

Freud, S. (1916b). "Introductory Lectures on Psycho-analysis: Part II, Dreams." *SE 15*, 81–239.

Freud, S. (1917[1916–1917]). "General Theory of the Neuroses." *SE 16*, 243–463.

Freud, S. (1921). "Group Psychology and the Analysis of the Ego." *SE 18*, 65–143.

Freud, S. (1925[1924]). "An Autobiographical Study." *SE 20*, 1–74.

Freud, S. (1930). "The Goethe Prize." *SE 21*, 205–212.

Freud, S. (1933a). "New Introductory Lectures, Lecture 29: Revision of the Theory of Dreams." *SE 22*, 7–30.

Freud, S. (1933b). "New Introductory Lectures, Lecture 31: Dissection of the Psychical Personality." *SE 22*, 57–80.

Freud, S. (1937). "Analysis Terminable and Interminable." *SE 23*, 209–253.

Freud, S. (1940[1939]). "An Outline of Psychoanalysis." *SE 23*, 139–207.

Gandini, L. (1996). "Educational and Caring Spaces." In C. Edwards, L. Gandini & G. Forman, *The Hundred Languages of Children: The Reggio Emilia Approach to Early Childhood Education*. Norwood, NJ: Ablex Publishing Co., 135–149.

Gershon, M.D. (1998). *The Second Brain*. New York, NY: Harper.

Government of Ontario. (2023). *Key Changes—Language, Grades 1 to 8*. Toronto: Queen's Printer. Retrieved from https://www.dcp.edu.gov.on.ca/en/key-changes-language

Granger, C. (2004). *Silence in Second Language Learning: A Psychoanalytic Reading*. Clevedon, UK: Multilingual Matters Ltd.

Gray, C. (2010). *The New Social Story Book*. Arlington, TX: Future Horizons Inc.

Greenspan, S.I. (1989). *The Development of the Ego: Implications for Personality Theory, Psychopathology, and the Psychotherapeutic Process*. Madison, WI: International Universities Press.

Greenspan, S.I. & Benderly, B.L. (1997). *The Growth of the Mind and the Endangered Origins of Intelligence*. Cambridge, MA: Perseus Books.

Greenspan, S.I. & Wieder, S. (1998). *The Child With Special Needs: Encouraging Intellectual and Emotional Growth*. Cambridge, MA: Da Capo Press.

Guillerault, G. (Ed.). (1997). *Francoise Dolto: Le Sentiment de soi, aux sources de l'image du corps*. Paris: Gallimard. (Original work published 1956–1957)

Gulati, S. (2003a). "Epilogue: When the Therapist is Deaf." In N.S. Glickman & S. Gulati (Eds.), *Mental Health Care of Deaf People: A Culturally Affirmative Approach*. Mahwah, NJ: Lawrence Erlbaum Associates, 349–371.

Gulati, S. (2003b). "Language Deprivation Syndrome." In N.S. Glickman & S. Gulati (Eds.), *Mental Health Care of Deaf People: A Culturally Affirmative Approach*. Mahwah, NJ: Lawrence Erlbaum Associates, 24–53.

Gulati, S. (2003c). "Psychiatric Care of Culturally Deaf People." In N.S. Glickman & S. Gulati (Eds.), *Mental Health Care of Deaf People: A Culturally Affirmative Approach*. Mahwah, NJ: Lawrence Erlbaum Associates, 33–107.

Guttmann, M.G. (2001). *The Enigma of Anna O: A Biography of Bertha Pappenheim*. Wickford, UK: Moyer Bell.

Halmos, C. (Ed.). (1994). *Françoise Dolto, Articles et conférences, II: Les Chemins de l'éducation*. Paris: Gallimard. (Original work published 1946–1989)

Halmos, C. (2000). «Un héritage qui dérange.» In F. Authier-Roux, *Madame Dolto*. Paris: Erès, 31–38.

Halmos, C. & Dolto, C. (Eds.). (1994). *Françoise Dolto, Articles et conférences, I: Les étapes majeures de l'enfance*. Paris: Gallimard. (Original work published 1946–1988)

Hamelin, A. (Producer) & Rabaté, F. (Director). (2011). «Grandir à petits pas» [Video]. *Le Monde en Face avec Carole Gaessler*. France: Les Films Grains de Sable. Retrieved from www.youtube.com/watch?v=skxuanPsBis

Hepper, P.G. (2013). "The Developmental Origins of Laterality: Fetal Handedness." In *Developmental Psychobiology*, *55*(6): 588–595.

Hertrich, I., Mathiak, K. & Ackermann, H. (2016). "The Role of the Cerebellum in Speech Perception and Language Comprehension." In P. Mariën & M. Manto (Eds.), *The Linguistic Cerebellum*. Amsterdam: Elsevier, 33–50.

Herz, R. (2007). *The Scent of Desire: Discovering Our Enigmatic Sense of Smell*. New York, NY: William Morrow.

Higashida, N. (2007/2013). *The Reason I Jump: One Boy's Voice from the Silence of Autism* (KA Yoshida & D. Mitchell, Trans.). London: Sceptre.

Higashida, N. (2017). *Fall Down Seven Times, Get Up Eight* (D. Mitchell & KA Yoshida, Trans.). London: Sceptre.

Hoffman, E. (1989). *Lost in Translation: A Life in a New Language*. New York, NY: Penguin Books.

Hyltenstam, K. & Viberg, Å. (1993). "Linguistic Progression and Regression: An Introduction." In K. Hyltenstam & Å. Viberg (Eds.), *Progression and Regression in Language*. New York, NY: Cambridge University Press, 3–36.

Ito, M. (2011). *The Cerebellum: The Brain for an Implicit Self.* Upper Saddle River, NJ: Pearson Education Inc.

Johnson, E. Pauline (Tekahionwake). (1917/2022). *Flint and Feather: The Complete Poems of E. Pauline Johnson (Tekahionwake)*. [Reprint of the Leopold Classic Library.] Toronto: The Musson Book Company Ltd.

Jones, E. (1953/1982). *The Life and Work of Sigmund Freud, Vol. 1*. New York, NY: Basic Books.

Kahneman, D. (2011a). *Système 1, Système 2. Les deux vitesses de la pensée*. Paris: Clés des champs.

Kahneman, D. (2011b). *Thinking, Fast and Slow*. Toronto: Anchor.

Kanner, L. (1946/1973). "Irrelevant and Metaphorical Language in Early Infantile Autism." In L. Kanner, *Childhood Psychosis: Initial Studies and New Insights*. New York, NY: John Wiley & Sons, 45–50.

Kanner, L. (1949). "Problems of Nosology and Psychodynamics of Early Infantile Autism." In *American Journal of Orthopsychiatry*, 19(3): 416–426.

Katz, L. (1996). "What can we Learn from Reggio Emilia?" In C. Edwards, L. Gandini & G. Forman, *The Hundred Languages of Children: The Reggio Emilia Approach to Early Childhood Education*. Norwood, NJ: Ablex Publishing Co., 19–37.

Kedar, I. (2011a, 13 March). "Emotional Overflow." Ido in Autismland: Monthly Archives [Blog]. Retrieved from http://idoinautismland.com/?m=201103

Kedar, I. (2011b, 21 March). "Exercise is Good for Fighting Autism." Ido in Autismland: Monthly Archives [Blog]. Retrieved from http://idoinautismland.com/?m=201103

Kedar, I. (2011c, 25 March). "Crying in My Heart." Ido in Autismland: Monthly Archives [Blog]. Retrieved from http://idoinautismland.com/?cat=98

Kedar, I. (2011d, 25 March). "Noticing Our Blessings and Defeating Our Sorrows." Ido in Autismland: Monthly Archives [Blog]. Retrieved from http://idoinautismland.com/?cat=160

Kedar, I. (2011e, 20 December). "Hills in Seismic Country." Ido in Autismland: Monthly Archives [Blog]. Retrieved from http://idoinautismland.blogspot.com/search/label/nature

Kedar, I. (2012). *Ido in Autismland*. Los Angeles, CA: Sharon Kedar.

Kedar, I. (2018). *In Two Worlds: A Novel*. Houston, TX: Double Buck Publishing.

Kedar, I. (2019, 11 October). "Silent Advocates." Ido in Autismland: Monthly Archives [Blog]. Retrieved from http://idoinautismland.com/?m=201910

Kedar, I. (2020, 6 July). "On Early Reading." Personal Communication [Facebook].

Kouki, É. (Ed.). (2005). *Françoise Dolto: Parler de la solitude*. Paris: Mercure de France. (Original work published 1975–1985)

Kouritzin, S.G. (1999). *Face[t]s of First Language Loss*. Mahwah, NJ: Lawrence Erlbaum Associates.

Lane, H. (1984). *When the Mind Hears: A History of the Deaf.* New York, NY: Vintage Books.

Laplanche, J. & Pontalis, J.-B. (1967/2004). *Vocabulaire de la psychanalyse*. Paris: Quadrige/Presses Universitaires de France.

Ledoux, M.-H. (2006). *Dictionnaire raisonné de l'oeuvre de Françoise Dolto*. Paris: Payot.

Lee, C. (2022, 23 January). "Do Children Learn Better in Forest Schools?" BBC Future. Retrieved from www.bbc.com/future/article/20220105-how-asia-fell-in-love-with-forest-schools

Le Point. (2012, 6 novembre). «Le secrétariat du Père Noël fête ces 50 ans et ouvre mardi.» Retrieved from www.lepoint.fr/societe/la-poste-ouvre-mardi-le-traditionnel-secretariat-du-pere-noel-17-11-2014-1881861_23.php

Le Point. (2014, 17 novembre). «La poste ouvre mardi le traditionnel secrétariat du Père Noël.» Retrieved from www.lepoint.fr/societe/la-poste-ouvre-mardi-le-traditionnel-secretariat-du-pere-noel-17-11-2014-1881861_23.php#11

Lévy, D.M. (Ed.). (2002). *Parler juste aux enfants: Entretien de Françoise Dolto & D. M. Lévy*. Paris: Mercure de France. (Original work published 1978–1988)

Littner, N. (1974). "An Intuitive Clinician but a Poor Theoretician." *APA: Psychcritiques, 19*(8): 616–617.

Loersch, C. & Payne, K.P. (2014). "Situated Inferences and the What, Who, and Where of Priming." In D.C. Molden (Ed.), *Understanding Priming Effects in Social Psychology*. New York, NY: The Guilford Press, 142–156.

Mahler, M.S. (1965). "On Early Infantile Psychosis: The Symbiotic and Autistic Syndromes." *Journal of the American Academy of Child Psychiatry, 4*(4): 554–568.

Malaguzzi, L. (1996). "History, Ideas, and Basic Philosophy: An Interview with Lella Gandini." In C. Edwards, L. Gandini & G. Forman, *The Hundred Languages of Children: The Reggio Emilia Approach to Early Childhood Education*. Norwood, NJ: Ablex Publishing Co., 41–89.

Malandrin, M.-H. & Schauder, C. (Eds.). (2009). *Françoise Dolto: Une psychanalyste dans la cité: L'aventure de la Maison verte*. Paris: Gallimard.

Manier, C. & Kouki, É. (2003). *Françoise Dolto: La vague et l'océan, Séminaire sur les pulsions de mort (1970–1971)*. Paris: Gallimard.

Marette, F. (1940). *Psychanalyse et pédiatrie: Le complexe de castration, étude générale et cas cliniques*. Paris: Amédée Legrand.

Miller, A. & Eller-Miller, E. (1989). *From Ritual to Repertoire: A Cognitive-Developmental Systems Approach with Behavior-Disordered Children*. New York, NY: John Wiley & Sons.

Molden, D.C. (2014). "Understanding Priming Effects in Social Psychology: What is 'Social Priming' and How Does it Occur?" In D.C. Molden (Ed.), *Understanding Priming Effects in Social Psychology*. New York, NY: The Guilford Press, 3–13.

Montessori, M. (1913/2017). *Pedagogical Anthropology*. New York, NY: Frederick A. Stokes & Company, republished by Createspace Independent Publishing Platform.

Montessori, M. (1914). *Dr. Montessori's Own Handbook* (D.M.M. Marchioness Guerrieri-Gonzaga, Trans.). New York, NY: Frederick A. Stokes Company Publishers.

Montessori, M. (1949/2010). *The Montessori Series, Volume I: The Absorbent Mind* (C.A. Claremont, Trans.) Amsterdam: Montessori-Pierson Publishing Company.

Mukhopadhyay, T.R. (2000). *Beyond the Silence: My Life, the World and Autism*. London: The National Autistic Society.

Mukhopadhyay, T.R. (2003). *The Mind Tree: A Miraculous Child Breaks the Silence of Autism*. New York, NY: Arcade Publishing.

Mukhopadhyay, T.R. (2005). *The Gold of the Sunbeams and Other Stories*. New York, NY: Arcade Publishing.

Mukhopadhyay, T.R. (2008). *How Can I Talk if My Lips Don't Move?* New York, NY: Arcade Publishing.

Mukhopadhyay, T.R. (2012). *I'm Not a Poet But I Write Poetry: Poems from My Autistic Mind*. Bloomington, IN: Xlibris Corp.

Mukhopadhyay, T.R. (2015a). *Plankton Dreams: What I Learned in Special Ed.* London: Open Humanities Press.

Mukhopadhyay, T.R. (2015b). "Tito: #Autism is My Destiny." [News Feature, 18 February 2015]. *Art of Autism.* Retrieved from http://the-art-of-autism.com/tito-autism-is-my-destiny/

Mundy, P.C. (2016). *Autism and Joint Attention: Development, Neuroscience, and Clinical Fundamentals.* New York, NY: The Guilford Press.

Nasio, J.-D. (1987/1998). «Débat: Solange Nobécourt, Jean-Pierre Dreyfuss, Françoise Dolto.» In J.D. Nasio (Ed.), *Le silence en psychanalyse*, Paris: Désir/Payot, 207–212.

Nobécourt, É. (Producer). (2008a). *Dolto par Dolto, No.1* [DVD]. France: MK2.

Nobécourt, É. (Producer). (2008b). *Dolto psychanalyste, No.2* [DVD]. France: MK2.

Nobécourt, É. & Simonetta, B. (Producers). (1978). *Françoise Dolto: Les enfants d'abord* [Film]. France: Arte France

Nobel Prize Outreach. (2022). "Nominations for the Nobel Prize in Physiology or Medicine." Retrieved from www.nobelprize.org/prizes/facts/facts-on-the-nobel-prize-in-physiology-or-medicine/#:~:text=In%20the%20nomination%20database%2C%20you,or%20Medicine%2C%20but%20never%20awarded

Notre Famille. (2015). «Les plus belles lettres écrites au Père Noël: Texte de Françoise Dolto au dos de la carte postale» [Image]. Retrieved from www.vosquestionsdeparents.fr/dossier/1054/lettres-au-pere-noel

Nowell, A. (2021). *Growing Up in the Ice Age: Fossil and Archaeological Evidence of the Lived Lives of Plio-Pleistocene Children.* Oxford: Oxbow Books.

Nuwer, R. (2014, 5 June). "Languages: Why We Must Save Dying Tongues." BBC. Retrieved from www.bbc.com/future/article/20140606-why-we-must-save-dying-languages

Onondaga Nation. (2022). "Wampum." [Otgó'ä]. Retrieved from www.onondaganation.org/culture/wampum/

Pappenheim, B. ["Anna O"]. (1888/2008). *In the Junk Shop and Other Stories* (R. Latimer, Trans.). Riverside, CA: Ariadne Press.

Pappenheim, B. (1924/1986). *Le travail de Sisyphe.* Paris: Des femmes.

Parten, M.B. (1932). "Social Participation among Pre-school Children." *The Journal of Abnormal and Social Psychology, 27*(3): 243–269.

Pavlenko, A. (2005). *Emotions and Multilingualism.* New York, NY: Cambridge University Press.

Pavlenko, A. (2014). *The Bilingual Mind (and What it Tells Us About Language and Thought).* Cambridge: Cambridge University Press.

Percheminier, C. (Ed.). (1991). *Françoise Dolto: Correspondance, 1913–1938.* Paris: Hatier.

Pérez-Foster, R.M. (2004). "Assessing the Psychodynamic Function of Language in the Bilingual Patient." In R.M. Pérez-Foster, M. Moskowitz & R.A. Javier (Eds.), *Reaching Across Boundaries of Culture and Class: Widening the Scope of Psychotherapy.* Lanham, MD: Jason Aronson, 243–263.

Pérez-Foster, R.M., Moskowitz, M. & Javier, R.A. (Eds.). (2004). *Reaching Across Boundaries of Culture and Class: Widening the Scope of Psychotherapy.* Lanham, MD: Jason Aronson.

Perrin, M. (2015). "Introduction." In M. Perrin (Ed.), *Affinity therapy: Nouvelles recherches sur l'autisme.* Rennes: Presses Universitaires de Rennes, 11–20.

Piaget, J. (1962). "Secondary Symbolism in Play, Dreams, and 'Unconscious' Symbolism." In J. Piaget, *Play, Dreams and Imitation in Childhood*, New York, NY: W.W. Norton & Company, 169–214.

Pinker, S. (1994). *The Language Instinct: How the Mind Creates Language*. New York, NY: HarperCollins.

Potin, Y. (Ed.). (2008). *Françoise Dolto: Archives de l'intime*. Paris: Gallimard.

Rankin, B. (1996). "Curriculum Development in Reggio Emilia: A Long-Term Curriculum Project about Dinosaurs." In C. Edwards, L. Gandini & G. Forman, *The Hundred Languages of Children: The Reggio Emilia Approach to Early Childhood Education*. Norwood, NJ: Ablex Publishing Co., 189–211.

Ribowski, N. [Producer]. (1987/2004). *Apostrophes, Les grands entretiens de Bernard Pivot: Françoise Dolto*. [Television Documentary, 2 novembre 1987]. Paris: Gallimard/ Institut National de l'Audiovisuel.

Rimland, B. (1964). "Chapter 8: Ideas for Research." In S.M. Edelson (Ed.) (1964/2015). *Infantile Autism: The Syndrome and Its Implications for a Neural Theory of Behavior* by Bernard Rimland, Ph.D. (50th Anniversary Edition). London: Jessica Kingsley Publishers, 174–184.

Roudinesco, É. (1982). *La bataille de cent ans: Histoire de la psychanalyse en France, Volume 1: 1885–1939*. Paris: Éditions Ramsay.

Roudinesco, É. (1986). *La bataille de cent ans: Histoire de la psychanalyse en France, Volume 2: 1925–1985*. Paris: Éditions du Seuil.

Saint-Onge, K. (2013). *Bilingual Being: My Life as a Hyphen*. Montreal: McGill Queen's University Press.

Saint-Onge, K. (2019). *Discovering Françoise Dolto: Psychoanalysis, Identity and Child Development*. London: Routledge.

Sapir, E. (1915/1949). "Abnormal Forms in Nootka." In D.G. Mandelbaum (Ed.), *Selected Writings of Edward Sapir in Language, Culture and Personality*. Berkeley, CA: University of California Press, 179–196.

Sapir, E. (1917). "The Blind Man." *Dreams and Gibes*. Boston, MA: The Gorham Press.

Sapir, E. (1921/1971). *Language: An Introduction to the Study of Speech*. London: Rupert Hart-Davis.

Sapir, E. (1925/1949). "Sound Patterns in Language." In D.G. Mandelbaum (Ed.), *Selected Writings of Edward Sapir in Language, Culture and Personality*. Berkeley, CA: University of California Press, 33–60.

Sapir, E. (1931/1949). "Communication." In D.G. Mandelbaum (Ed.), *Selected Writings of Edward Sapir in Language, Culture and Personality*. Berkeley, CA: University of California Press, 61–82.

Sapir, E. (1933). "The Psychological Reality of Phonemes" (M. Dalimier, Trans.). *Journal de psychologie normale et pathologique*, *30*: 247–265. Retrieved from http://ksw.shoin.ac.jp/spaelti/classes/Grad_Ling_105/files/Sapir.pdf

Sapir, E. (1933/1949). "Language." In David G. Mandelbaum (Ed.), *Selected Writings of Edward Sapir in Language, Culture and Personality*. Berkeley, CA: University of California Press.

Schauer, M. & Elbert, T. (2010, January). "Dissociation Following Traumatic Stress." *Zeitschrift für Psychologie/Journal of Psychology*, 218(2): 109–127.

Sellin, B. (1995). *In Dark Hours I Find My Way: Messages from an Autistic Mind* (A. Bell, Trans.). London: Victor Gollancz. [Also published as Sellin, B. (1995). *I Don't Want to be Inside Me Anymore* (A. Bell, Trans.). New York, NY: Basic Books.]

Strachey, J. (1900). "Editor's Introduction." In S. Freud (J. Strachey, Trans). *SE 4*, xii–xxii.

Suskind, R. (2014). *Life Animated: A Story of Sidekicks, Heroes, and Autism*. New York, NY: Kingswell.

Taylor, M. (1999). *Imaginary Companions and the Children Who Create Them*. New York, NY: Oxford University Press.

Trevarthan, C. (2011). "The Generation of Human Meaning: How Shared Experience Grows in Infancy." In A. Seemann (Ed.), *Joint Attention: New Developments in Psychology, Philosophy of Mind and Social Neuroscience*. Cambridge, MA: The MIT Press, 73–113.

Truax, B. (1978/1999). *Handbook for Acoustic Ecology*. World Soundscape Project. Vancouver, BC: Simon Fraser University and ARC Publications. Retrieved from www.sfu.ca/sonic-studio-webdav/handbook/Binaural_Hearing.html

Tustin, F. (1981). *Autistic States in Children*. London: Routledge & Kegan Paul Ltd.

UNESCO. (2011). *Atlas of the World's Languages in Danger*. Retrieved from https://unesdoc.unesco.org/ark:/48223/pf0000187026

UNESCO. (2022). *World Atlas of Languages (Summary Document)*. Retrieved from https://unesdoc.unesco.org/ark:/48223/pf0000380132

Union of Ontario Indians. (2013). "An Overview of the Indian Residential School System." North Bay, ON: Nipissing First Nation. Retrieved from www.anishinabek.ca/wp-content/uploads/2016/07/An-Overview-of-the-IRS-System-Booklet.pdf schools

United Nations. (2022, 2 March). "COVID-19: Depression, Anxiety Soared 25 Per Cent in a Year." Retrieved from https://news.un.org/en/story/2022/03/1113162

Waters, J. (2013). "Chapter Two: Talking in Wild Outdoor Spaces: Children Bringing Their Interests to Their Teachers in Wales." In S. Knight (Ed.), *International Perspectives on Forest School: Natural Spaces to Play and Learn*. London: SAGE Publications Ltd. Retrieved from https://sk.sagepub.com/books/international-perspectives-on-forest-school/n2.xml

Wien, C.A. (2008). "Emergent Curriculum." In *Emergent Curriculum in the Primary Classroom: Interpreting the Reggio Emilia Approach in the Schools*. New York, NY: Teachers College Press, 5–16.

Wilson, D.A. & Stevenson, R.J. (2006). *Learning to Smell: Olfactory Perception from Neurobiology to Behavior*. Baltimore, MD: The Johns Hopkins Press.

Wing, L. (1976). "The Principles of Remedial Education for Autistic Children." In L. Wing (Ed.), *Early Childhood Autism: Clinical, Educational and Social Aspects*, 2nd Ed., Oxford: Pergamon Press, 197–220.

Winnicott, D.W. (1945). "Primitive Emotional Development." *The International Journal of Psychoanalysis*, *26*: 137–143.

Winnicott, D.W. (1956/1992). "Primary Maternal Preoccupation." In *Collected Papers: Through Paediatrics to Psycho-Analysis*. London: Tavistock Press & Routledge, 300–303.

Winnicott, D.W. (1968/1986). "Sum I Am." In C. Winnicott, R. Shepherd & M. Davis (Eds.), *Home is Where We Start From: Essays by a Psychoanalyst*. New York, NY: W.W. Norton & Company, 55–64.

Winnicott, D.W. (1971). "Transitional Objects and Transitional Phenomena." In D.W. Winnicott, *Playing and Reality*. London: Routledge, 1–25.

World Health Organization. (2022, 2 March). "COVID-19 Pandemic Triggers 25% Increase in Prevalence of Anxiety and Depression Worldwide." Retrieved from www.who.int/news/item/02-03-2022-covid-19-pandemic-triggers-25-increase-in-prevalence-of-anxiety-and-depression-worldwide

Wurzburg, G. & Biklen, D. [Producers]. (2011). "Wretches & Jabberers" [Motion Picture]. Washington, DC: State of the Art Inc. Retrieved from www.wretchesandjabberers.org/

Index

Note: Page references with "n" denote endnotes.

absence 26, 56, 119, 200, 205
adaptability (adaptation) 31, 178, 190
"aerial life" 56; *see also* birth
Aesop 120–121, 208–209
affect *see* unconscious affect
affective 11, 43; economy 17, 26, 31, 56; environment 33–34; life 15, 37; quanta 25, 65, 83–86, 94, 166, 177–179; securitization 56, 193, 201, 212, 217, 227; similitude 49, 67–69, 138, 152, 211; *see also* affective circulation; affective investment(s); unconscious affect
affective circulation 59, 63, 90n7, 166, 188; continuity of 45, 55, 66, 75, 118–120, 200; impeded 10n12, 175, 177, 179; and mother tongue 176, 180, 224; pathways 56, 92, 166; restituting 33, 40, 64, 191, 201, 223; as securing 216, 219; sustaining 15, 38, 68, 167, 182, 204; and triangulation 76, 86; *see also* unconscious affect
affective investment(s) 16–17, 44, 59, 64, 136–137, 169, 173; archaic 14, 43, 61, 118, 200; in common objects 66, 210; facilitating continuity with 24, 221, 224; as lured 15–16, 43, 55, 57, 83, 87, 144, 212; in objects of reality 7, 16–17, 24, 30, 177, 203; in objects of dream-work 86, 118; pathways 49, 58, 221; perseverated 28, 93; in phonemes 87, 120, 122, 139, 167, 170, 174, 176; and security 48, 56; and witness 177, 209; *see also* reinvestment; unconscious affect
affectivity 5, 34n24, 48, 62
affinity (affinities) 112n150, 147, 169
alphabet 60, 122, 149–150, 186
amygdala 32
animal(s) 96, 121, 140–148, 155n77, 214; critical period in 69; olfaction in 32; and projection (identification) 67, 187, 209; in stories 74n226, 209; *see also* nature
"Anna O." 10n12, 177, 185–186; *see also* Bertha Pappenheim
anonymity (anonymous) 4, 43, 150, 212–217
anxiety 20n2, 28–32, 77, 100–108, 149–150; anxiogenic 15, 75, 158, 190, 192–193; anxious 45–46, 86, 95, 101, 103–105, 151; and audition (tempering) 56, 58; chronic 96, 157; in common terminology 91–92; contagion of 92, 101, 108n8; and COVID-19 194n9; excessive 5, 16, 95, 101, 108, 164, 169, 183, 187, 223; existential 19, 30, 38, 83, 94–96, 189; and fear 176; and L2 176–177, 181; as language 14; mortifying 30, 158; mother's 25, 32, 42, 83, 92, 101; and pleasure 18, 148–150, 170; reduced by affective liberation 63, 87–89, 138, 145, 167–168, 210, 221; reduced by exiting regression 95, 224; reduced by nature 142, 148, 158, 170, 214, 216; reduced by phonemes 67, 173–174, 183; reduced by reading 158, 170, 187; reduced by writing 149–153, 157, 160; and regression 75, 77, 86, 88, 190; as resistance

28; as result not cause 37, 46, 69, 77, 145; and social stories 192–193; as symptom 6, 10n12, 94, 103–106, 129, 142, 166–168, 223
après-coup 65, 196; *see also* dream-work
archaic 22–24; affect 23, 58, 60–62, 64, 85, 165, 190, 193, 219; audition in 55, 65, 138, 181, 214; continuity with 18, 170, 215; desire in 37, 67; development in 19, 81, 95, 118, 165–166, 169–170, 218n27, 222–224; dream-work 18–19, 26–28, 37, 44–48, 57, 63, 83–85, 118–120, 145, 193, 215, 223; echoes 46, 61–64, 85, 158–159, 182–187, 189–193, 203–205, 211–214, 219–225; environment 56, 144, 199, 220, 223; and experience of surviving 23, 32, 48, 56, 62; fixation in 37; heritage 22, 31, 55, 58, 61, 142; history 23, 49, 59, 167, 180, 193, 215, 219; as idiosyncratic 179; image 15; in individuation 62, 205, 210; instinct in 89n6, 42; investment(s) 14, 17, 43, 61, 63, 65, 77, 167–168, 193; landmarks 60; and language acquisition 180–182, 204, 219; learning in 32–34, 181, 224; libidinal organization of 23, 29; moorings 9, 129, 218; and nature 147, 169, 210–217; object relations 14–18, 23, 45–49, 51n44, 59, 69, 76, 84, 92, 118, 170, 189, 211–212, 223; parents (blurred) in 17–18, 42, 53n98, 82, 137; passivity in 40–42, 83, 144, 181, 188, 213, 215; pathways 49; permanent 18, 26, 59–60, 64, 158, 167; phonemes in 40, 56, 58–61, 85–86, 158, 167–168, 171n14, 173–175, 181–189, 198–199, 219–224; pleasure 17, 23, 63, 66, 131; and "positions" of self 159, 168; register 17; reserves 85; rhythmic exchanges in 22; security 15, 30, 47, 50, 57, 60–63, 87–88, 146, 158, 166–168, 175, 201, 215; stage 8, 14–16, 22–25, 28–34, 37–39, 65–67, 75–77, 81–82, 87–88, 222–224; subbasement of life 23; symbolic satisfaction 23, 45, 49; -syntonic 186, 200, 214, 223; system of expression 23; terrain 69, 87, 89, 124, 126, 212, 223, 225; and transference 33–34, 38–39, 48, 63, 141, 200–201; truth 59; witness 17, 25, 63, 200–201, 205, 210
archaic triangular situation (triangulation): and affective circulation 41, 50, 55, 61, 75–76, 83, 86, 138; and associations 76, 158, 169; and common objects 39, 66, 84, 141; blurry (fluid) 17, 33, 53n98, 63, 82, 150; constructed unconsciously 38; development 84–85, 137, 186; as dream-work 45–46; as first learning 38, 84–85; and identification 188; idiosyncratic 63; in individuation 38; and instinct 22, 89n6; and nature 169, 214–215, 217; and Oedipus 16, 75, 82, 166; and passivity 42; as permanent inscription 17, 39–40, 56, 58, 64–67, 76, 88, 138, 159, 168; and phonemes 17, 77, 117, 158–159, 168, 189, 203–205, 220, 222–224; and reading 62, 186, 192; as relation not structure 75, 167; reversibility in 62, 64, 67; and "third" 38; and transference 41, 45; and unconscious security 40, 153, 157–158, 165–166, 189; and witness 67; and writing 89, 199; *see also* archaic
Arnulf, Isabelle 197, 202, 206n15
art 64–65, 164, 204
association(s): in affective transfers 34, 76–77, 82–85, 107; to archaic object(s) 15–17, 43, 159, 200; and dream-work 33, 125, 137; in homonymic play 197– 198; in luring to reality 77, 190, 212; in multilingualism 20n16; "narcissistic organo-emotional representative associations" 23; in nature 145–146, 158, 212–216; in networks for displacement 44, 50, 57, 113, 167, 170, 177, 179; to new object(s) 15, 77, 87, 138, 169; in olfaction 32; in parallel play 141; and phonemes 58–60, 76, 93, 115–117, 138–139, 158, 166–167, 173–179, 187, 193, 204; to prior object(s) 14, 18, 34, 48, 85, 118, 137; as process 17, 19, 32; proliferations of 17, 116–118, 137, 158, 166–168, 188–189;

in reading 60–61, 186, 189; in regression 94, 102, 121, 175, 190; in symbolization 47–49, 86, 132, 180, 223; and "third" 16, 38–42; unconscious 13, 17, 118, 175, 188; and witness 64, 170, 177, 183, 193, 201, 217; word 14, 18, 49, 113, 120, 123, 182, 197–199; in writing 197–199, 203
associative: activation 60; branch(ing) 26; coherence 60–61; displacements 26; distance 14, 17, 31, 49, 60, 76–77, 83, 158, 167, 177, 223; emotional arousal as 21; history 182; mechanism 137; memory 60; networks 59–60, 158, 166, 181; object(s) 26, 188, 212; in olfaction 32; in passive education 33; pathways 30–32, 47–49, 55–56, 61, 66, 77, 83–84, 87, 94; (as) play 123, 138, 140–141; proliferations 76; relations 76–77, 84, 86, 145, 169, 174, 183; *see also* associative thinking
associative thinking 48–49, 60, 82, 123, 174; and affect 8, 92, 176, 179, 204–205; and literacy 187–188, 196–201; and nature 210–216, 220; ontogeny 2, 32, 138, 178, 202, 224–225; and passivity 89, 113, 121, 141, 145; and phonemes 88, 158–159, 166–169, 173, 179–183, 201–202, 219, 224
audition (auditory) 57, 181, 199–201; development 25, 31, 41–43, 55–56, 65, 75, 82, 132, 165–166, 169; and dream-work 41, 60, 132, 166, 199, 227; and environment 9, 18, 175–176, 188, 201–202, 225; and habituation 43; influence 113–135; as language reception 177; "like eating" 58; in luring to reality 55–58, 99, 166, 180–182, 198; of mother's environment 33, 119; and nature 145, 148; in parallel play 141; precocious 9, 40–43, 56–57, 75, 82, 113–119, 138, 165–169, 177–178; in pre-conscious learning 4, 8, 13, 127; reliance on 127–129, 132, 157, 166, 223; return (echo) 127–131; role in continuity 18, 160; in symbolization 87–89, 115, 128; in tempering anxiety 56; and triangulation 39, 141; and witness 152; and words 68, 138–140, 182; and writing 199
auto-: auto-conservation 20n16; auto-formation 178; auto-maternting 63, 68; auto-recovery 63, 67, 180, 198; *see also* self-autobiography 5, 101, 109n36, 110n47, 110n49, 174, 177, 185, 190, 193n5, 195–197, 206n18
awaken(ing) 3, 18, 24–29, 68, 149, 152, 176–177, 191, 198, 213, 221

Barr, Martin W. 186, 192
Bastian, Henry Charlton 182
Berthold, Paul 185–186; *see also* Bertha Pappenheim
bilingual(ism) 155n77, 170, 173–177, 219
Binet, Alfred 47
biological 13, 21, 57, 84, 137, 175
birth: as liberation 55; maturation (later) 8, 13, 82–85, 155n77; maturation (prior) 24, 32, 43, 81, 113, 118, 165, 218n27; and name 117, 175–176, 215; and nature 211; and «reconnaissance» 70n17, 133n23; and survival 56; as transition 7, 15, 23, 27, 60, 118, 169; *see also* umbilical castration
boundaries of self 4, 31, 214
brain 13–14, 21–25, 32, 42, 48, 96, 100–102
branch(es) 6, 26, 44, 50, 77, 126, 144, 146, 225; *see also* pathway(s)
bridge(s) 9, 18, 126, 224; Mute Bridge 1–4, 9, 226; words as 121, 183, 219
Bridgman, Laura 202, 206n38
Brison, Susan 174, 176

call: of archaic 24, 85, 123, 214; beyond 46; code of 18, 63; to read 191–193; up 40, 177, 213
castration(s): anxiety 28, 30; complex 30; oral (weaning) 14; symboligenic 28; umbilical (birth) 14, 18, 28–29, 39, 56, 81, 165, 218n27
cathexis 41, 87
cerebellum 47–48
Charcot, Jean-Martin 197
choral clinics 40, 164
classroom(s) 6, 34, 123, 159, 163, 182, 188, 204, 215, 221n2; *see also* education

co-: "co-being" 56; co-birth 133n23; co-constructed 191; co-creating 219; "co-existential" 56; co-experience 68–70, 76, 82–84, 90n7, 137, 145, 157, 165–168, 181–189, 201, 210; co-living 33, 141; «co-moi papa-maman» 33; co-presence 125; co-witnessing 66; *see also* indissociable
coma(tose) 3, 44, 59
condensation 61–62, 83; and archaic triangulation 44–46, 82; "condensation-work" 49; and displacement 7, 15, 17, 23, 49, 53n96, 82, 196; and literacy 196–199; *see also* dream-work
confirmation(s) 32, 70n17, 77, 139, 174, 177, 202; *see also* proof of life
conservation 20n16, 21–36; of energy 83, 93–94, 96; of health 15, 46; and nature 121; and unconscious security 34; *see also* instinct of conservation
consciousness 10n9, 29, 100, 113–117, 165, 168–169, 221; altered 188; coming to reality 2, 18, 24, 38, 48, 50n2, 56, 59; developing gradually 3, 14, 18, 21–22, 27, 49, 178; and learning 3–4, 9, 221, 224; and literacy 192, 203; losing 44, 47; and motor acts (speech) 94, 177; and nature 212; and phoneme 57, 117, 167, 198; unaware 2, 21, 23, 37, 41, 50, 65, 114, 141, 159, 167–168, 174
consolation(s) 55, 57, 130, 139, 159, 216
contagion (contamination) 92, 101, 108n8, 163
continuity: affective 34, 45–48, 56–57, 64, 76–84, 93, 118, 137–145, 190; with archaic objects 17–18, 56, 64, 86, 170, 215–217; and associative thinking 119; and audition 141; between dream-work and thought 19, 47, 59, 65, 67, 131, 165, 198–200, 223; discontinuity 39, 63; as existential security 15, 34, 45, 50n2, 60, 104, 180; and nature 215–220; and witness 66, 212; and writing 220
COVID-19 163, 187, 194n9
creativity 48, 121, 126; *see also* art
critical period (in learning) 69, 155n77, 190
Darwin, Charles 195–197, 200, 205, 206n1, 224
Darwin, Francis 195, 199
daydream(ing) 157, 169; and literacy 125, 131, 186–187, 202; and nature 6, 88, 120–121, 144–145, 213, 216, 226; and symbolization 47, 106–107, 123, 131; and unconscious security 88, 124–126, 130, 139, 145; and words 19, 121, 142–143, 187; *see also* dream(s); dream-work
Deaf (deafness) 9n8, 52n74, 70n2, 153, 176, 200, 202, 206n38
defence 81, 91–112; energy saving 96; fragile ego 88, 90n10, 201; "hide" 43, 46; in infants 15, 75, 220; language as 176–177, 179; mutism as 69; passive 42, 69; as regression 11–15, 45–46, 75, 88–96, 108, 128–131, 150–157, 169, 177, 192, 201, 211–215, 223–224; sleep as 44; *see also* regression
dependence 28, 46, 67, 93, 151; fusional 127, 149–150, 188, 201; in passivity 76, 142, 157, 192, 204, 209, 217; on regression 46, 128, 131, 150, 201, 221; *see also* fusion; regression
differentiation 23, 39; *see also* individuation
diffusion 13, 26, 76, 83–87, 94, 158, 176, 189, 200, 209; *see also* displacement
displacement(s) 27, 29–30, 82–83, 106, 153, 168, 196, 214; by association(s) 13, 17, 26, 38, 82, 92, 138; and condensation 7, 15, 17, 23, 26, 44, 49, 53n96, 77, 82, 113, 196; as movement 43, 148; and primary processes 24, 44; and transference 24, 33; *see also* diffusion
Doidge, Norman 45
Dolto, Catherine 11, 12n4
dormant 45, 76, 117, 126; *see also* sleep(ing)
drawings 64, 211, 220; *see also* art
dream(s) 19, 23–28, 35n56, 41–42, 47–49, 67, 147, 213, 226; and archaic 22–27, 143–145, 167–168, 193; and art 64; and audition 127, 132; at boundary to reality 4, 7, 19,

25, 59, 69, 85, 95, 120, 126, 188; dream-content 50; dreamed "other" 17, 33, 76, 85, 159, 187; dream-life 25, 146; dreamscape 26, 29, 147; and echoes 27, 64, 139; as evidence 3–4, 20n7, 110n49; and externalization 25; fetal 18–19, 227; first 17; and fixation 29; and flower-doll 68; as guarantors of survival 26; journals 200–202; objects of 14, 18, 24–26, 165, 212, 227; on phonemes 183; as pleasure 17–18, 27, 33, 94, 130–137, 139, 151, 166, 202; and reading 60; state 28, 152; and symbolization 47, 49–50, 140; as system of expression 23; and wish to sleep 27, 49, 165; and witness 157; and word association 113; words as things 49; work of 7, 17; world 27; *see also* dream-work

dream-work 7, 23, 30, 37, 44–49, 53n96, 61, 75–76, 82–85, 165, 223; *après-coup* 65, 196; and archaic objects 19, 25–26, 34, 48, 51n44, 62–63, 83, 118, 131, 223, 226; archaic parents of 17, 39, 53n98, 137; and archaic triangulation 33, 38, 40, 42, 63, 82, 85, 137, 167; and associations 33, 56, 84, 94, 166, 169, 202–204; as consolation 55, 69; fluidity of 22, 62; idiosyncratic 49; in infants 24–25, 28, 31, 37, 40–45, 60, 76, 83; invested objects of 16, 18, 58, 77; and language 17–18, 64, 82, 127, 192, 199, 227; and liquid objects 14–16, 19, 24, 45, 49, 55, 60, 82–84; and nature 70, 215–217; and "other" 67, 84, 88; and passivity 31, 41, 131–132, 145, 177; and phonemes 59, 113, 158, 202, 223, 226; and pleasure 28, 106, 130, 152, 159; and reading 63, 70, 90n11, 158, 167, 187–188, 192; and regression 44, 92, 151; and reparation 66, 93, 158, 210–211, 213–214; reversal in 64–65; as self-securing 43, 46, 56–57, 66, 68; and symbolization 19, 47, 60, 82, 98, 110n49, 120, 137, 181, 192, 202; in transition to reality 86, 98, 118, 205; as unconscious relation 16; and wish to live 23; and witness 212; words as things in 58; and writing 196–197, 199–201; *see also* dream(s)

echo(es) 18, 63, 138–139, 183, 190, 205, 210, 217, 219–227; of archaic investments 43–48, 61–64, 85, 120, 182–191, 203, 211–214; of archaic security 57, 63, 127, 155n77, 193, 197, 213; of dreams 27, 140, 193; echolalia 10n12, 182, 186, 188; echo-location 139, 201; and hearing 139–140; and name 172–184; and nature 4, 6, 147–148, 208–218; and "other" (position of self) 127, 131, 138, 141, 153, 189, 199–201, 210, 214, 225; and phonemes 58–61, 87, 120, 138, 153, 155n77, 165–168, 173–175, 186–189, 199–203; and reading 61, 125, 158, 168, 170, 185–194; and speech 90n10, 191, 202; and thought 68, 196; and triangulation 140, 159, 189, 202–203; and witness 66, 85, 199–200; and writing 142, 147, 157, 170, 195–207; *see also* archaic; resonance

education (educate, educator) 8, 34, 36n85, 88, 155n77, 163–165, 182, 204, 216; and autists 98, 123–128, 153; passive 8, 31–34, 120–128, 220–224; in reparation (health) 169–170, 182, 204, 215–224; *see also* learning; teaching

ego 47, 88, 90n10, 119, 201, 220

Eisenberg, Rita B. 57

emotional (emotion) 57, 60–62, 104–105, 197, 219; activity 50, 165, 200; arousal 21; and bilingualism 174; capacities 8, 47–48, 84; climate 40; and common interest 38–39, 62; constitution 65, 127, 158; development 60–62, 81–88, 158, 173, 182, 192; "emotional and mental" 19, 37, 62, 158, 166, 179, 187–188, 198, 200–201, 209, 223–26; health 31, 68, 138; and indissociable "other" 76, 118, 137; and individuation 137, 157; journey between worlds 7; life 7–8, 10n9, 20n7, 22, 38–39, 44–48,

58–63, 69–75, 81–88, 95, 113–115, 120–125, 130–136, 165–167, 173–179, 198; motivation 30, 115; "organo-emotional representative associations" 23; and regression 44, 77, 95; resonance 25, 58; situation 2, 19, 199, 212; systems 29; unconscious 20n2, 26; theory of 33; trajectory 222; transition 55, 58, 118; world(s) 26, 29, 166, 171n14, 197, 219
enteric nervous system 24
environment(al) 3, 8, 26, 30–34, 36n85, 45, 83, 182; "all-providing" 33, 76, 84, 88, 127, 144–145, 158, 169–170, 181, 189, 213, 217, 223; and archaic objects 25, 41, 70, 82, 178, 186, 199, 220; and association 102, 132, 174, 220; and audition 9, 24–25, 93, 176, 181, 200–203, 225; changes 56, 100, 116–118, 126, 139, 145, 180; and contamination 42–43, 92; in education 163, 215–217, 220, 224; and literacy 61–63, 70, 87, 123, 187–188, 191–193, 197, 200–205; in luring to reality 46, 190, 193, 224; mother as 16, 39, 41, 44, 49, 82, 84; and nature 68, 70, 88, 209, 211–216, 220, 223; and passivity 59, 93, 120, 126–127, 183, 215; and regression 96–98; and securitization 168, 180–181, 187–190, 197, 203, 227; and transference 25, 38, 68; *see also* nature
evolution(ary) 21, 30, 45, 91
existential: anxiety 19, 28, 30, 38, 94, 96, 136, 189; security 15, 45, 50, 173, 175, 193; threat 83, 91, 95
exterior 30, 46, 55–59, 145–150, 168–170, 214; exteriorization 66–70, 77, 88, 142–147, 153; *see also* liberate; vent(ing)

fable(s) 61, 143, 208–209
facilitated (facilitation) 6, 30, 34, 117, 125, 152, 188, 203–205, 213–219
Facilitated Communication 6, 206n40
fairy tales 61, 125
father's tongue 14, 172, 180
fear 3, 14, 18, 32, 42, 90n13, 91, 102–104, 190, 197
fetal (fetus): development 18–19, 31, 37–39, 42–43, 47, 55, 57, 227; dreams 19; epoch 23, 60; habituation 42; life 32; "parasitic fetal stage" 49; "purée of significance" 41; sonority 210
filiation(s) 50, 108n13, 174, 177, 186, 193
finger(s) 5, 128, 151, 202; *see also* hand
first days (weeks) 9, 22, 27, 29, 31, 66, 69, 83
first language (L1) *see* language; *see* mother tongue
fixation 28–30; archaic 37, 45, 118; libidinal 45; and regression 93, 211–213; in therapy 112n150
"flight or fight" 43, 46, 91–92; *see also* "freeze"
flower(s) 67, 130, 211; flower-doll («poupée fleur») 9n4, 67–68, 209–211, 217n4; *see also* nature
food 33, 58, 93, 129, 140, 208–209; and dream-work 25, 201; familiar 8, 27–28; oral stage 15, 28; phonemes as 18, 41, 58, 118, 182; and thinking 69, 179, 201; "third" as 16; *see also* provision
forest 4, 6, 24, 146, 148, 208–217, 220; forest school(s) 216, 218n45; *see also* trees
freedom 10, 99, 102, 104, 142, 157, 160, 188, 211, 216; *see also* liberty
"freeze" 91–92, 95; *see also* hide; regression
Freud, Sigmund 61, 75, 82, 92–93, 113, 186, 197, 200, 225–227; on affect 2–8, 10n12, 20n2, 25, 29–32, 34n24; on "arrogance of consciousness" 221; on art 65; on associative thought 48, 197; on continuity 18–19, 50; on dream-work 17, 23, 25, 27, 49, 64; on fixations 28; on frontier of biological and psychological 69; on identification 62; on inertia 27; on instincts 21–22, 63, 214; on libidinal organization 15; and Montessori 177; on pleasure 29, 33, 41, 55–56, 63, 193, 228; on preconscious 10n9; on psychosexual stages 13–14; on reading 60–61, 187; on regression 20n7, 30, 44, 69; on self-preservation 20n16; slips 3;

and "third" 40, 62; on transference 24–25, 57–58; on venting 67, 177; watery metaphors 44; on writing 196–197, 203
fusion(al): in autobiography 10; and indissociability 120, 141, 201, 204; partial 142; and passivity (dependence) 126–127, 149–151, 169, 188, 192, 201; and transference 62; *see also* indissociable

going-becoming («allant-devenant») 37, 50n2
grammar 117, 119, 139, 192
Gray, Carol 192, 194n30
Greenspan, Stanley 30, 47, 61

habituation 4, 42–43; habitus 28, 43, 82, 97
hallucinatory (hallucinate) 41, 56
hand(s) 6, 31, 63–67, 98–106, 123–131, 140–144, 149–152, 195, 202–203, 226; *see also* finger(s)
heal(ing) 33, 39–40, 84; *see also* reparation
health 121, 172, 194n9, 216; and affect 13, 31, 68, 77, 83, 181, 225–226; and archaic history 219–226; and consciousness 3, 21; and conservation of resources 15–16, 46; inter-relational 22, 42; and psychosexual maturation 16, 28–31, 210; *see also* heal(ing); reparation
Herz, Rachel 32
hide 43, 46, 95–96, 103, 105, 117; *see also* "freeze"; regression
Higashida, Naoki 5, 10n13, 90n15, 109n30, 205; on anxiety 103–106, 149–150; on daydreaming 130–132; on exteriorization 143; on fusion 127–128, 150–152; on individuation 100–102, 152–153; on love of language 121–122; on non-initiation 129–130; on passion for reading 123–124; on passivity 126–129; on phonemes in associative thinking 121; on reality (space-time) 98–100; on regression 96–98; on revitalizing energy 143–154; on securitizing provision 146–147; on self-calming 145–146; on stims (venting) 106–108; on witness 149; on word and letter play 122–123
Hoffman, Eva 173, 183n9
homonym(s) 70n17, 133n23, 142, 154n26, 155n62, 175, 197–200, 206n18, 219; *see also* phoneme(s)

identification 62, 67–68, 118, 139, 141, 186, 188, 20–211
idiosyncratic: archaic situation 63; associations 116; history 22–24, 40, 44, 139, 179; inscription 14; libidinal organization 23, 49; phonemes 59, 61, 86, 93, 115, 119, 131, 186, 222; witness 212
imaginary companions 187, 189
indissociable: affect and thinking 48; archaic parents 16, 48, 166–167; associations 200, 210; dream of provision 166; fluid environment 31– 34; individuation 119, 138, 166; infant-mother 17, 31–33, 37, 84, 92, 118–119, 137, 145, 165; "like-me" 40, 49, 62, 82, 117, 137; "me-mymother" 26, 31, 38, 55, 66–67; presence 58, 118, 168, 218n27; "second" 63, 165; *see also* fusion; "other"
individuation 38, 66, 188, 221; challenge of 88, 92, 96–103, 119, 124–125, 144–152, 160, 192, 223; and echoes 189, 193; gradual 76, 84, 119, 137, 204, 210; and nature 170, 209–210, 213–214; and passivity 125–132, 157; and phonemes 199, 201, 219, 224; and reading 120, 124–125, 158, 170; as securing 169, 205, 210; and "third" 39–41; triangulated 137, 139, 152, 198, 201, 205, 217; and voice 159; and writing 8, 87, 142, 157–159, 170, 200–205, 220–223; *see also* differentiation
infans 9, 227
infant's learning style 9, 224
initiation 120, 132; *see also* non-initiation
inscription 8–9, 30, 195, 227n11; of affect 14, 25, 82, 137, 189; of archaic 23, 33, 37, 76, 85, 159, 167; and phoneme 40, 57, 64–65, 117, 139, 159, 167, 189, 197, 222, 225; and security 34, 37, 68, 141
instinct of conservation 21–27, 210; in auto-recovery 180, 201, 213, 221;

dominance in early life 2, 19–23, 42, 55, 87–88, 89n6, 91, 223; driving language acquisition 9, 85–87, 175, 180, 222; driving primary processes 82–87, 93, 144–147, 165, 213–217; in self-regulation 16, 30, 67, 77, 87–88, 93–94, 166–167, 175, 191–193, 210–214, 221–222; *see also* instinct(s)
instincts 3, 61–63, 115, 129, 168; theory of (Freud) 20n2, 20n16, 21–29, 41–44, 61–69, 214
interhuman: affective circulation 63, 191; communication 93, 150, 217; exchanges 119,137; interactions 118; language 93, 118; languaged affects 60; relations 77
Ito, Masao 47

Johnson, E. Pauline (Tekahionwakeh) 172
joint attention 39, 49, 66; *see also* object(s)

Kahneman, Daniel 21–22, 44, 60
Kanner, Leo 133n25, 210
Kedar, Ido 5, 10n13, 109n27, 109n30, 134n66, 216; on anxiety 103–106, 149–150; on daydreaming 130–132; on exteriorization 143; on fusion 127–128, 150–152; on individuation 100–102, 152–153; on love of language 121–122; on non-initiation 129–130; on passion for reading 123–124; on passivity 126–129; on phonemes in associative thinking 121; on reality (space-time) 98–100; on regression 96–98; on revitalizing energy 143–154; on securitizing provision 146–147; on self-calming 145–146; on stims (venting) 106–108; on witness 149; on word and letter play 122–123
kindergarten 184n55, 188; *see also* classroom; education; learning; teaching
Klein, Melanie 53n98
Kouritzin, Sandra 174

Lacan, Jacques 9n4
landmark(s) 9, 17, 56, 60, 108n13, 212, 226
language(s): acquisition 9, 85, 116–117, 202, 219–225; attrition 41, 59, 173–182, 219; bath 57, 199, 201–204; first 173–175, 179–183, 192; love 120–122, 132, 169; migration 59, 183; second 59–61, 155, 155n77, 158, 174–183, 184n49, 192, 219; *see also* mother tongue
languaged 56, 60, 95, 108n13, 119, 176
latent 13, 64, 77, 95, 115, 119, 138, 159, 167, 198
learn(ing) (learner) 2–9, 24, 43, 52n74, 97, 141–143, 155n7, 163–170, 196–198, 200–209, 220–224; and affect 34, 47, 138, 170–179, 180, 193, 224; and archaic triangulation 31–34, 38n15, 138, 181, 189–198, 219–227; and association 26, 34, 121, 138, 180, 193; and autists 97, 101–102, 107, 127, 153, 155n77, 186, 191; and common interest 40, 49, 140–141; continuous 120, 128–132; and dream-work 47, 188; earliest 6–8, 31–33, 75, 170–178, 222–225; and environment 26, 33, 182, 215; idiosyncratic 182–183; and language 66–68, 85, 117, 155n77, 159, 169, 172–182, 184n49, 186, 202, 219–227; and literacy 169, 189; passive 31, 33, 120, 126, 128, 220, 224; pre-conscious 8–9, 43, 85, 170, 221–224; and reading 6, 123–125, 134n66, 189, 192, 205; recovering 164, 169; universal design for learning (UDL) 8, 224; and writing 88–96, 101, 150–153, 155n77, 200–204, 220; *see also* critical period; education; infant's learning style; teach(ing)
letter play *see* play
liberate (liberation) 29, 123, 131, 150; of affect 8, 14, 29, 65, 83, 138, 152, 166, 187; birth as 55; in decreasing anxiety 167, 170; difficulty with 83, 166; drive for 94, 107; and flower-doll 67; and literacy 142, 193, 197, 203, 210; and nature 214, 216; need for 61; pathways for circulation 30, 66, 77, 166; and words 67–68, 173–178; *see also* exteriorization; vent(ing)
libidinal (libido) 15, 20n7, 29, 33, 34n24, 44, 68; dynamic 30; energy 165; evolution 30, 45; fixation 45; history 68; investment 45; organization 23, 28; position 29, 93; regression 45; stages 28; wealth 23

library 87, 89, 185–193
"like-me" 33–34, 36n106, 40–41, 49, 62–63, 82–84, 117, 129, 137; *see also* similitude
limbic system 32
liminal (liminality) 31, 120, 131, 148, 165–166, 188, 213
liquid object 20n3; as dream objects 14, 19, 24, 31, 45, 49, 55–56, 60, 84; and literacy 61; and names 18; and phonemes 14, 18, 137, 227; *see also* object
literacy 8, 39, 59, 63, 121, 164, 169, 181, 193, 223–224; *see also* reading; writing
liturgical language(s) 86, 180; *see also* language(s)
lure(s) (luring): by archaic echoes 43, 120, 175–176; by association to archaic 46, 77, 86, 94, 116, 131, 190; by audition 55–57, 59–60, 87, 139, 158, 167, 175–176, 179, 187, 193; difficulty finding 169, 186–187, 190, 193; and exiting regression 16, 29; to follow 144, 158; for forward investments 27, 46, 82, 144, 167, 189; in literacy 189–191; mediating 57; and nature 215–216; in passivity 15, 58, 87, 190; to reality 16–17, 29–33, 83, 93, 118, 130–131, 168, 175–175, 212; self-luring 201

Mahler, Margaret 15, 44
«Maison vertes» 154n24, 210
maternal 39, 42, 53n98, 59, 69, 119; object 118
mediating: ideas 40; lures 57; object(s) 56–59; *see also* object(s)
memoir(s): autism 5, 89, 112n150; language 173, 183n9
me-mymother («moi-mamère») 16, 22, 26, 31, 33, 37–38, 48, 55, 63, 65–66
me-notme 125
metaphor (metonymy) 2, 44, 58, 61, 128
mimicry 67, 69
mobility (immobility) 33, 43, 91–92; *see also* movement
Montessori, Maria 177–179, 184n35, 190, 202, 215–216, 221
Morgenstern, Sophie 164
mother tongue 121, 155n62, 155n77, 180; and associative thinking 167–169, 179, 219, 223; attrition 41, 59, 170–173, 179, 183; defenses 174–175; environment 8; function(s) of 8, 176; idiosyncratic 59; integrating with child 119, 178; and literacy 61, 86, 158; and mother 17, 59, 68; phonemes 7, 26, 58, 68, 75, 84–86, 158, 174–176, 223–224; as securing 68, 223–224; as source of lures 18, 58, 84–86; pathways 60; in unconscious symbolization 117; *see also* language(s); phoneme(s)
motherify («mamaïsé») 34; motherification 68
movement 5, 211; affective 26, 46; consciousness (speech) 10n12, 83, 86, 129, 153, 169, 202, 221; difficulty initiating 126, 130, 144, 203, 217; and dream-work 82; and flower-doll 67; to follow 37, 144–145, 211, 214–217; and habituation 42; instincts initiating 63, 214; as language 122; laryngeal 119; and literacy 149; and nature 67, 144, 212–217; prenatal development of 47–48; as proof of life 148; in self-regulation 107; unconscious activity as 37; *see also* displacement
Mukhopadhyay, Tito 5, 10n13, 109n30, 109n36, 110n47, 110n49, 181, 206n41; on anxiety 103–106, 149–150; on daydreaming 130–132; on exteriorization 143; on fusion 127–128, 150–152; on individuation 100–102, 152–153; on love of language 121–122; on non-initiation 129–130; on reading 123–124; on passivity 126–129; on phonemes in associative thinking 121; on reality 98–100; on regression 96–98; on revitalizing energy 143–154; on securitizing provision 146–147; on self-calming 145–146; on stims 106–108; on witness 149; on word and letter play 122–123
multilingual(ism) 20n16, 121, 182; *see also* language
mute (mutism) 21, 28, 42, 69, 74n199, 121, 128, 202, 225; as challenge to venting 69–70, 181–182; and

defence 94, 106, 182; "de-muting" 64, 181; *infans* 9, 215; mute but listening 27, 169; mute but thinking 19, 50, 88, 108, 169; and nature 4, 213; and passivity 43, 69, 97, 217; symptomatic 10n12, 68, 87, 96, 103, 175–181; and writing (right to write) 10, 142, 149, 153; *see also* silence

name 169, 172–183, 186–186, 198–199, 211, 224–226; anonymity 213; associations with 18, 211; changing 170, 175–176, 179–183, 188; of child 26, 52n74, 117, 122, 159, 175–180, 215, 219; of father 26; and literacy 188; of mother 14; of mother's other 25, 31; and phonemic play 198–199
narcissism (narcissistic): joy 58; mode of being 57; "narcissistic organo-emotional representative associations" 23; primary 27, 68, 175; projection of 67
nature 90n12, 157, 169–170, 208–217; all-providing 144–147, 158, 169, 212–217; and associative thinking 214; and dream-work 220; externalizing affect 143–147; in reparation 209–210, 212–217, 223–224; securing 4, 68, 142, 147, 158–160, 212–217; sounds 144–145; and witness 67, 144–146, 158, 212–217; world (natural) 4, 8, 88, 96, 140, 143, 217; *see also* environment
negative(ly) 26, 43, 73n131, 92, 177
neutral sites 212–213 *see also* nature
Nobel 21, 196–197
node(s) 44–45, 62, 113, 214; *see also* association; associative; pathway(s)
non-initiation 126–127, 129–130, 132; *see also* initiation
non-speaking 10n10, 150, 227; *see also* speaking
nonverbal 171n13; and anxiety 6, 108, 142, 149, 176, 189–191; and archaic security 131, 186; and audition 132, 148; author(s) 5; autism 6, 8, 10n10, 69, 75, 77, 81, 88–89; and education 155n77, 170, 219–220; and fear 104; Freud on 10n12; and individuation 142, 183, 200–203; and language attrition 181; and literacy 88, 90n11, 189–193, 219; and love of language 121–122, 129, 189; and nature 142, 160, 210, 216–217; and passivity 121–124, 132, 150, 176, 201–204; and precocious reading 87; presume competence 81, 89, 108, 121, 130, 157–165, 169, 193, 202–203, 223; and reality (space-time) 98, 120; and regression 96–97, 157, 176, 180, 183, 188–190, 201, 221, 223–224; and venting 108, 189, 219; and writing 88, 142, 150, 155n77, 159, 169, 200–205
note-taking *see* transcription
Nowell, April 25
nursery rhymes 186

object(s) 14–15, 23–31, 39–41, 53n98, 92, 67, 102, 132, 140–141, 170–174, 185–189; abundant (in language) 18, 60, 83–84, 113, 165–168, 223; archaic 14–23, 45–51, 58–59, 69–77, 84, 92, 118, 170, 189, 212–215, 223; and association 15, 30–34, 44–50, 76–84, 86–94, 116–118, 138–145, 169, 179–188, 190–198, 200–203, 210–217, 221; auditory 128, 138–140, 166, 198, 213; beloved 14–15, 27–29; co-experienced 38, 62–68, 76, 84–86, 125–129, 137–145, 150–157, 165–168, 181–189, 200–201, 210–211; and development 38, 44, 55, 75, 82, 118, 128, 137, 177, 190; of dream-work 14–18, 23–31, 37, 45–51, 75, 137, 165, 210–212, 227; earliest (first) 33, 117, 166; and echoes 18, 46, 131–140, 189, 203, 210; and enclaves 30, 39, 43, 59, 76, 179; exterior 145–146; facilitating investments 7, 14–19, 23–28, 48–49, 55–59, 82–87, 94–95, 117–118, 124, 138, 169; fields of 66, 82, 92, 137; and fixation 16–18, 26–34, 39–46, 76–85, 83, 93–96, 116–118, 210; and Freud 20n7, 29–30, 62; and fusion 127–129, 144, 150–157; idiosyncratic 14, 24–25, 34–37, 41–49, 68, 131, 141, 187–188, 216;

inheriting affect 14, 23, 34–37, 50, 82–83, 200, 224; interior 145–146; invested 14–18, 27, 64–70; liquid 14–19, 20n3, 24, 31, 41–49, 55–61, 82–84, 137, 227; and literacy 60–63, 123–125, 131–132, 157, 170, 185–189, 220; lost 15–19, 42–46, 83, 96, 116, 139; in luring 43, 82, 158, 167, 177, 187–190; mediating 56–59; and mother's environment 16–18, 25, 30–38, 55–56, 75–76, 92, 118–120, 132–137, 165, 211–216, 224; in nature 7, 158, 169, 210–216; and passivity 15, 31, 41–43, 55, 75, 83, 92, 128, 211–215; phonemes as 7, 58, 76, 82–87, 94, 113–119, 137–141, 157, 166, 185–189, 198–200, 223–227; as provision 14, 144, 166, 201, 210, 216; and regression 42–49, 76, 83–86, 145, 179, 190, 223; repetitive 18, 27, 93, 127; and security 56, 82–85, 132–137, 145–150, 167–169, 193, 200, 210, 219–221; suitable (new) 13–16, 118, 150, 168–170; and symbolization 49–55, 82, 120–123, 186, 203, 221; and third 16, 33–38, 63, 76, 82–85; and transference 23–26, 37–38, 68, 86; transitional 40, 51, 51n44, 57; triangulated 32–33, 65–66, 76, 85, 131, 138–145, 165–167, 199, 209–212, 223; word as 14, 33, 40, 57, 123–124, 177, 188

Oedipus (Oedipal): complex 22, 38, 75, 82; "larval" 22; triangle (triangulation) 16, 38, 138, 166

olfaction (olfactory) 31–32

ontogeny of thought 2, 82–84, 119, 176, 223–224

oral castration *see* castration

oral stage: archaic foundations 18, 23–24, 55–62, 87; audition 55; babble 18–19, 87; call and response 18; cathexis 87–88; encounter with reality 25, 66, 87; fixations 28–29; inaugurated by umbilical castration 56, 81, 165; influence of unconscious 39; object relations 16, 62; passivity 41, 59, 62, 83, 218n27; permanent mark of 28; pleasure 27–29; prior to 14–15, 222; regression 16, 18–19, 24, 83, 87; speech 83, 87–88; transition from archaic 26–27, 30, 58–59, 62, 66, 95, 218n27

organic 47, 126, 136, 144, 212–213, 217, 220

"other" 23, 40, 56, 62–64, 70, 76, 125, 137–140, 166–168, 227; all-providing 76, 165; and association 76, 166; auditory 129, 131; differentiating self 39, 84; of dream-work 86, 137, 145; first 33, 119; good-enough 143, 145, 151, 158, 167, 170, 212; indissociable 37–39, 61–67, 75–76, 119, 127, 133n23, 137–138, 150–158, 165–168, 200, 210; "is and is not self" 101, 124, 127, 131, 137– 138, 159, 192; (m)other 17, 38, 42, 85, 89n6, 119, 137, 165, 167, 175; mother's (significant) 14, 25, 31, 39, 82; and passivity 76, 127–136, 142–144, 150–151, 157, 166, 169, 209; and "second" 63; securing 124, 127; similar-enough 34, 64–68, 84–85, 139, 151–152, 165–167, 188, 205, 210–211; and "third" 33, 38; trusted 48, 124, 141–142, 152, 160, 205; words as 17; *see also* indissociable

Pappenheim, Bertha 10n12, 177, 185–186, 193n7

parallel play *see* play

parasympathetic system 45–46

Parten, Mildred 140

parturition 26, 31, 39, 46; *see also* birth

passive (passivity) 19, 41–44, 51n45, 125–132, 144; absorption of nutrients 15, 215; and affective continuity 34; dependence (fusion) 5, 16, 69, 75, 143–144, 150, 158, 169, 175, 181, 201, 223; dominance in archaic 15; dream-like state 40, 120, 152; education (learning) 8, 31, 33–34, 120, 151, 188, 203, 220, 224; and environment (objects) 93, 183, 192, 219, 223; and flower-doll 67–68; and intention (difficulty) 143; and language 180; and literacy 192–193; and nature 158; position 26; and priming 57; and reading 158; receptivity 92, 121, 124, 166, 177, 213, 221; recipient 181; and

regression 46, 69, 76, 88, 145, 164, 169, 176–177, 192, 213, 217; and repetition 16; and speech (challenge) 68–69; and transition to oral stage 18, 59, 62, 77, 83–85, 183, 218n27; and transition to reality 209, 213; and waiting (for lures) 58, 87, 144, 190; and witness 211, 217
paternal 39, 42, 53n98
pathway(s): affective 62, 167; archaic roots 49–50, 56, 158; associative 30–32, 47–49, 55–56, 61–66, 76–77, 83–84, 87, 92, 220–221; circulatory 179, 189; constrained 46, 86, 94, 166, 173; and differentiation 39–41; for displacements 26, 44, 87, 94, 190; and literacy 63, 190, 201–203; and mother tongue 60; and nature 212, 214, 217; proliferation 138, 166; recovering 89, 223; and resorption 43, 48, 58–59, 77, 83, 166–168; for survival 14; and "third" 42–43; *see also* branch(es)
Pavlenko, Aneta 174, 176–177
perception 34, 39, 62, 91; and dream-work 82, 168; gradual development 7, 17, 23, 25, 31, 38, 44, 47, 75, 83–84, 137, 166; sound woven with body 55, 117, 119; *see also* proprioception
Pérez-Foster, RoseMarie 174
phantasm(s) 55–56, 58, 69, 118, 168
phoneme(s) 7, 39–40, 51n44, 56–60, 120–124, 125–132, 171n14, 193; and anxiety 67–68; and associative thinking 76, 113–121, 130, 158–159, 166–174, 182–187, 193–199, 201–203, 214–223; in clinic 64, 198, 211; definition 4, 9, 40, 51n44, 57–60, 75, 82, 114–116, 166, 170, 179, 223–227; in development 19, 40, 58, 137, 155n77, 170, 191, 219–223; and dream-work 17, 62, 82–84, 113, 183, 187, 201–202, 223; and "duty of testimony" 65; in echo 61, 85, 120, 138–140, 153–159, 165–168, 189, 197–199, 201–203, 205, 219–227; and education 3, 180–182; idiosyncratic 59, 61–62, 86–87, 93, 119, 131, 157, 168, 186, 188; immune to conscious effort 168, 181–182, 185; and indissociable "other" 76, 84, 133; and language loss 60, 170, 179, 182–183; and "like-me" 62, 84, 117, 189; in linguistics 9n7, 114–116; as liquid object 14, 132, 227; and liturgical languages 86; as mediating objects 26, 57–59, 76, 85, 118, 155n77, 173–175, 181–185, 193, 211; and name 117, 169, 175–176, 179, 185, 198–199; and passivity 87, 116, 120, 179–180, 190–193; and phonemic play 70n17, 123, 133n23, 141, 154n5, 155n62, 179–181, 193n5, 198–199, 205, 219–220; and phonemic overlaps 86, 175; preserving 179–180; and primary narcissism 57–58; and reading 61–62, 86–87, 119, 158, 168–170, 181–185, 190–192, 223; and regression 94, 175–179, 187–190; and reparation 40, 88, 93, 60, 181, 223; repetitions 4, 39, 58–62, 75, 84–87, 166–169, 179–180, 200–201, 220; and "second" 63, 192; and second language 158, 174–175, 179, 192; as securitization 58, 76, 176, 182, 190, 224; and suggestion 59, 70n17, 117, 133, 181, 198–199; as sustenance 58, 63; and symbolization 117, 131; and "third" 76, 85; and transference 58–62, 167; and triangulation 59, 76–77, 117, 133, 141, 157–159, 166–167, 186–189, 201–210, 222–224; and unconscious affect 7–8, 14–18, 58–59, 76–77, 85, 119, 157, 167, 174, 179–183, 223; uttered 18, 83, 86, 119, 155n77, 159, 175, 204; valuation of 11, 18, 132, 224; and writing 63–65, 119, 141–142, 159, 169–175, 181–185, 197–199, 202–205; *see also* homonym(s); mother tongue
phonics 181, 221n2
Piaget, Jean 13, 47, 89
picture exchange communication system (PECS) 181, 184n54
play 127, 193; associative 138, 213; dream-work as 196, 200; of echoes 64, 142, 159; homonymic 142, 175, 197, 200, 206n18; letter 120–123; and literacy 142, 159,

196, 205, 219; and nature 143, 213–216, 226; parallel 140–142, 204; phonemic 70n17, 123, 133n23, 141, 154n5, 155n62, 179–181, 193n5, 198–199, 205, 219–220; physical 102, 129, 188; symbolic function 47–48; and toys 102, 144, 155n77; unconscious 159, 199, 211; word 4, 58, 113, 120–123, 132, 142, 147, 159
pleasure 7, 33, 141, 199, 204; affective returns to self 136, 138, 168, 181; anxiety 77, 142, 146, 149, 168, 187; archaic 15, 23, 47, 68, 131; as continuous circulation 41; displeasure 7; and dream-work 26, 28, 130, 143; echoes as 139, 142, 187; exchanges of 15, 17–18; and indissociable "other" 26, 40, 56; and language 115, 121–122, 181, 198; as liberation 152, 168; and nature 152, 158, 170, 217; oral stage 27–28; and reading 189, 196; as securing 47, 115, 147, 217; shifting objects of 28; and speaking 155n77; survival as 17, 47; and symbolic function 47; and thought 97, 126; unconscious 24, 60, 93, 141, 216; and wish to sleep 29; and writing 149–150
precocious 49, 69–70, 222; experiences with phonemes 115, 170; learning 4–5, 31–34; reading 63, 87, 157–159, 169, 190, 193, 219; stage 23, 28, 45; symbolization 50, 117; *see also* audition
pre-conscious 21, 31, 68, 118, 137, 155n77; audition 169, 227; development 226–227; learning 4–5, 8–9, 10n9, 85, 170, 224; symbolization 82, 89n6, 113, 115, 137
preconscious 10n9, 21, 31, 43, 75, 82
pregenital stages 33
premature (prematurity) 7, 46, 57, 218n27
pre-self 33, 75–76, 82–85, 90n7, 117, 137, 141, 157–159, 165–169
presence 40, 108, 125–127; author's 62; conditions of 56, 119, 200; dreamed 33, 76, 85, 145, 159, 187; as finding self 103, 152; in language 40; and mother 18, 39, 119, 212; and nature 6, 139, 148; and "other" 1–2, 8, 150–152, 155n77, 160, 166, 169, 191, 205, 223; securing 56–58, 61–67, 90n7, 124–127, 146–147, 167, 177, 201–205; unconscious 62; and witness 143, 201
presentification (presentify) 40, 55–58, 77, 83, 118, 125, 149, 210, 223
primary: anxiety 30; audition as 127; defence 88, 91–93, 201; education 155n77; function (discharging affect) 27; influence on associative thinking 89; influence of instinct of conservation 21; mechanisms of dream-work 82; mode of human learning 3, 8; "narcissistic mode of being" 57; narcissism 27, 68, 175; obstacle 103; prior to consciousness 24, 50; processes 5, 24–25, 88, 106–108, 120, 125, 128, 138, 145, 168, 226; reservoir 89; source of security 214
priming 57, 67
progression 4–6, 65, 86–93, 169, 193, 201, 210–213; and affect 28, 44, 55, 83–84, 118, 155, 177; and consciousness 7, 18, 48, 56–59, 87, 151, 165, 173–182; and individuation 142, 149–151, 210, 221–224; iterations of self 186–188, 210; and language 19, 87, 95, 155, 177; and literacy 89, 125; normative 92, 118, 169, 190; physiological 69, 77, 83, 86; of psychosexual maturation 16–18, 29, 42, 86, 93, 105, 201, 223; and regression 42–46, 77, 118, 137, 151, 191, 201, 210; resuming 85–89, 93–95, 137, 191, 201–205, 210–212; and triangulation 2, 50, 85, 117, 169, 212, 223
projective identification 67–68, 85; *see also* identification
prolonging («prolongement») 64, 138; *see also* fusion; indissociable
pronoun(s) 86, 119, 159, 192; in third person 96–97, 101–104, 109n36, 110n47, 127, 133n25, 192
proof of life 42, 76, 136, 147, 158–159, 165, 189, 210, 217; confirmation as 150
proprioception: 59, 82, 91; gradual 7, 17, 23, 25, 31, 38, 44, 47, 75, 82–84, 137, 166; *see also* perception
prosopography 89

provision 82, 136, 146, 166, 216; environmental 76, 144, 147, 158, 181–187, 192, 216; phonemes as 61, 139, 143, 158, 186–192; *see also* food; proof of life
psychobiography 72n125
psychosexual: development (maturation) 13–14, 29, 42, 56; and anxiety 28; archaic stage 8, 14–15, 17, 23–24, 28–32, 38, 75–76, 81–88, 165; gradual progress 18, 23, 26, 37–38; regression in 15–16, 29–31, 39–46, 75; role of phonemes 19, 177; sequelae of instincts 21; stages 13, 23, 27, 30–31, 177; unconscious affect as fuel 13, 16–17, 24, 30–31, 82–86, 94, 165–169
pulsion(al) 20n16, 30, 34n24, 60, 67–68

reactions: "chain reactions of de-structuration" 45; defensive 91; «réactions affectives» 26
reading: as archaic-syntonic 186, 200; and association 115, 121, 188, 199; and chain of custody 186; and dream-work 19, 60–63, 158, 167, 170, 187–188, 220; and echoes 159, 168, 170, 186, 193, 205, 219, 224; and education 164, 170, 188–193, 203–204; freely 8, 61, 86, 158, 192–193, 220; Freud on 60; hyperlexia 73n131; and individuation 124–125, 139; and language (L1 versus L2) 192; and nature 147, 215, 224; note-taking from 195–199, 203–204; passion 120–125, 132, 187–189; power 2; precocious 9n4, 60–63, 87–89, 121–128, 133n51, 134n66, 157–160, 168, 189–193, 219–220; refusal 193; as reparative 61, 67, 88, 159, 187–189, 192–193, 205, 223; rereading 65, 189, 197–199, 203–204; returning archaic affects 60–65, 70, 168, 170, 175, 192–193; as securing 124, 170, 175, 187, 189–193, 224; silent 220; transference in 61, 65, 95, 120, 192, 199–200; *see also* literacy
reanimating: "archaic faith" 213; archaic triangulation 44, 62, 76, 153–159, 170, 193, 215, 220–223
receptivity 41–42, 69, 92, 124, 127–128, 177, 213, 221
reconnaissance 15, 56, 64, 70n17, 154n5, 204, 209, 211–212
refinding 143, 187; archaic objects 17, 45, 76, 84, 137, 168, 189, 193; and literacy 168, 187, 189; self 45
refuge(s) 42, 67, 94–97, 102, 106–108, 151–152, 159
Reggio Emilia 36n85, 204, 206n43, 215
register 17, 38, 41, 70, 76–77, 95, 139, 159, 167, 171n14, 183
regression (regressive) 45–48, 81, 96–102, 151, 173–177, 190, 203, 212, 226; as affect impeded 30, 42–48, 59, 95; to anonymity 43; and anxiety 15, 75–78, 83–86, 93–95, 108, 167, 183, 190; and archaic 15, 44–45, 62, 78, 83, 118; autism as 11, 43, 62, 66, 78, 81, 87–88, 157, 160, 165, 169, 219, 223; at birth 15; in conserving health 15, 83, 96, 175; by contamination 92; dependence on 46, 150, 157, 169, 188, 192, 201, 221; desolidarizing 45; as de-structuration 45; as "dynamic involution" 42; enduring 94; exiting 15–17, 33, 43, 46, 60, 137, 170, 190, 205, 211, 221; and fear 44; as first defence 11–15, 46, 69–75, 85–88, 90n13, 93–96, 128–131, 177, 213–220, 223–224; and fixation 186, 191, 193, 211–213; and flower-doll 68, 211; as "freeze" 92–93; Freud on 20n7; and insecurity in reality 49–50, 93, 151, 191, 212, 223; and language loss 173, 180–181; libidinal 45; and literacy 187–188, 190, 205; momentary 45; and nature 210–217, 220; and non-individuation 92, 119, 127, 144, 189, 204, 223; and non-initiation 69, 78, 83, 87, 107, 202, 226; oral stage 18–19, 24, 62, 87; as "organizing silence" 69; and passivity 26, 43, 69, 145, 190–192, 201, 212; position 50, 127, 190, 192, 205, 220; precocious 70; to prior object relations 17, 26, 59, 66–68, 177; process of 15; as "refolding" 46; as refuge 152; reliance on 8–9, 75, 90n10,

93–95, 102–108, 150, 157, 169, 223; as reparative 45; as securing 68, 76, 88, 93, 191, 212; as "stagnant dynamic situation" 46; and symbolization 63, 68, 83, 221; temporary 46, 92, 180, 186, 191, 204; as withdrawal 93, 105, 128, 151, 159; *see also* "freeze"; hide
reinvestment 16, 18, 26, 30, 39, 43, 45–46, 59, 77, 83, 189, 227; *see also* affective investment(s)
relay 25, 60, 64, 84; *see also* affective circulation
reparation 93–95, 213; archaic echoes as 61, 66, 93, 201; and education 169, 182, 191–193, 201, 224; and flower-doll 67–68; instinct of conservation 180, 201, 221; and language 181–182, 191–193, 201; literacy as 8, 66–67, 88–89, 151, 159, 182, 191–197, 201, 223; nature as 66–67, 209–217, 220; and phonemes 93, 198, 201; of regression 45–46; and witness 93, 223; *see also* healing
repetition (repetitive): associations 31, 166; echoes 138; experiences 8, 22, 25, 42, 44, 48, 82, 137, 139, 192; habitus 43; and literacy 60, 199, 227; and name 175; in nature 140; over-determination 87, 90n11; and passivity 16, 18, 30, 127, 227; perseveration 83, 86, 93, 103, 106–107, 112n150, 151, 188; phonemes 4, 39, 57–62, 75, 82–87, 139, 159, 166–169, 180, 199, 201, 220–227; and primary processes 106–107; and regression 46; and "third" 39; and words 18, 127, 188, 192, 199, 204
reservoir(s) 3, 13, 21, 23, 29, 89
residential school(s) 172–175
resistance (resistant) 4, 28, 44, 62, 122, 203
resonance (resonate): affectivity in 48, 62–64, 159; of archaic peace 63, 213, 225; of archaic triangular situation 67, 159, 200, 225; emotional 25, 58; and flower-doll 67; interhuman 191, 198; in literacy 62, 167; and name 175; and nature 147; as play 159; with words 60–62; *see also* echo(es)
resorptive (resorb, resorption) 16, 42–43, 77, 83, 166, 168, 225
resurge(nce) 45, 181
retreat(ing) 43, 96–98, 100–108, 124–128, 131, 146, 217; *see also* withdrawal
reverberation (reverberate) 138, 225; *see also* echo(es); resonance
reversibility (reversible, reversal) 6, 13, 46, 62–68, 131, 133n25, 169, 202, 210; *see also* fusion
rhythm(ic) 7, 13, 22, 119–120, 176, 212, 214, 217, 220, 227
right to write 9, 142, 160; *see also* writing
Rimland, Bernard 46
river(s) 143, 172–173; Humber 1–7, 96, 102, 120, 125–126, 142, 148, 224–227, 227n11; libido as 17
road: of learning 34; of listening 41, 56, 58–59; as pathway 43; *see also* pathway(s)
Roudinesco, Élisabeth 20n16, 224

Sapir, Edward 114–117, 132n1
scent *see* olfaction
"second": associated with self (blur) 17, 63; indispensable 33; indissociable 16, 40, 75; and "like-me" 40–41, 63; and "me-mymother" 16, 63; and security 40–42; and texts 63; and "third" 16–17, 56, 61; and transference 33; and triangulation 40; *see also* "third"
second language (L2) *see* language
securitization 34–43, 49, 90n10, 168, 180, 197, 213; and affect 26, 45, 56, 143–145, 189; archaic 26, 40, 153–157, 215, 224; de-securitizing 175–176; and dream-work 46, 92, 200; and language 58, 175–176, 180, 204, 224; and literacy 87–89, 158, 168, 197; as proof of life 37, 147; as provision 143–146; in reality 26, 49, 56, 68, 82–85, 175, 189, 200; and witness 85, 158; *see also* security
security 28, 37, 47, 65–68, 176, 217; affective 47, 56, 66, 93, 137, 152, 167, 181–187, 193, 201, 210–217, 223–227; archaic 18, 30, 50, 56–63, 131, 146, 158, 166–168, 201, 223; assurance of 40, 93, 95, 186, 187; de-securing 177, 191; and

dream-work 43–45, 57, 64–68, 76, 88–93, 118, 124, 159–168, 177, 212, 223; and echoes 127, 170, 189–193, 205, 223; existential 15, 32, 45, 50, 56, 173, 175, 193; and fusion 127, 169; habitus of 28, 97; and language 18, 56–58, 68, 94, 122, 140, 158, 168, 175, 179, 186–191, 205; and literacy 120–125, 132, 142, 147, 151, 170, 187–191, 220; loss 50, 83, 93, 177, 211; and luring 83, 87; maternal and paternal 39, 42, 53n98, 119; and nature 8, 67–68, 142–147, 216–217, 220; and passivity 217, 221; as pleasure 115, 181, 217; and provision 14, 18, 56, 76, 129, 139, 193, 204, 210; of refuge 97–98, 151, 215–217; and wish 23, 108; and witness 56–58, 61, 85, 124, 137, 146–147, 167, 177–183, 191, 200–205, 212; *see also* securitization; unconscious security
self-: self-calming 106, 143–146; self-feeding 18, 63, 201; self-luring 201; self-observation 196–197, 203, 210; self-preservation 7, 16, 20n16, 21–22, 43–50, 55–59, 67–68, 223–225; self-provision 157, 170; self-securing 43–45, 57, 66–68, 73n131, 138–142, 157–160, 166–170, 188–193, 205, 220–223; self-triangulation 153; *see also* auto-; self-regulation
self-regulation: of affect 30, 77, 88, 138, 166–169, 190, 201, 224; in development 2, 8, 29, 108, 138, 187, 191; and instinct of conservation 77, 166, 175, 193, 210, 213–214, 221; and language 95, 120, 167, 175, 180, 223; and literacy 88, 190–193; and nature 142, 145; *see also* auto-
Sellin, Birger 5, 10n13, 109n30, 133n51, 191; on anxiety 103–106, 149–150; on daydreaming 130–132; on exteriorization 143; on fusion 127–128, 150–152; on individuation 100–102, 152–153; on love of language 121–122; on non-initiation 129–130; on passion for reading 123–124; on passivity 126–129; on phonemes in associative thinking 121; on reality (space-time) 98–100; on regression 96–98; on revitalizing energy 143–154; on securitizing provision 146–147; on self-calming 145–146; on stims (venting) 106–108; on witness 149; on word and letter play 122–123
sensory 18, 24–26, 32, 40, 48, 60, 75, 91, 106, 127
Sign language 10n10, 52n74, 153, 176, 182, 200, 202
silence (silent) 4, 14, 22, 42–43, 60, 222; and associative thinking 60, 200; and dream-work 132, 146, 213; language loss 179, 182; in nature 4, 88, 126, 142–143, 147, 212, 215–217, 220; organizing 69, 213; reading 193, 220; and regression 9, 43, 94, 131–132, 150, 220; retreat 97– 98, 124, 128, 130–131, 146; securing 97, 215, 220; as trap 151–153, 159; and voice 13, 142–143; *see also* mute
similitude ("similar") 34, 48, 62, 76, 138; and affect 48–49, 62–65, 141, 151, 167, 201; good-enough 64–68, 85, 93, 139–141, 152, 210–211; in identification 205, 210; and language (phoneme) 139–140, 167–168; and literacy 65, 149–152; and nature 209–215; in play 140–144; reconnaissance of 48, 62–67, 88; and recovery 68, 137, 188, 205; «semblable» 36n106, 90n7; in triangulation 140–145, 165–166, 188, 205; unconsciously 65, 84, 93, 138, 158, 188, 211, 223; *see also* witness
sleep(ing) 3, 13, 41–47, 59, 103, 120, 152, 174–178, 186, 197; as defence 44–45; and dreams 67, 127, 193; in and out of 19, 31, 43, 49; and nature 96–97, 147; as reparation 67, 147, 213; wish to 27, 29; *see also* dormant
slips: of the fingers 202; of the pen 196, 199; of the tongue 3, 44, 49
social stories 192, 194n30
solitude 4, 43, 56, 64, 69, 94–95, 150, 213
sonar (sonority) 9, 55–58, 116, 155n77, 169, 176–180, 210–211, 227
speak(ing) 68, 69, 155n77, 169, 176, 186, 190; babble 18, 51n44, 87; development of 119, 131, 153, 155n77, 202; and phonemes 167,

175, 198, 202; and pronouns 119, 192; thinking then speaking 6, 202, 225; writing as-if 88, 149, 157–159, 176, 202; *see also* non-speaking; speech
species (human) 8, 30, 91,136–138; as communicative 13–14, 95, 119, 178, 191, 226–227; role of unconscious in 86, 95, 221; survival 21, 221, 225
speech 4, 16, 25, 57–60, 69, 75, 121, 155n77, 177, 182; as conscious act 5, 68–69, 77, 83–88, 90n10, 94–96, 108, 115, 169, 177, 202, 221, 226; as defence 90n10, 94–96; difficulty 6–9, 10n12, 97, 102, 107, 119–121, 223; and flower-doll 67; and individuation 40, 86, 119, 160; inner 176, 202; latent 95; and thought 19, 50, 115, 223; writing as substitute 87, 153–159, 204; *see also* speaking
"spoken or written" (speak or write) 119, 138–139, 159, 167, 175–176, 191, 197, 201, 205
stim(s) 103, 106–108 112n150, 131
Strachey, James 35n56, 226
suggestion (suggestibility) 59, 70n17, 94, 117, 132n17, 139, 154n5, 155n62, 198–200, 216
Suskind, Ron 112n150
syllable(s) 4, 9, 57, 75, 128, 189, 225; syllable-type unit(s) 75, 82, 166; *see also* phoneme(s)
symbolic 23, 45–50, 53n98, 57, 115–117, 147, 204; father 17, 39–41, 61–63, 84–85, 137
symboligenic castration(s) *see* castration(s)
symbolism 4, 47–50, 114–117, 144
symbolization 7, 19, 47–50; and audition (phonemes) 117, 128; and dream-work 120, 131, 169; pre-conscious 82, 89n6, 113,115, 137; and thought 68, 86, 157, 169

talking cure 33, 40, 67, 167, 185
Taylor, Marjorie 187–189
teach(ing) (teacher) 6–8, 24, 81, 155n77, 163–164, 170–172, 181; and autism 106, 122–129, 182; and common objects 140–141; Dolto as 70, 164–165, 170, 219–227; and environment 31, 36n85, 143, 215–217; and literacy 87, 181, 191–193, 202–205; *see also* education; learn(ing)
"third" 16, 38–43, 61–63, 138, 215; and dream-work 40–41, 63, 76; and father 38–39, 41, 85; and "like-me" 33–34, 40, 82; and mother 16, 38–39, 85; phonemes as 40, 76, 85; in presentification 43, 56, 76; and "second" 17, 38–42, 56; and self 17, 38–39; as word 33, 39–40, 56; *see also* "second"
touch: in autism 104, 151–152, 203; as evocative 62, 116, 189, 214, 217; in fetus 47 48; "human" 136
trace(s) 14, 23, 37, 59–67, 72n125, 93–95, 148–150, 197, 204; of affective history 14–18, 25–27, 60–61, 77, 87, 158, 169, 189, 222; echoes as 139, 142; idiosyncratic 119; in latent register 77, 95, 142; lost 172, 175; and phonemes 88, 142, 175, 189; in pronouns 159; in texts 65–70, 87, 95, 142, 189
transcription (transcribe, transcribing) 195–205; and dream-work 199–206; and echoes 203–206; in education 155n77, 170, 204–205, 220; and phonemes 199; in reparation 201–206; *see also* writing
transfer: affect 13–18, 23–31, 34, 44, 58, 77, 82–86, 93, 107, 212, 223; anxiety 101; stims 107
transference 19, 23–26, 38–41, 58–65, 68, 75, 198; and affective liberation 29, 33, 46, 64, 94; of archaic relations 23, 26, 37, 58, 63–64; immune to conscious control 33, 68; and language 39–41, 57–58, 63, 174; and nature 68, 211; in texts 61, 63, 87, 119, 192, 193n5, 200
translation 5, 10n13, 20n16, 50n3, 70n17, 72n104, 185, 197, 206n15, 208, 225–227; and autists 121–122, 152; consciousness as 19; "lost in" 173; of pulsional energy 30, 67; of wish to survive 93
tree(s) 6–7, 24, 126, 136, 142–145, 172, 208, 220; and flower-doll 209; as securing 142–147, 208, 214; and symbolization 99, 131, 145–147, 208, 214; as witness 67, 74n226, 209–211; *see also* nature

Trevarthen, Colwyn 47–48
triangulation(triangular) *see* archaic triangular situation
Tustin, Frances 197, 201

umbilical castration *see* castration
unconscious 14–15, 20n2, 36n85, 114, 137, 140, 169, 186, 200; activity 2, 24–25, 37, 48, 75, 178, 221; aspect 9, 222; association(s) 13–17, 47, 61, 115, 118, 175, 188–189; capacities 3, 8, 22–24, 41, 67, 204; circulation 2, 18–19, 61, 94, 175, 177, 214, 221, 223; continuity 56, 60, 186, 223; current 43, 95, 118; defence(s) 88, 201, 223; desire 34, 55; development 165, 179; dream-work 19, 205; echoes 18, 85, 87, 120, 159, 170, 205; encounter(s) 34, 62; energy 13, 23, 30, 34n24; experience(s) 59, 85, 167, 191–193, 200, 205, 209–210, 218n27, 219; history 15, 23, 119, 139; ideation 3, 50; identification 67, 118; image 60, 72n81; influence 3, 8, 191, 196; inheritance 31, 55; investment(s) 15, 18, 70, 77, 88, 176, 198; language 25, 65; life 3, 22, 32, 82, 118, 165; material 199, 20n7; mechanism 10n9, 23–24, 210; pleasure 24, 93, 168, 216; recognition 90n7, 138, 143, 151–152, 197; reconnaissance 64–65, 209, 211–212; register 76, 139; relation(s) 18, 82, 85; remains 3, 21; reparation 62, 68, 93, 193, 214, 220–223; reserves 28–29, 179, 226; resource 159, 217; reversibility 64, 68; role 7–8, 77, 178, 191; roots 22, 116, 119, 224; scaffolding 47, 221; state 2, 7, 15, 22, 27–28, 50n2, 223; thinking 3, 50; traces 14, 18, 175, 197; transference 14, 37, 45, 211; transits 65, 93, 189; triangulation 19, 38, 65, 76, 113, 117, 140–141, 145, 157, 166–167, 223; wish 41, 50, 56; work 157, 169–170, 182, 190, 192, 198, 217; *see also* unconscious affect(s); unconscious process(es); unconscious security
unconscious affect(s) 13, 20n2, 25, 34n24, 94, 158, 183, 190–192, 205, 211–212, 221–224; and association 18, 77, 84, 205, 219; circulation of 8, 14–17, 27–33, 37–44, 59–67, 77–84, 95, 115–120, 145, 157, 166–168, 173–181, 190; continuity of 93, 137, 212, 219–224; displacement 26, 33, 83, 94; idiosyncratic 24, 63, 86; inheriting 14, 18, 64, 82, 189; investments 14–18, 43, 49, 59, 83, 95, 168, 223; and language (words, phonemes) 7, 14, 60–61, 76, 120, 138, 152–157, 166–169, 171n14, 173–182; liberating 65–67, 152, 170; reservoirs (sources) 13, 16, 23, 30, 83–85, 94, 158, 166, 174, 183; and symbolization 48, 219; transfer(ence) of 13–18, 25–26, 34, 62, 77, 94, 223; withdrawn (resorbed, trapped) 15–16, 26, 42–45, 77, 83, 168, 181; *see also* unconscious
unconscious process(es) 14, 24, 48; and affect 15–19, 24–26, 49, 142, 151–153, 188, 193; and archaic 27, 33–41, 55, 60–65, 76, 84–85, 137, 168, 182, 193, 217; and development 7–8, 24–26, 32–37, 47–48, 56–65, 84–88, 141, 157, 166–168, 178, 189–193, 221–224; and displacement 17, 23–27, 42, 55–61, 76, 82–87, 138, 168, 183; and education 8, 24, 170, 178, 190, 196, 215–222; immune to conscious effort 65, 82, 168–170, 182, 203, 211, 221; influence of 3, 32, 197–199, 223–225; and language acquisition 9, 85, 108, 153, 159, 180–181, 199, 219–225; and literacy 61, 67, 86–87, 158, 168, 190–193; and nature 67, 210–214, 220; and passivity 15, 46, 83, 92–93, 158, 167, 182–190, 219; and phonemes 18, 23, 40, 55–58, 68, 86, 115–119, 166–168, 173–181, 183–191; restorative 41, 86, 153–159, 168–170, 178–181, 183–188, 191–193, 201–204, 210–214, 220–224; and survival 14–18, 21–22, 82, 108, 165, 192–193, 201, 222; and symbolization 19, 47–51, 59–61, 86–88, 113, 140–145, 188, 196–197; and triangulation 16–17,

33, 49, 61–67, 70–76, 84–85, 90n7, 137–145, 151–157, 165–167, 188; *see also* unconscious
unconscious security (securing, securitizing, securitization) 23–26, 65–68, 82, 151–159, 169, 188; and affective continuity 66, 76, 152, 180; and archaic triangulation 15–17, 41–42, 64, 76, 88, 141, 159, 168, 214, 223; and association 14, 43, 55–60, 137–138, 180–182, 219; and dream-work 16, 47–48, 144, 214; and language (phonemes) 7–9, 58, 76, 85, 118, 179–180, 182–183, 219; and luring to reality 92–93, 168; as self-preservation 7, 33–37, 42, 55, 58, 214; *see also* unconscious
UNESCO 182, 222

vent(ing) 67–70, 83, 103–108, 138, 175; *see also* exteriorization; liberate
vision (visual) 6–8, 55, 59, 65, 122, 129, 139–141, 152, 165, 204, 215
vocabulary 2, 50n3, 58, 60, 179, 183, 220, 226; *see also* phonemes; provision
voice 39, 98, 127–131, 147–152, 180, 215; gradual discernment 31, 56–58, 82, 166; as mediating lure 57–60; mother's 14–18, 25–26, 84, 98, 175; own (echo) 68, 139, 142, 147, 153, 159, 175, 190
Von Hameln, Glückel 186, 193n7; *see also* Bertha Pappenheim

weaning *see* oral castration
Wing, Lorna 203, 206n41
Winnicott, Donald 50n2, 51n44
wish 23, 28, 130, 187; and desires 97, 101, 104–105, 122, 129; energy of 41, 56; fulfilment 49–50, 56, 63, 226; to live 22–23, 27, 37, 47, 55–56, 93, 165; to sleep 27, 29; *see also* dream-work
withdraw(al) (withdrawing): and anxiety 103, 179; as a defence (regression) 42–46, 92–94; dependence on 46, 83, 92–97; to dream-work 30, 44–46, 69, 151; and individuation 66, 83, 102; and passivity 46, 69, 77, 164, 213, 217; to preserve affect 13–16, 20n7, 42–48, 59, 77, 167; as retreat (refuge) 96–103, 131; and solitude 96–100; to thought 97–100; *see also* regression
witness 4, 32, 63–69, 76, 88, 89n6, 148–154, 170–173, 181–188, 200–201, 211–212; and affect 137, 181–183, 186–193, 200–201, 210–212, 217–223; archaic 17, 25; in clinic 40, 51n31, 164; Dolto as 22, 222; and flower-doll 209–212; good-enough 64–65, 170, 209–210; and individuation 68–69, 181–188, 217; listener as 64–67, 198; and literacy 62–70, 158, 168–170, 186–193, 201–210, 223; lost 69–70, 170, 210–212, 218n27; and nature 67, 70, 143–147, 169–170, 209, 211–220; in similitude 76, 84–87, 90n11, 93, 120, 137–139, 143–147, 151–152, 167–168; and triangulation 65–67, 85, 141, 157–159, 168, 177, 186–189, 198–203, 209, 217–224; *see also* similitude
word association *see* association(s)
writing 141, 197; and affect 65, 70, 87, 153; and anxiety 89, 149–153, 170; in auto-recovery 63–68, 88–89, 151, 159; and echoes 139, 142, 170, 202–205, 223–224; in education 155n77, 202–205, 220, 221n2; independent 88, 149–153, 157–159, 220; and individuation 8, 149–153, 159, 186, 200–205, 220–223; as pleasure (play) 149, 205; as self-triangulation 153, 200, 202; as speech 87, 90n10, 142–149, 153–159, 181, 200–205; in third person 96, 101, 110n47; and traces 65, 67, 147; and witness 63–64, 87, 142, 149, 152, 170, 223; *see also* literacy; transcription